AF442665

Mechanisms of Intestinal Inflammation: Implications for Therapeutic Intervention in IBD

FALK SYMPOSIUM 133

Mechanisms of Intestinal Inflammation: Implications for Therapeutic Intervention in IBD

Edited by

R. Duchmann
Medizinische Klinik I
Charité – Universitätsmedizin Berlin
Campus Benjamin Franklin
D-12200 Berlin, Germany

J. Schölmerich
Innere Medizin I
Klinikum der Universität
Regensburg
D-93042 Regensburg, Germany

R. S. Blumberg
Brigham and Women's Hospital
GI Division
75 Francis Street
Boston, MA-2115-6195, USA

W. Strober
National Institutes of Health
NIAID, Bldg. 10, Room 11N 238
Mucosal Immunity Section
Bethesda, MD 20892-1890, USA

M. F. Neurath
Innere Medizin I
Klinikum der Universität
Langenbeck Str. 1
D-55131 Mainz, Germany

M. Zeitz
Medizinische Klinik I
Charité – Universitätsmedizin Berlin
Campus Benjamin Franklin
D-12200 Berlin, Germany

Proceedings of Falk Symposium 133 (New Findings on Pathogenesis and Progress in Management of Inflammatory Bowel Diseases, Part I) held in Berlin, Germany, June 10–11, 2003

KLUWER ACADEMIC PUBLISHERS
DORDRECHT / BOSTON / LONDON

Library of Congress Cataloging-in-Publication Data is available.

ISBN 0-7923-8787-2

Published by Kluwer Academic Publishers, BV
P.O. Box 17, 3300 AA Dordrecht, The Netherlands.

Sold and distributed in North, Central and South America
by Kluwer Academic Publishers,
101 Philip Drive, Norwell, MA 02061, USA.

In all other countries, sold and distributed
by Kluwer Academic Publishers, Distribution Center,
P.O. Box 322, 3300 AH Dordrecht, The Netherlands.

Printed on acid-free paper

Contents

CONTENTS

List of Principal Contributors

RS Blumberg
Brigham and Women's Hospital
GI Division
75 Francis Street
Boston, MA 02115-6195
USA

R Duchmann
Medizinische Klinik I
Charité – Universitätsmedizin Berlin
Campus Benjamin Franklin
Hindenbergdamm 30
D-12200 Berlin
Germany

CO Elson
University of Alabama at Birmingham
Division of Gastroenterology and
 Hepatology
703 19th Street South, ZRB 633
Birmingham, AL 35294-0005
USA

IJ Fuss
National Institutes of Health
NIAID
Bldg 10, Room 11N 242
Mucosal Immunity Section
Bethesda, MD 20892-1890
USA

A Hamann
Rheumatologie
Universitätsklinikum Charité
Humboldt-Universität zu Berlin
Schumannstr. 21/22
D-10117 Berlin
Germany

F Heller
Medizinische Klinik I
Universitätsklinikum Benjamin Franklin
 der Freien Universität Berlin
D-12200 Berlin
Germany

JC Hoffmann
Medizinische Klinik I
Charité – Universitätsmedizin Berlin
Campus Benjamin Franklin
Hindenbergdamm 30
D-12200 Berlin
Germany

W Holtmeier
Medizinische Klinik II
Klinikum der Johann Wolfgang
 Goethe-Universität Frankfurt
Theodor-Stern-Kai 7
D-60590 Frankfurt
Germany

A Kitani
National Institute of Health
Mucosal Immunity Section
Laboratory of Clinical Investigation
 NIAID
Bldg 10, 11N 242
10 Center Drive
Bethesda, MD 20892-1890
USA

TT MacDonald
University of Southampton
School of Medicine
Southampton General Hospital
Mailpoint 813, Level E, South Block
Southampton SO16 6YD
UK

J Maul
Medizinische Klinik I
Charité – Universitätsmedizin Berlin
Campus Benjamin Franklin
Hindenburgdamm 30
D-12200 Berlin
Germany

WF Müller
GBF – Gesellschaft fur
 Biotechnologische Forschung mbH
Experimentelle Immunologie
Mascheroder Weg 1
D-38124 Braunschweig
Germany

MF Neurath
Innere Medizin I
Klinikum der Universität
Langenbeckstr. 1
D-55131 Mainz
Germany

F Obermeier
Innere Medizin I
Klinikum der Universität Regensburg
D-93042 Regensburg
Germany

S Pettersson
Division of Molecular Pathology
Karolinska Institutet
MTC – Division of Gastroenterology
S-17177 Stockholm
Sweden

F Powrie
University of Oxford
Sir William Dunn School of
 Pathology
South Parks Road
Oxford OX1 3RE
UK

J Reimann
Department of Medical Microbiology
 and Immunology
University of Ulm
Helmholtzstr. 8/1
D-89081 Ulm
Germany

M Rescigno
Department of Experimental
 Oncology
European Institute of Oncology
Via Ripamonti 435
I-20141 Milan
Italy

G Rogler
Klinik und Poliklinik für
 Innere Medizin I
Klinikum der Universität Regensburg
D-93042 Regensburg
Germany

J Schölmerich
Klinik und Poliklinik für
 Innere Medizin I
Klinikum der Universität Regensburg
D-93042 Regensburg
Germany

B Siegmund
Medizinische Klinik I
Charité – Universitätsmedizin Berlin
Campus Benjamin Franklin
Hindenburgdamm 30
D-12200 Berlin
Germany

U Steinhoff
Max Planck Institute for Infection
 Biology
Schumannstr. 21/22
D-10117 Berlin
Germany

W Strober
National Institutes of Health
NIAID
Bldg 10, Room 11N 238
Mucosal Immunity Section
Bethesda, MD 20892-1890
USA

E Suri-Payer
Abteilung Immungenetik
Tumorimmunologie
Deutsches Krebsforschungszentrum
Im Neuenheimer Feld 280
D-69120 Heidelberg
Germany

J Wehkamp
Department of Internal Medicine I
Robert-Bosch-Krankenhaus
Klinische Pharmakologie
Auerbachstr. 110
D-70376 Stuttgart
Germany

BM Wittig
Medizinische Klinik I
Charité – Universitätsmedizin Berlin
Campus Benjamin Franklin
Hindenburgdamm 30
D-12200 Berlin
Germany

M Zeitz
Medizinische Klinik I
Charité – Universitätsmedizin Berlin
Campus Benjamin Franklin
Hindenburgdamm 30
D-12200 Berlin
Germany

Preface

In recent years considerable progress has been achieved in regard to our understanding of the induction and modulation of the immune response in the intestinal mucosa. It is clear that this mucosal immune reaction is predominantly steered by certain T-cell populations, which are characterized by their cytokine secretion profile. Less known are the conditions under which the uptake and processing of a specific antigen lead to a particular immune response, whether it be protective, tolerant or inflammatory. However, here again distinct progress has been made in our understanding of this. Equally significant for the immune regulation in the gut appears to be so-called innate immunity. Every shift of the equilibrium in the highly regulated mucosal immune reaction is accompanied by an inflammatory reaction and destruction of the mucosa. In nearly all cases, this inflammatory response is dependent on the presence of a bacterial intestinal flora.

The goal of the Falk Symposium No. 133 in Berlin was to summarize the present knowlege in the area of the unspecific and specific immune reaction in the gut, to record the gaps in our knowledge and, in particular, to present the possibilities of targeted intervention. The link to inflammatory bowel diseases – Crohn's disease and ulcerative colitis – was always in focus. For this, an international panel of basic scientists, clinical researchers and clinicians was summoned, also to record the problems which can originate through modulation of the immune reaction possible today, and to recognize gaps in our knowledge that need to be filled by research efforts in the future. In this sense, there was an intensive, joint discussion with all participants, who, from different perspectives, have an interest in IBD research and in the clinical management of these diseases. This book collects the presentations of the speakers and provides a timely and thorough insight into the scientific work done by international experts in this field. The editors are very grateful to the speakers, moderators and discussants for their willingness to participate and present their most recent data, and particularly to the Falk Foundation for their generous support.

R. Duchmann, R. Blumberg, M. Neurath, J. Schölmerich,
W. Strober, M. Zeitz

Section I
Handling of luminal antigens I:
Innate immunity

1
Toll-like receptors (TLRs) in inflammatory bowel disease

G. ROGLER, H. HERFARTH, J. SCHÖLMERICH
and M. HAUSMANN

INTRODUCTION

The intestinal mucosa forms the primary barrier against the multitude of bacteria in the intestinal lumen. During diseases or conditions in which this barrier becomes leaky, the adaptive and innate immune systems collaborate to defend the attacked organism[1–5]. The immediate and effective recognition of bacterial products is of great importance for defence against bacterial infections and for the maintenance of body integrity and health[6]. Besides adaptive immune mechanisms involving antigen presentation and a T- or B-cell response innate immune mechanisms are necessary for immediate immune responses[2,5,7–12]. A feature of the inborn or innate immune system is the rapid recognition of bacterial wall components such as lipopolysaccharide (LPS) of Gram-negative bacteria[13–15], recognition of peptidoglycans[5,16–19], the most important stimulating component of Gram-positive bacteria and of lipoproteins which are produced by all bacterial pathogens[20–24]. In addition, bacterial DNA as another indicator of bacterial invasion must be rapidly recognized, and this must be followed by appropriate immune responses[25–31].

For a long time LPS has been known to activate macrophages and induce cytokine production in numerous cells followed by an inflammatory response[32–42]. Other bacterial products, such as flagellin[43–46] or bacterial DNA (CpG motifs)[26,28,47,48] also activate mononuclear immune cells. In 1998, first evidence was published showing that the molecules that mediate the rapid surface recognition of such bacterial products are the so-called Toll-like receptors (TLRs)[49–54]. TLRs are transmembrane proteins of the interleukin-1 (IL-1) receptor superfamily, which are characterized by a cytoplasmatic Toll IL-1 receptor

"

domain or TIR domain[1,55–59]. A defect in response to LPS in two different mouse strains has been localized to mutations in the TLR4, which is homologue to the *Drosophila* toll gene[49]. The human Toll-like receptor TLR4 is able to bind LPS together with MD-2 and CD14, and to induce cellular signalling as a response to bacterial LPS[5,6,13,15,25,60–68].

EVIDENCE FOR A ROLE OF TLRs IN INTESTINAL GENE EXPRESSION

The role of bacteria and bacterial products during the induction and chronification of inflammatory bowel disease has been shown impressively during recent years. Balfour Sartor's group and others proved that certain bacterial strains such as *Bacteroides* can induce or aggravate colonic inflammation in models such as HLA-B27 rats or IL-10 knockout mice[69–79]. Raising IL-2 knockout mice (or IL-10-deficient mice, HLA-B27 transgenic rats and other animal models of IBD) in a germ-free environment protects them from developing colitis, indicating the essential role of bacteria for the pathophysiology of inflammation in these models[73]. It is intriguing to assume that this important role is mediated by a surface receptor for bacterial products such as the Toll-like receptor family[9]. On the other hand, we know from a number of different laboratories, such as Martin Kagnoff's[80–89] or Dan Podolsky's group[90–92], that bacteria can interact with intestinal epithelial cells and induce the secretion of a number of cytokines or chemokines. Even in the normal intestinal mucosa, however, bacteria play an essential role in regulating gene expression in epithelial cells. In an impressive experiment, Lora Hooper, Jeff Gordon and co-workers showed that colonization of animals held under germ-free conditions with just one definite bacterial strain did induce a rapid change in gene expression[93,94]. The gene expression profile in epithelial cells from animals colonized with that bacterium showed an up-regulation of more than 20 genes[93,94]. As one example, colipase was dramatically induced in intestinal crypts compared to villi. In a recent study it was demonstrated that colonization of TLR4 knockout mice results in differences in gene expression pattern compared to wild-type mice colonized with the same bacteria: especially a lack of induction of PPARgamma expression was found in colonized mice devoid of functional TLR4 (Lps(d)/Lps(d) mice)[95]. This is interesting, as PPARgamma is thought to be a mainly anti-inflammatory transcription factor and to counteract NFκB activation in epithelial cells and macrophages[96–102]. Therefore an impaired signal transduction via TLRs could lead to a decreased protection of the intestinal barrier or epithelial cells. On the other hand, it may be assumed that mutations in TLRs could be associated with a lack of inflammatory responses to bacterial overgrowth.

WHICH TLRs MAY PLAY A ROLE DURING IBD?

So far, most investigations have focused on the expression of TLR2 and TLR4 during intestinal inflammation[91,103–110] (Figure 1). Recent attention has been paid to TLR9[48], but TLR3[90,91] and TLR5[111] may be of importance. TLR1 and TLR6 form heterodimers with TLR2 and may therefore contribute to changes in intestinal gene expression[112,113] (Figure 1). Heterodimers of TLR1/TLR6 and TLR2 are receptors for lipopeptides, lipoarabinomannan, peptidoglycan, zymosan, and heat-shock proteins[113] (Figure 1). Especially the latter point may be of interest in IBD as a strong up-regulation of heat-shock proteins has been reported. TLR3 homodimers bind double-stranded RNA[114–116]. TLR4, the classic LPS receptor, associates with MD2 and CD14 to bind lipopolysaccharide[49,117–121], heat-shock proteins[122–125], and fibronectin[126,127]. TLR5 has been demonstrated to be a receptor for flagellin, which is an important component of the flagella of many pathogenic bacteria[43,111,128–130]. As mentioned, the ligands for TLR9 are so-called CpG motifs, which are much more frequent in bacterial DNA compared to vertebrate DNA[27,30,48,131–133] (Figure 1). In addition, the CpG motifs are much less menthylated compared to human DNA. Via the signal transduction pathways involving MyD88, IRAK or NIK a number of mediators are induced that could play a role in IBD, such as tumour necrosis factor, IL-6 and interferon β[33,55,65,134–141] (Figure 2). In addition, as a response to a ligation

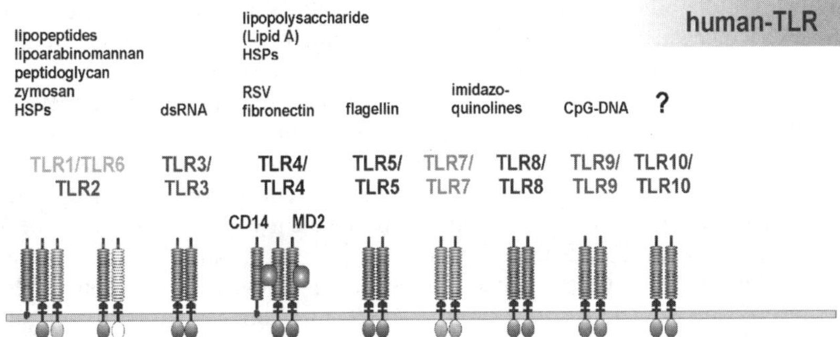

Figure 1   Human TLRs and their ligands

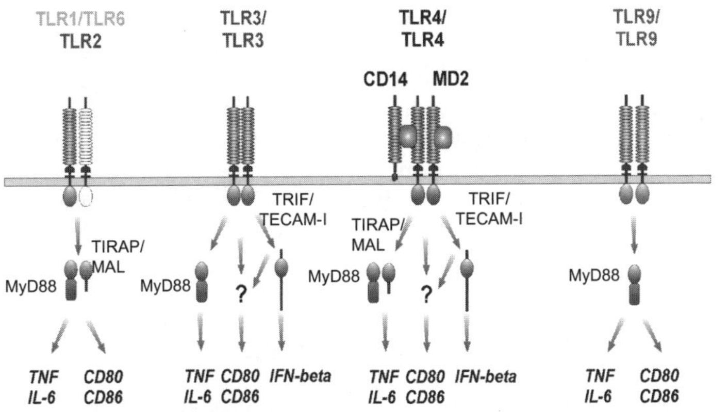

Figure 2   Intracellular signalling via different TLR and typical effector molecules

of TLR2, TLR3 and TLR4, as well as TLR9, an up-regulation of CD80 and CD86 has been observed[43,137,142,143] (Figure 2). Both are co-stimulatory molecules and necessary to induce a T-cell response and expansion. If CD80 and CD86 are absent, tolerance is induced[144–149].

PATHOPHYSIOLOGICAL ROLE OF TLRs IN MODELS OF COLITIS

Based on these theoretical considerations is there evidence for a role of TLRs in IBD? In a paper by Hornef and co-workers it was clearly demonstrated that LPS is internalized in murine intestinal epithelial cells and co-localizes after 10 or 30 min with TLR4 in the Golgi region of intestinal epithelial cells[150]. Much attention has been paid to the role of TLRs in intestinal epithelial cell (IEC) functions[90–92,104,109,110,151,152]. However, so far the physiological role of TLRs for IEC is not clear and more data are needed to be sure of the importance of TLRs in IEC physiology.

The responses of mice and humans to LPS are largely different; therefore results on TLR4 expression are not easy to transfer from mouse models to humans. On the other hand, effects of TLR9 might be more similar in mice and humans. However, there is discussion about whether the application of DNA containing CpG motifs into models of colitis ameliorates or exacerbates colitis[153,154]. Data from Florian Obermeier et al. indicate that this largely depends on the time point of application[154] (also unpublished observations). Application of CpG motifs after the onset of disease dramatically worsened weight loss, overall survival and the histology of the animals in different mouse models of colitis. Cytokine secretion from lamina propria mononuclear cells supported the development of colitis. In contrast, application of CpG motifs before the onset of colitis may be protective (unpublished observations). In the DSS (dextran sulphate sodium) model, as well as in the CD4$^+$/CD62L$^+$ transfer model, pretreatment of either DSS-treated animals or the donor animals for the transplanted T cells was followed by an amelioration of colitis. This down-regulation or amelioration of colitis might be induced by regulatory T cells that are induced by the pretreatment with CpG motifs. This is also a window to a new treatment option that could be used in IBD during phases of remission.

The role of TLR9 during *acute* inflammation may be different. In TLR9 knockout mice treated with DSS a reduced survival rate and an increased weight loss was observed. On the other hand, there was less infiltrate in the mucosa and less cytokine secretion compared to wild-type mice. This indicates that TLR9 may be involved in the recruitment of the early infiltrate in acute DSS colitis, and that a lack of this infiltrate may be deleterious for the animals, for example, due to a missing stimulus for repair of damaged epithelia.

DATA ON TLR EXPRESSION IN HUMAN IBD

Dan Podolsky's group was the first to report a change in TLR expression on intestinal epithelial cells during IBD. Elke Cario and co-workers reported that

TLR3 is down-regulated and TLR4 is up-regulated on the epithelial cells in patients with Crohn's disease[90]. When we investigated TLR expression we found that TLR2 (Figure 3) and TLR4 expression (Figure 4) was virtually absent in non-inflamed mucosa[105]. In patients with Crohn's disease and active ulcerative colitis TLR2- (Figure 3) and TLR4- (Figure 4) positive cells were detected in the lamina propria. A few positive cells were also found in patients with diverticulitis. When we isolated CD33-positive cells (intestinal macrophages) from the mucosa of controls and patients with Crohn's disease a lack of expression of both TLRs on the surface of intestinal macrophages isolated from control mucosa was evident[105]. On macrophages isolated from Crohn's disease patients a population expressing TLRs and a population without expression could be demonstrated, indicating a heterogeneity of macrophages in the diseased mucosa. Investigating mRNA expression of TLR1, TLR2, TLR3, TLR4 and TLR5 a specific pattern was found. Whereas TLR1, TLR2, TLR3, TLR4, and TLR5-mRNA were all expressed on monocytes we could not amplify any of the transcripts from control mucosa macrophages[105]. In macrophages isolated from Crohn's disease patients expression of TLR2, TLR4 and TLR5 was detected. This clearly indicates that macrophages isolated from the diseased mucosa are not simply monocytes, but already lost TLR1 and TLR3 expression and underwent a certain differentiation. Another possibility would be an induction of TLR2, TLR4 and

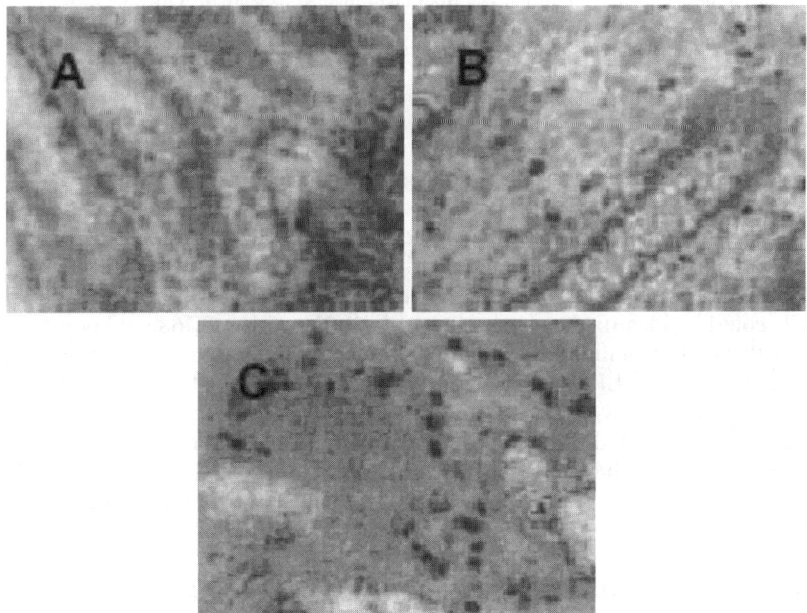

Figure 3   Immunohistochemical detection of TLR2 in control mucosa and inflamed mucosa. **A**: No cells containing TLR2 were detectable in control mucosa from non-inflamed patients. **B**: In Crohn's disease cells with TLR2 were detectable in the lamina propria. **C**: In ulcerative colitis cells with TLR2 were detectable in the lamina propria (original magnification× 400)

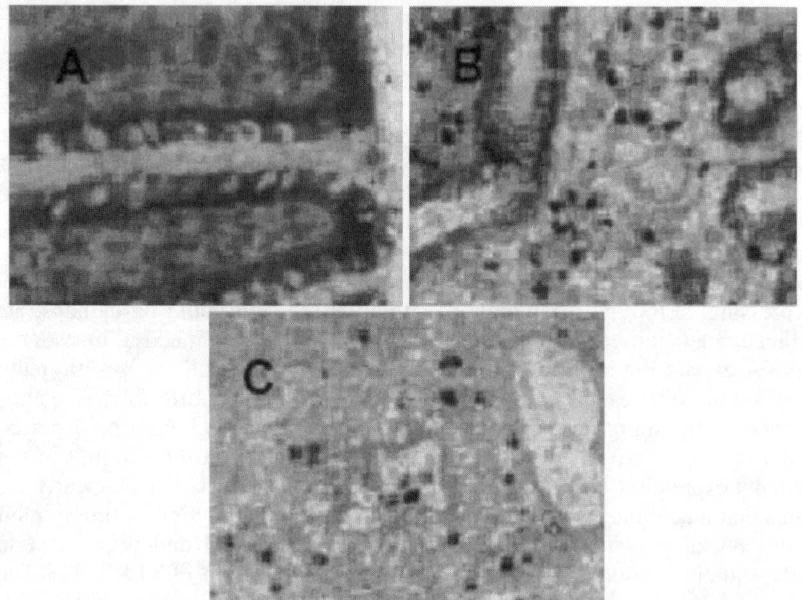

Figure 4   Immunohistochemical detection of TLR4 in the inflamed mucosa. **A**: No cells containing TLR4 were detectable in control mucosa from non-inflamed patients. **B**: In Crohn's disease cells with TLR4 were detectable in the lamina propria. **C**: In ulcerative colitis cells with TLR4 were detectable in the lamina propria (original magnification× 400)

TLR5 in the resident macrophage population. Our data so far do not allow us to conclude whether there is an impaired differentiation of blood monocytes in Crohn's disease or an induction of the transcripts in the resident macrophage population. However, the data clearly indicate that TLR2 and TLR4 are expressed on the same cells. By double immunohistochemistry the TLR-expressing cells could be identified as macrophages (staining with a CD68 antibody as well as with the TLR antibodies) (Figure 5). When we isolated the cells and incubated them with LPS with a concentration of 10 ng/ml only macrophages isolated from actively inflamed Crohn's disease mucosa secreted IL-1. Macrophages isolated from control mucosa and Crohn's disease mucosa without any inflammation did not react with IL-1 secretion to LPS stimulation[105]. This indicates that TLR expression is necessary for an LPS response on those cells.

TLRs IN IBD – WHAT HAVE WE LEARNED SO FAR?

It is too early to draw any definite conclusions from the data that have been obtained on the regulation and expression of TLRs in IBD. Their role for monocyte activation is clear. However, it is still unclear whether they play an essential and specific role during the pathophysiology of IBD. Recent reports (so far

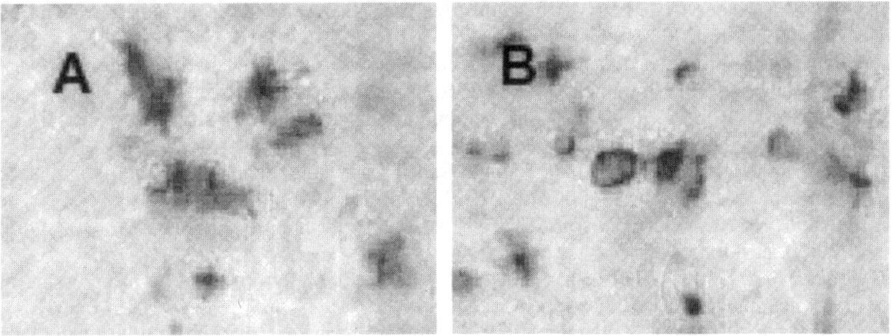

Figure 5   Identification of the cell types containing TLR2 in the inflamed mucosa. Cellular markers were stained in a first step by anti-CD68. TLR2 was stained in a second step. Positive cells were visualized with NovaRED and benzidine dihydrochloride (BDHC) reaction product. TLR2 could be co-localized in macrophages from a Crohn's disease patient (**A**) and a ulcerative colitis patient (**B**) (original magnification× 400)

unpublished) suggest that single nucleotide polymorphisms may change the function of TLRs, and that certain polymorphisms are more frequent in Crohn's disease patients than in controls. These results are still somewhat contradictory, and further studies are awaited.

So far it is clear that the innate immune system is predominant for host–bacteria interactions in the gut. Pattern recognition receptors are important for differential responses. TLR signalling obviously induces common and distinctive genes, and the regulation of TLR expression is differentially changed in the inflamed mucosa. In addition, modulation of TLR responses might be an interesting approach for tolerance maintenance or re-induction of remission. Further data certainly will be of interest and relevance for the understanding of the pathophysiology of IBD.

References

1. Beutler B, Rehli M. Evolution of the TIR, tolls and TLRs: functional inferences from computational biology. Curr Top Microbiol Immunol. 2002;270:1–21.
2. Werling D, Jungi TW. Toll-like receptors linking innate and adaptive immune response. Vet Immunol Immunopathol. 2003;91:1–12.
3. Modlin RL. Mammalian toll-like receptors. Ann Allergy Asthma Immunol. 2002;88:543–7.
4. Hacker G, Redecke V, Hacker H. Activation of the immune system by bacterial CpG-DNA. Immunology. 2002;105:245–51.
5. Beutler B, Poltorak A. Sepsis and evolution of the innate immune response. Crit Care Med. 2001;29:S2–7.
6. Imler JL, Hoffmann JA. Toll and Toll-like proteins: an ancient family of receptors signaling infection. Rev Immunogenet. 2000;2:294–304.
7. Ruland J, Mak TW. Transducing signals from antigen receptors to nuclear factor kappaB. Immunol Rev. 2003;193:93–100.
8. Triantafilou M, Brandenburg K, Gutsmann T et al. Innate recognition of bacteria: engagement of multiple receptors. Crit Rev Immunol. 2002;22:251–68.
9. Kanai T, Ilyama R, Ishikura T et al. Role of the innate immune system in the development of chronic colitis. J Gastroenterol. 2002;37(Suppl. 14):38–42.
10. Henneke P, Golenbock DT. Innate immune recognition of lipopolysaccharide by endothelial cells. Crit Care Med. 2002;30:S207–13.

11. Opal SM, Huber CE. Bench-to-bedside review: Toll-like receptors and their role in septic shock. Crit Care. 2002;6:125–36.
12. Uthaisangsook S, Day NK, Bahna SL et al. Innate immunity and its role against infections. Ann Allergy Asthma Immunol. 2002;88:253–64.
13. Heumann D, Roger T. Initial responses to endotoxins and Gram-negative bacteria. Clin Chim Acta. 2002;323:59–72.
14. Ingalls RR, Heine H, Lien E et al. Lipopolysaccharide recognition, CD14, and lipopolysaccharide receptors. Infect Dis Clin N Am. 1999;13:341–53.
15. Kaisho T, Akira S. Critical roles of Toll-like receptors in host defense. Crit Rev Immunol. 2000;20:393–405.
16. Armant MA, Fenton MJ. Toll-like receptors: a family of pattern-recognition receptors in mammals. Genome Biol. 2002;3:3011.
17. Mattsson E, Persson T, Andersson P et al. Peptidoglycan induces mobilization of the surface marker for activation marker CD66b in human neutrophils but not in eosinophils. Clin Diagn Lab Immunol. 2003;10:485–8.
18. Michelsen KS, Aicher A, Mohaupt M et al. The role of toll-like receptors (TLRs) in bacteria-induced maturation of murine dendritic cells (DCS). Peptidoglycan and lipoteichoic acid are inducers of DC maturation and require TLR2. J Biol Chem. 2001;276:25680–6.
19. Maldonado C, Trejo W, Ramirez A et al. Lipophosphopeptidoglycan of *Entamoeba histolytica* induces an antiinflammatory innate immune response and downregulation of toll-like receptor 2 (TLR-2) gene expression in human monocytes. Arch Med Res. 2000;31:S71–3.
20. Birchler T, Seibl R, Buchner K et al. Human Toll-like receptor 2 mediates induction of the antimicrobial peptide human beta-defensin 2 in response to bacterial lipoprotein. Eur J Immunol. 2001;31:3131–7.
21. Modlin RL. Activation of toll-like receptors by microbial lipoproteins: role in host defense. J Allergy Clin Immunol. 2001;108:S104–6.
22. Sieling PA, Modlin RL. Activation of toll-like receptors by microbial lipoproteins. Scand J Infect Dis. 2001;33:97–100.
23. Aliprantis AO, Yang RB, Mark MR et al. Cell activation and apoptosis by bacterial lipoproteins through toll-like receptor-2. Science. 1999;285:736–9.
24. Brightbill HD, Libraty DH, Krutzik SR et al. Host defense mechanisms triggered by microbial lipoproteins through toll-like receptors. Science. 1999;285:732–6.
25. Ahmad-Nejad P, Hacker H, Rutz M et al. Bacterial CpG-DNA and lipopolysaccharides activate Toll-like receptors at distinct cellular compartments. Eur J Immunol. 2002;32:1958–68.
26. Klinman DM, Takeshita F, Gursel I et al. CpG DNA: recognition by and activation of monocytes. Microbes Infect. 2002;4:897–901.
27. Chuang TH, Lee J, Kline L et al. Toll-like receptor 9 mediates CpG-DNA signaling. J Leukoc Biol. 2002;71:538–44.
28. Krieg AM. CpG motifs in bacterial DNA and their immune effects. Annu Rev Immunol. 2002;20:709–60.
29. Wagner H. Interactions between bacterial CpG-DNA and TLR9 bridge innate and adaptive immunity. Curr Opin Microbiol. 2002;5:62–9.
30. Takeshita F, Leifer CA, Gursel I et al. Cutting edge: role of Toll-like receptor 9 in CpG DNA-induced activation of human cells. J Immunol. 2001;167:3555–8.
31. Dalpke AH, Frey M, Morath S et al. Interaction of lipoteichoic acid and CpG-DNA during activation of innate immune cells. Immunobiology. 2002;206:392–407.
32. Grimm MC, Pavli P, Van de Pol E et al. Evidence for a CD14+ population of monocytes in inflammatory bowel disease mucosa – implications for pathogenesis. Clin Exp Immunol. 1995;100:291–7.
33. Tsan MF, Clark RN, Goyert SM et al. Induction of TNF-alpha and MnSOD by endotoxin: role of membrane CD14 and Toll-like receptor-4. Am J Physiol Cell Physiol. 2001;280:C1422–30.
34. Dobrovolskaia MA, Vogel SN. Toll receptors, CD14, and macrophage activation and deactivation by LPS. Microbes Infect. 2002;4:903–14.
35. Smith PD, Smythies LE, Mosteller-Barnum M et al. Intestinal macrophages lack CD14 and CD89 and consequently are down-regulated for LPS- and IgA-mediated activities. J Immunol. 2001;167:2651–6.
36. Tobias PS, Ulevitch RJ. Lipopolysaccharide binding protein and CD14 in LPS dependent macrophage activation. Immunobiology. 1993;187:227–32.

37. Chow CW, Grinstein S, Rotstein OD. Signaling events in monocytes and macrophages. New Horiz. 1995;3:342–51.
38. Schutt C. CD14. Int J Biochem Cell Biol. 1999;31:545–9.
39. Sweet MJ, Hume DA. Endotoxin signal transduction in macrophages. J Leukoc Biol. 1996;60:8–26.
40. Kitchens RL. Role of CD14 in cellular recognition of bacterial lipopolysaccharides. Chem Immunol. 2000;74:61–82.
41. Landmann R, Muller B, Zimmerli W. CD14, new aspects of ligand and signal diversity. Microbes Infect. 2000;2:295–304.
42. Su GL. Lipopolysaccharides in liver injury: molecular mechanisms of Kupffer cell activation. Am J Physiol Gastrointest Liver Physiol. 2002;283:G256–65.
43. Means TK, Hayashi F, Smith KD et al. The Toll-like receptor 5 stimulus bacterial flagellin induces maturation and chemokine production in human dendritic cells. J Immunol. 2003;170:5165–75.
44. Moors MA, Li L, Mizel SB. Activation of interleukin-1 receptor-associated kinase by gram-negative flagellin. Infect Immun. 2001;69:4424–9.
45. Liaudet L, Deb A, Pacher P et al. The flagellin-TLR5 axis: therapeutic opportunities. Drug News Perspect. 2002;15:397–409.
46. Szabo C. Role of flagellin in the pathogenesis of shock and acute respiratory distress syndrome: therapeutic opportunities. Crit Care Med. 2003;31:S39–45.
47. Krug A, Rothenfusser S, Selinger S et al. CpG-A oligonucleotides induce a monocyte-derived dendritic cell-like phenotype that preferentially activates CD8 T cells. J Immunol. 2003;170:3468–77.
48. Ashkar AA, Rosenthal KL. Toll-like receptor 9, CpG DNA and innate immunity. Curr Mol Med. 2002;2:545–56.
49. Poltorak A, He X, Smirnova I et al. Defective LPS signaling in C3H/HeJ and C57BL/10ScCr mice: mutations in Tlr4 gene. Science. 1998;282:2085–8.
50. Kirschning CJ, Wesche H, Merrill Ayres T et al. Human toll-like receptor 2 confers responsiveness to bacterial lipopolysaccharide. J Exp Med. 1998;188:2091–7.
51. Yang RB, Mark MR, Gray A et al. Toll-like receptor-2 mediates lipopolysaccharide-induced cellular signalling. Nature. 1998;395:284–8.
52. O'Neill LA, Greene C. Signal transduction pathways activated by the IL-1 receptor family: ancient signaling machinery in mammals, insects, and plants. J Leukoc Biol. 1998;63:650–7.
53. Rock FL, Hardiman G, Timans JC et al. A family of human receptors structurally related to *Drosophila* Toll. Proc Natl Acad Sci USA. 1998;95:588–93.
54. Chan VW, Mecklenbrauker I, Su I et al. The molecular mechanism of B cell activation by toll-like receptor protein RP-105. J Exp Med. 1998;188:93–101.
55. Bowie A, O'Neill LA. The interleukin-1 receptor/Toll-like receptor superfamily: signal generators for pro-inflammatory interleukins and microbial products. J Leukoc Biol. 2000; 67:508–14.
56. Dunne A, O'Neill LA. The interleukin-1 receptor/Toll-like receptor superfamily: signal transduction during inflammation and host defense. Sci STKE. 2003;2003(171): re 3.
57. Eto A, Muta T, Yamazaki S et al. Essential roles for NF-kappa B and a Toll/IL-1 receptor domain-specific signal(s) in the induction of I kappa B-zeta. Biochem Biophys Res Commun. 2003;301:495–501.
58. Martin MU, Wesche H. Summary and comparison of the signaling mechanisms of the Toll/interleukin-1 receptor family. Biochim Biophys Acta. 2002;1592:265–80.
59. O'Neill L. The Toll/interleukin-1 receptor domain: a molecular switch for inflammation and host defence. Biochem Soc Trans. 2000;28:557–63.
60. Mancek M, Pristovsek P, Jerala R. Identification of LPS-binding peptide fragment of MD-2, a toll-receptor accessory protein. Biochem Biophys Res Commun. 2002;292:880–5.
61. Gomi K, Kawasaki K, Kawai Y et al. Toll-like receptor 4–MD-2 complex mediates the signal transduction induced by flavolipin, an amino acid-containing lipid unique to Flavobacterium meningosepticum. J Immunol. 2002;168:2939–43.
62. da Silva Correia J, Ulevitch RJ. MD-2 and TLR4 N-linked glycosylations are important for a functional lipopolysaccharide receptor. J Biol Chem. 2002;277:1845–54.
63. Kawasaki K, Akashi S, Shimazu R et al. Mouse toll-like receptor 4. MD-2 complex mediates lipopolysaccharide–mimetic signal transduction by Taxol. J Biol Chem. 2000;275:2251–4.

64. Shimazu R, Akashi S, Ogata H et al. MD-2, a molecule that confers lipopolysaccharide responsiveness on Toll-like receptor 4. J Exp Med. 1999;189:1777–82.
65. Dziarski R, Gupta D. Role of MD-2 in TLR2- and TLR4-mediated recognition of Gram-negative and Gram-positive bacteria and activation of chemokine genes. J Endotoxin Res. 2000;6:401–5.
66. Oshikawa K, Sugiyama Y. Gene expression of Toll-like receptors and associated molecules induced by inflammatory stimuli in the primary alveolar macrophage. Biochem Biophys Res Commun. 2003;305:649–55.
67. Kirschning CJ, Schumann RR. TLR2: cellular sensor for microbial and endogenous molecular patterns. Curr Top Microbiol Immunol. 2002;270:121–44.
68. Sato S, Nomura F, Kawai T et al. Synergy and cross-tolerance between toll-like receptor (TLR) 2- and TLR4-mediated signaling pathways. J Immunol. 2000;165:7096–101.
69. Rath HC, Schultz M, Freitag R et al. Different subsets of enteric bacteria induce and perpetuate experimental colitis in rats and mice. Infect Immun. 2001;69:2277–85.
70. Veltkamp C, Tonkonogy SL, De Jong YP et al. Continuous stimulation by normal luminal bacteria is essential for the development and perpetuation of colitis in Tg(epsilon26) mice. Gastroenterology. 2001;120:900–13.
71. Sartor RB. Colitis in HLA-B27/beta 2 microglobulin transgenic rats. Int Rev Immunol. 2000;19:39–50.
72. van Tol EA, Holt L, Li FL et al. Bacterial cell wall polymers promote intestinal fibrosis by direct stimulation of myofibroblasts. Am J Physiol. 1999;277:G245–55.
73. Schultz M, Tonkonogy SL, Sellon RK et al. IL-2-deficient mice raised under germfree conditions develop delayed mild focal intestinal inflammation. Am J Physiol. 1999;276:G1461–72.
74. Rath HC, Wilson KH, Sartor RB. Differential induction of colitis and gastritis in HLA-B27 transgenic rats selectively colonized with *Bacteroides vulgatus* or *Escherichia coli*. Infect Immun. 1999;67:2969–74.
75. Rath HC, Ikeda JS, Linde HJ et al. Varying cecal bacterial loads influences colitis and gastritis in HLA-B27 transgenic rats. Gastroenterology. 1999;116:310–19.
76. Sellon RK, Tonkonogy S, Schultz M et al. Resident enteric bacteria are necessary for development of spontaneous colitis and immune system activation in interleukin-10-deficient mice. Infect Immun. 1998;66:5224–31.
77. Sartor RB. The influence of normal microbial flora on the development of chronic mucosal inflammation. Res Immunol. 1997;148:567–76.
78. Sartor RB. Role of the enteric microflora in the pathogenesis of intestinal inflammation and arthritis. Aliment Pharmacol Ther. 1997;11(Suppl. 3):17–23.
79. Rath HC, Herfarth HH, Ikeda JS et al. Normal luminal bacteria, especially *Bacteroides* species, mediate chronic colitis, gastritis, and arthritis in HLA-B27/human beta2 microglobulin transgenic rats. J Clin Invest. 1996;98:945–53.
80. Maaser C, Kagnoff MF. Role of the intestinal epithelium in orchestrating innate and adaptive mucosal immunity. Z Gastroenterol. 2002;40:525–9.
81. Eckmann L, Kagnoff MF. Cytokines in host defense against *Salmonella*. Microbes Infect. 2001;3:1191–200.
82. Kagnoff MF, Eckmann L. Analysis of host responses to microbial infection using gene expression profiling. Curr Opin Microbiol. 2001;4:246–50.
83. Izadpanah A, Dwinell MB, Eckmann L et al. Regulated MIP-3alpha/CCL20 production by human intestinal epithelium: mechanism for modulating mucosal immunity. Am J Physiol Gastrointest Liver Physiol. 2001;280:G710–19.
84. Elewaut D, DiDonato JA, Kim JM et al. NF-kappa B is a central regulator of the intestinal epithelial cell innate immune response induced by infection with enteroinvasive bacteria. J Immunol. 1999;163:1457–66.
85. Yang SK, Eckmann L, Panja A et al. Differential and regulated expression of C-X-C, C-C, and C-chemokines by human colon epithelial cells. Gastroenterology. 1997;113:1214–23.
86. Eckmann L, Stenson WF, Savidge TC et al. Role of intestinal epithelial cells in the host secretory response to infection by invasive bacteria. Bacterial entry induces epithelial prostaglandin h synthase-2 expression and prostaglandin E2 and F2alpha production. J Clin Invest. 1997;100:296–309.
87. Kagnoff MF, Eckmann L. Epithelial cells as sensors for microbial infection. J Clin Invest. 1997;100:6–10.

88. Rasmussen SJ, Eckmann L, Quayle AJ et al. Secretion of proinflammatory cytokines by epithelial cells in response to *Chlamydia* infection suggests a central role for epithelial cells in chlamydial pathogenesis. J Clin Invest. 1997;99:77–87.
89. Huang GT, Eckmann L, Savidge TC et al. Infection of human intestinal epithelial cells with invasive bacteria upregulates apical intercellular adhesion molecule-1 (ICAM)-1) expression and neutrophil adhesion. J Clin Invest. 1996;98:572–83.
90. Cario E, Podolsky DK. Differential alteration in intestinal epithelial cell expression of toll-like receptor 3 (TLR3) and TLR4 in inflammatory bowel disease. Infect Immun. 2000;68:7010–17.
91. Cario E, Rosenberg IM, Brandwein SL et al. Lipopolysaccharide activates distinct signaling pathways in intestinal epithelial cell lines expressing Toll-like receptors. J Immunol. 2000;164:966–72.
92. Cario E, Brown D, McKee M et al. Commensal-associated molecular patterns induce selective toll-like receptor-trafficking from apical membrane to cytoplasmic compartments in polarized intestinal epithelium. Am J Pathol. 2002;160:165–73.
93. Hooper LV, Wong MH, Thelin A et al. Molecular analysis of commensal host–microbial relationships in the intestine. Science. 2001;291:881–4.
94. Hooper LV, Falk PG, Gordon JI. Analyzing the molecular foundations of commensalism in the mouse intestine. Curr Opin Microbiol. 2000;3:79–85.
95. Dubuquoy L, Jansson EA, Deeb S et al. Impaired expression of peroxisome proliferator-activated receptor gamma in ulcerative colitis. Gastroenterology. 2003;124:1265–76.
96. Mann DA, Smart DE. Transcriptional regulation of hepatic stellate cell activation. Gut. 2002;50:891–6.
97. Delerive P, Fruchart JC, Staels B. Peroxisome proliferator-activated receptors in inflammation control. J Endocrinol. 2001;169:453–9.
98. Chinetti G, Fruchart JC, Staels B. Peroxisome proliferator-activated receptors (PPARs): nuclear receptors at the crossroads between lipid metabolism and inflammation. Inflamm Res. 2000;49:497–505.
99. Ricote M, Huang JT, Welch JS et al. The peroxisome proliferator-activated receptor (PPARgamma) as a regulator of monocyte/macrophage function. J Leukoc Biol. 1999;66:733–9.
100. Ricote M, Li AC, Willson TM et al. The peroxisome proliferator-activated receptor-gamma is a negative regulator of macrophage activation. Nature. 1998;391:79–82.
101. Glass CK. Potential roles of the peroxisome proliferator-activated receptor-gamma in macrophage biology and atherosclerosis. J Endocrinol. 2001;169:461–4.
102. Cunard R, Ricote M, DiCampli D et al. Regulation of cytokine expression by ligands of peroxisome proliferator activated receptors. J Immunol. 2002;168:2795–802.
103. Ortega-Cava CF, Ishihara S, Rumi MA et al. Strategic compartmentalization of toll-like receptor 4 in the mouse gut. J Immunol. 2003;170:3977–85.
104. Melmed G, Thomas LS, Lee N et al. Human intestinal epithelial cells are broadly unresponsive to Toll-like receptor 2-dependent bacterial ligands: implications for host–microbial interactions in the gut. J Immunol. 2003;170:1406–15.
105. Hausmann M, Kiessling S, Mestermann S et al. Toll-like receptors 2 and 4 are up-regulated during intestinal inflammation. Gastroenterology. 2002;122:1987–2000.
106. Naik S, Kelly EJ, Meijer L et al. Absence of Toll-like receptor 4 explains endotoxin hyporesponsiveness in human intestinal epithelium. J Pediatr Gastroenterol Nutr. 2001;32:449–53.
107. Fusunyan RD, Nanthakumar NN, Baldeon ME et al. Evidence for an innate immune response in the immature human intestine: toll-like receptors on fetal enterocytes. Pediatr Res. 2001;49:589–93.
108. Backhed F, Meijer L, Normark S et al. TLR4-dependent recognition of lipopolysaccharide by epithelial cells requires sCD14. Cell Microbiol. 2002;4:493–501.
109. Abreu MT, Arnold ET, Thomas LS et al. TLR4 and MD-2 expression is regulated by immune-mediated signals in human intestinal epithelial cells. J Biol Chem. 2002;277:20431–7.
110. Abreu MT, Vora P, Faure E et al. Decreased expression of Toll-like receptor-4 and MD-2 correlates with intestinal epithelial cell protection against dysregulated proinflammatory gene expression in response to bacterial lipopolysaccharide. J Immunol. 2001;167:1609–16.
111. Gewirtz AT, Navas TA, Lyons S et al. Cutting edge: bacterial flagellin activates basolaterally expressed TLR5 to induce epithelial proinflammatory gene expression. J Immunol. 2001;167:1882–5.
112. Wyllie DH, Kiss-Toth E, Visintin A et al. Evidence for an accessory protein function for Toll-like receptor 1 in anti-bacterial responses. J Immunol. 2000;165:7125–32.

113. Wetzler LM. The role of Toll-like receptor 2 in microbial disease and immunity. Vaccine. 2003;21(Suppl. 2):S55–60.

114. Heinz S, Haehnel V, Karaghiosoff M et al. Species-specific regulation of Toll-like receptor 3 genes in men and mice. J Biol Chem. 2003;278:21502–9.

115. Sarkar SN, Smith HL, Rowe TM et al. Double-stranded RNA signaling by Toll-like receptor 3 requires specific tyrosine residues in its cytoplasmic domain. J Biol Chem. 2003;278:4393–6.

116. Alexopoulou L, Holt AC, Medzhitov R et al. Recognition of double-stranded RNA and activation of NF-kappaB by Toll-like receptor 3. Nature. 2001;413:732–8.

117. Beutler B. LPS in microbial pathogenesis: promise and fulfilment. J Endotoxin Res. 2002;8:329–35.

118. Beutler B. TLR4 as the mammalian endotoxin sensor. Curr Top Microbiol Immunol. 2002;270:109–20.

119. Beutler E, Gelbart T, West C. Synergy between TLR2 and TLR4: a safety mechanism. Blood Cells Mol Dis. 2001;27:728–30.

120. Beutler B, Du X, Poltorak A. Identification of Toll-like receptor 4 (Tlr4) as the sole conduit for LPS signal transduction: genetic and evolutionary studies. J Endotoxin Res. 2001;7:277–80.

121. Beutler B, Poltorak A. Positional cloning of Lps, and the general role of toll-like receptors in the innate immune response. Eur Cytokine Netw. 2000;11:143–52.

122. Vabulas RM, Ahmad-Nejad P, da Costa C et al. Endocytosed HSP60s use toll-like receptor 2 (TLR2) and TLR4 to activate the toll/interleukin-1 receptor signaling pathway in innate immune cells. J Biol Chem. 2001;276:31332–9.

123. Ohashi K, Burkart V, Flohe S et al. Cutting edge: heat shock protein 60 is a putative endogenous ligand of the toll-like receptor-4 complex. J Immunol. 2000;164:558–61.

124. Asea A, Rehli M, Kabingu E et al. Novel signal transduction pathway utilized by extracellular HSP70: role of toll-like receptor (TLR) 2 and TLR4. J Biol Chem. 2002;277:15028–34.

125. Vabulas RM, Ahmad-Nejad P, Ghose S et al. HSP70 as endogenous stimulus of the Toll/interleukin-1 receptor signal pathway. J Biol Chem. 2002;277:15107–12.

126. Okamura Y, Watari M, Jerud ES et al. The extra domain A of fibronectin activates Toll-like receptor 4. J Biol Chem. 2001;276:10229–33.

127. Vink A, Schoneveld AH, van der Meer JJ et al. *In vivo* evidence for a role of toll-like receptor 4 in the development of intimal lesions. Circulation. 2002;106:1985–90.

128. Mizel SB, Snipes JA. Gram-negative flagellin-induced self-tolerance is associated with a block in interleukin-1 receptor-associated kinase release from toll-like receptor 5. J Biol Chem. 2002;277:22414–20.

129. Hayashi F, Smith KD, Ozinsky A et al. The innate immune response to bacterial flagellin is mediated by Toll-like receptor 5. Nature. 2001;410:1099–103.

130. Gomez-Gomez L, Boller T. Flagellin perception: a paradigm for innate immunity. Trends Plant Sci. 2002;7:251–6.

131. Hemmi H, Takeuchi O, Kawai T et al. A Toll-like receptor recognizes bacterial DNA. Nature. 2000;408:740–5.

132. Bauer S, Kirschning CJ, Hacker H et al. Human TLR9 confers responsiveness to bacterial DNA via species-specific CpG motif recognition. Proc Natl Acad Sci USA. 2001;98:9237–42.

133. Lee J, Chuang TH, Redecke V et al. Molecular basis for the immunostimulatory activity of guanine nucleoside analogs: activation of Toll-like receptor 7. Proc Natl Acad Sci USA. 2003;100:6646–51.

134. Takeuchi O, Takeda K, Hoshino K et al. Cellular responses to bacterial cell wall components are mediated through MyD88-dependent signaling cascades. Int Immunol. 2000;12:113–17.

135. Wang Q, Dziarski R, Kirschning CJ et al. Micrococci and peptidoglycan activate TLR2→MyD88→IRAK→TRAF→NIK→KK→NF-kappaB signal transduction pathway that induces transcription of interleukin-8. Infect Immun. 2001;69:2270–6.

136. Takeuchi O, Akira S. Toll-like receptors; their physiological role and signal transduction system. Int Immunopharmacol. 2001;1:625–35.

137. Kaisho T, Akira S. Toll-like receptors and their signaling mechanism in innate immunity. Acta Odontol Scand. 2001;59:124–30.

138. Akira S, Hoshino K, Kaisho T. The role of Toll-like receptors and MyD88 in innate immune responses. J Endotoxin Res. 2000;6:383–7.

139. Fitzgerald KA, Palsson-McDermott EM, Bowie AG et al. Mal (MyD88-adapter-like) is required for Toll-like receptor-4 signal transduction. Nature. 2001;413:78–83.

140. Schilling D, Thomas K, Nixdorff K et al. Toll-like receptor 4 and Toll-IL-1 receptor domain-containing adapter protein (TIRAP)/myeloid differentiation protein 88 adapter-like (Mal) contribute to maximal IL-6 expression in macrophages. J Immunol. 2002;169:5874–80.

141. Adib-Conquy M, Moine P, Asehnoune K et al. Toll-like receptors-mediated TNF and IL-10 production differ during systemic inflammation. Am J Respir Crit Care Med. 2003;8:8.

142. Biragyn A, Ruffini PA, Leifer CA et al. Toll-like receptor 4-dependent activation of dendritic cells by beta-defensin 2. Science. 2002;298:1025–9.

143. Dabbagh K, Dahl ME, Stepick-Biek P et al. Toll-like receptor 4 is required for optimal development of Th2 immune responses: role of dendritic cells. J Immunol. 2002;168:4524–30.

144. Schweitzer AN, Sharpe AH. The complexity of the B7-CD28/CTLA-4 costimulatory pathway. Agents Actions Suppl. 1998;49:33–43.

145. Greenfield EA, Nguyen KA, Kuchroo VK. CD28/B7 costimulation: a review. Crit Rev Immunol. 1998;18:389–418.

146. Tamada K, Chen L. T lymphocyte costimulatory molecules in host defense and immunologic diseases. Ann Allergy Asthma Immunol. 2000;85:164–75.

147. Coyle AJ, Gutierrez-Ramos JC. The expanding B7 superfamily: increasing complexity in costimulatory signals regulating T cell function. Nat Immunol. 2001;2:203–9.

148. Kobata T, Azuma M, Yagita H et al. Role of costimulatory molecules in autoimmunity. Rev Immunogenet. 2000;2:74–80.

149. Carreno BM, Collins M. The B7 family of ligands and its receptors: new pathways for costimulation and inhibition of immune responses. Annu Rev Immunol. 2002;20:29–53.

150. Hornef MW, Frisan T, Vandewalle A et al. Toll-like receptor 4 resides in the Golgi apparatus and colocalizes with internalized lipopolysaccharide in intestinal epithelial cells. J Exp Med. 2002;195:559–70.

151. Suzuki M, Hisamatsu T, Podolsky DK. Gamma interferon augments the intracellular pathway for lipopolysaccharide (LPS) recognition in human intestinal epithelial cells through coordinated up-regulation of LPS uptake and expression of the intracellular Toll-like receptor 4-MD-2 complex. Infect Immun. 2003;71:3503–11.

152. Bocker U, Yezerskyy O, Feick P et al. Responsiveness of intestinal epithelial cell lines to lipopolysaccharide is correlated with Toll-like receptor 4 but not Toll-like receptor 2 or CD14 expression. Int J Colorectal Dis. 2003;18:25–32.

153. Rachmilewitz D, Karmeli F, Takabayashi K et al. Immunostimulatory DNA ameliorates experimental and spontaneous murine colitis. Gastroenterology. 2002;122:1428–41.

154. Obermeier F, Dunger N, Deml L et al. CpG motifs of bacterial DNA exacerbate colitis of dextran sulfate sodium-treated mice. Eur J Immunol. 2002;32:2084–92.

2
The γ/δ T-cell bridge: linking innate and acquired immunity

W. HOLTMEIER

INTRODUCTION

The innate and acquired immune systems are critical for the successful detection and elimination of infectious pathogens and tumours. There is now strong evidence that one of the crucial players involved in immune surveillance of the epithelium and regulation of innate and acquired immunity is the γ/δ T-cell population[1,2]. The epithelial-associated γ/δ T cells, which are abundant at mucosal surfaces, are ideally situated to contribute to the initial stages of the immune response. Subsets of γ/δ T cells were shown to recognize stress-induced self antigens which would enable a homogeneous population of γ/δ T cells to monitor multiple insults to the epithelium[3]. γ/δ T cells can be pro-inflammatory and kill infected cells or promote epithelial healing. Thus, γ/δ T cells are likely to consist of distinct subsets which carry out different functions depending on the stage of the immune response[4]. During the initiation stage of the immune response the γ/δ T cells can, by the production of proinflammatory cytokines, modulate the innate (natural killer cells and macrophages) and adaptive (α/β T cells, B cells) immune responses. During the late phase of the response, after the clearance of bacteria, γ/δ T cells release anti-inflammatory or immunoregulatory cytokines and promote tissue repair and cellular regeneration. In several animal models of colitis depletion of γ/δ T cells caused an exaggerated inflammatory response and an increased mortality. Thus, a malfunction or loss of intestinal γ/δ T cells, which down-modulate the inflammatory response, might explain the uncontrolled inflammation as seen in Crohn's disease or ulcerative colitis.

γ/δ T CELLS ARE ACTIVATED BY STRESS-INDUCED SELF ANTIGENS

As pathogens cross the physical barriers of the host, both the innate and acquired immune system are activated. γ/δ T cells which primarily live in epithelial tissues are thought to be crucial players involved in immune surveillance. Recent evidence suggests that they recognize stress-induced self antigens such as MICA/B (major histocompatibility complex class I chain-related A/B) which would enable many γ/δ T cells, carrying identical T-cell receptors (TCR), to monitor multiple insults to the epithelium (see Figure 1)[3,5–7]. This is in line with our own observations that γ/δ T cells are clonally expanded within mucosal surfaces[8–11] (see below) and the skin[12].

MICA and MICB are distant relatives of MHC class I molecules which have no role in antigen presentation[6]. These receptors are thought to function as signals of cellular distress since they are increasingly expressed in infected and transformed epithelial cells. Heat-shock proteins are known to induce the expression of MICA/B[13]. In healthy individuals the expression of MIC is restricted to the intestinal epithelium[13]. It remains unclear, however, whether this tissue

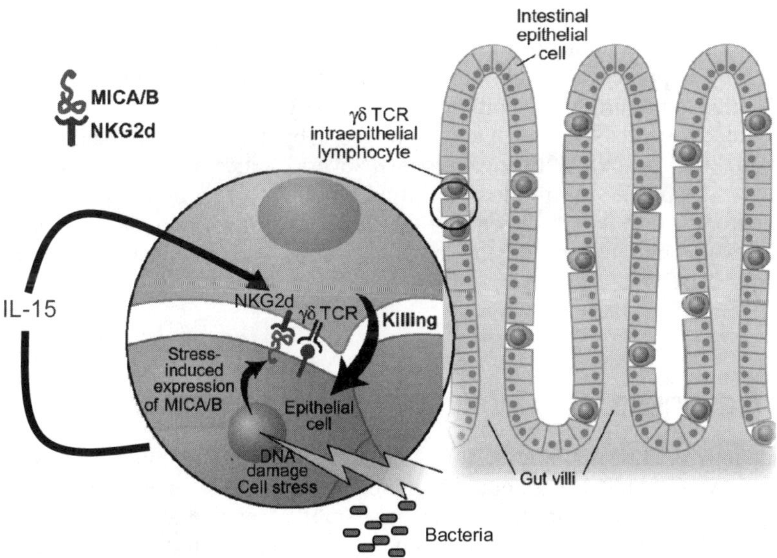

Figure 1   γ/δ IEL are activated by stress induced self-antigens (according to ref. 7). The epithelial lining of the gut is the prime target for pathogen invasion or tumour formation. These and other stress stimuli induce the expression of MICA/B in human epithelial cells. These receptors are non-classical class I molecules and have no role in antigen presentation. The ligand for MICA/B is NKG2d, which is expressed not only on natural killer cells but also on a subset of γ/δ T cells. An important cytokine in the induction of NKG2d is IL-15. The ligand for the γ/δ TCR is still unknown; however, recently it was shown that MICA is in direct contact not only with NKG2d but also with the γ/δ TCR itself. The activation of γ/δ T cells then leads to the killing of the infected or transformed epithelial cell

distribution is the result of permanent cellular stress or whether it may be induced by environmental factors.

The natural ligand of MICA/B is NKG2d, which is expressed on natural killer (NK) cells and CD8[+] α/β T cells but also on a subset of γ/δ T cells[14]. Interleukin 15 (IL-15), which is secreted by stressed epithelial cells, seems to be a key cytokine in the induction of NKG2d[15,16] and the activation of γ/δ T cells[17]. Interestingly IL-15 is overexpressed in the inflamed intestine of patients with inflammatory bowel disease (IBD)[15,18], suggesting an uncontrolled activation of the local inflammatory response. Intestinal γ/δ T cells which express the Vδ1 chain have been shown to recognize the stress-inducible MICA/B molecule[5,19]. Furthermore, peripheral γ/δ T cells expressing the Vδ2 chain were shown to be activated by MICA after infection with *Mycobacterium tuberculosis*[20]. A recent paper confirmed the notion that the γ/δ TCR itself directly binds to NKG2d[21]. Thus, MICA/B delivers both the TCR-dependent signal 1 and the NKG2d-dependent costimulatory signal 2 for a subset of γ/δ T cells. These dual receptor interactions of MIC might serve to preclude erroneous T-cell activation by crossreactive cell surface determinants[21].

The importance of stress-induced MICA is further illustrated by their recognition of tumour-infiltrating T cells[19,22]. Human NK cells and Vδ1[+] T cells bearing NKG2d receptors can lyse tumour cells which frequently express MICA[14,23]. Furthermore, mice lacking γ/δ cells are highly susceptible to multiple regimens of cutaneous carcinogenesis[24]. After exposure to carcinogens, skin cells express Rae-1 and H60, major histocompatibility complex-related molecules structurally resembling human MICA. *In vitro*, skin-associated NKG2d[+] γ/δ cells killed skin carcinoma cells by a mechanism that was sensitive to blocking NKG2d engagement. Several cancers seem to evade this immune response by producing large amounts of soluble MICA which binds to NKG2d. It was shown that this leads to a down-regulation of NKG2d and severe impairment of the responsiveness of tumour-antigen specific effector T cells[25].

MICA EXPRESSION IS INCREASED IN CROHN'S DISEASE

Immunoperoxidase staining of MICA in normal colon and colon from patients with active Crohn's disease could demonstrate that MICA expression in normal colon was weak and limited to the basal part of epithelial cells, whereas in Crohn's disease the entire epithelium was stained[26]. Furthermore, the same group could also show that MICA expression can be markedly increased by bacteria of the diffusely adherent *Escherichia coli* diarrhoeagenic group; furthermore, bacteria of this group could be isolated from patients with Crohn's disease[27,28]. Thus, it is possible that MICA is a pathogenic factor and autoimmune conditions such as Crohn's disease are triggered by bacterial infections[6]. MICA is a polymorphic molecule, but so far no primary allelic association with IBD or other autoimmune diseases has been identified[29]; nevertheless, some weak associations were described[30].

γ/δ T CELLS ARE ACTIVATED BY THE NON-POLYMORPHIC CD1 MOLECULE

During host infection, microbial antigens such as lipopolysaccharide (LPS) provide critical innate signals for dendritic cell (DC) maturation via cell surface Toll-like receptors[31]. However, maturation of DCs by microbial stimuli alone may promote a short-lived burst of IL-12 leading to an exhausted DC population unable to produce this cytokine upon subsequent encounter with naive T cells in the lymph node[32]. The ability of the host to successfully defend against microbial invasion is, therefore, dependent upon both innate signals provided by microbial products as well as T-cell signals (see Figure 2)[33].

Recent data demonstrate that a subpopulation of human Vδ1[+] γ/δ T cells can selectively stimulate dendritic cells to undergo maturation[32,34,35]. These γ/δ T cells recognize CD1c on the surface of immature DC[36]. CD1 molecules are known to present lipid and glycolipid complexes to T cells[37,38]. Importantly recognition of CD1c occurred in the absence of exogenous foreign antigens[33,36], implying reactivity against yet-to-be-identified self-lipids. Human γ/δ T cells bearing Vδ1

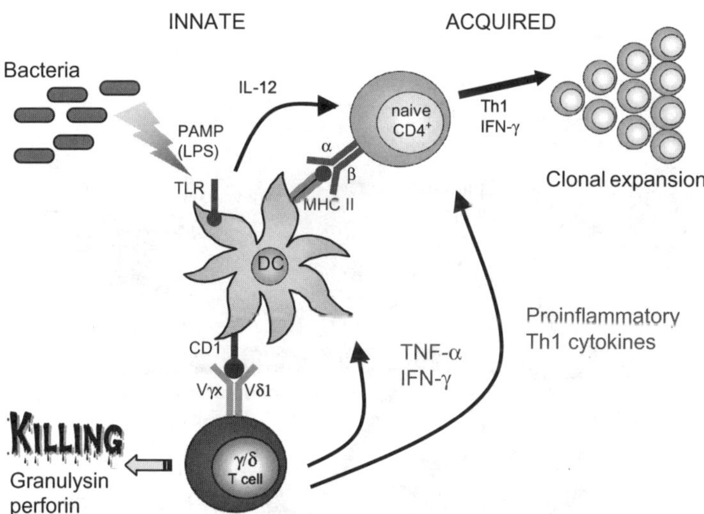

Figure 2 γ/δ T cells contribute to the initial stage of the immune response and act as a link between innate and acquired immunity. Bacterial products such as LPS activate dendritic cells by binding to Toll-like receptors (TLR). MHC class II molecules are up-regulated and present bacterial antigens to naive CD4 α/β T cells. In addition IL-12 is secreted and further activates naive CD4[+] T cells and drives them into a Th1 response and clonal expansion. However, the activation of dendritic cells by bacterial products alone is not sufficient to maintain the acquired immune response. It was shown that activated DC express CD1 which is recognized by the γ/δ TCR. Activated γ/δ T cells secrete proinflammatory cytokines such as IFN-γ and TNF-α, which mediate the maturation of dendritic cells and support the development of the acquired immune response. In addition activated γ/δ T cells have the ability to lyse neighbouring cells which are infected or transformed. The recognition of the non-polymorphic CD1 molecule provides the immune system with the capacity to rapidly respond to bacterial invasion

encoded TCRs account for the vast majority of γ/δ T cells in mucosal surfaces. Upon recognition of CD1c they secrete tumour necrosis factor alpha (TNF-α) and other proinflammatory factors that, together with microbial products such as LPS, induce immature DC to mature and to produce IL-12[32,34]. Furthermore, TNF-α and interferon gamma (IFN-γ), secreted by activated γ/δ T cells, provide the critical signals for Th1 polarization of naive CD4 T cells. In addition CD1c-specific γ/δ T cells contain bactericidal granulysin and can be cytotoxic[36]. Thus, γ/δ T cells are involved during the early stages of an immune response by interacting with immature DC and act as a link between innate and acquired immunity.

γ/δ IEL PROMOTE EPITHELIAL HEALING

Almost 10 years ago W. Havran suggested that intraepithelial γ/δ T cells function in repair of damaged epithelial tissues by secreting epithelial growth factors such as the keratinocyte growth factor (KGF)[35,39–41]. This finding is controversial since others could not find an increased secretion of KGF[42,43]. However, it was shown that at least activated, murine γ/δ T cells were capable of producing KGF[44]. In addition other protective factors such as connective tissue growth factor[45] or anti-inflammatory cytokines such as IL-10[46,47] were

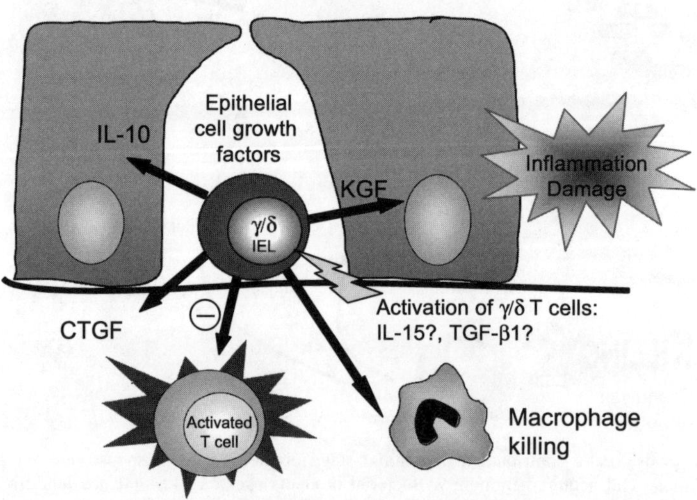

Figure 3 γ/δ T cells promote the repair of epithelial lesions. After the initial immune response which leads to inflammation and damage, subsets of γ/δ T cells are activated. It is not known if MIC or CD1 play a role in this activation but IL-15 and transforming growth factor TGF-β₁ are thought to be important. Activation of γ/δ T cells results in secretion of epithelial cell growth factors such as keratinocyte growth factor (KGF), and connective tissue growth factor (CTGF) and anti-inflammatory cytokines such as IL-10. Furthermore, γ/δ T cells can down-regulate the local inflammatory α/β T-cell response and killing of activated macrophages was demonstrated in a murine model. Thus, γ/δ T cells have anti-inflammatory properties and are capable of terminating an ongoing immune response

shown to be secreted by γ/δ T cells. Furthermore, several recent papers support the protective or regulatory role of γ/δ T cells in murine models of inflammatory diseases which lack γ/δ T cells[41,48–51] (see also below). Finally, the down-modulation of the inflammatory α/β T-cell response to bacterial infection[52] and the killing of activated macrophages were described[53]. Thus, γ/δ T cells are likely to have an important role in the termination of an ongoing immune response (Figure 3).

γ/δ T CELLS CONTRIBUTE TO DIFFERENT STAGES OF THE INFLAMMATORY IMMUNE RESPONSE

The findings of proinflammatory γ/δ T cells that kill cells and anti-inflammatory γ/δ T cells that promote healing are contradictory. A possible explanation might be that γ/δ T cells are not one homogeneous group of cells which have one function but consist of distinct subsets which contribute to different stages of the inflammatory response[4]. Support for this hypothesis comes from infectious disease models in which the kinetics of γ/δ T-cell responses and the TCR usage have been analysed (Figure 4).

For example, after infection of mice with the intracellular Gram-positive bacterium *Listeria monocytogenes* two waves of γ/δ T cells were observed[54,55]. The first wave, around day 3, is characterized by innate γ/δ T cells which are likely to have proinflammatory properties. Around this early period granuloma formation is observed at the sites of infection, which is essential for the containment of bacteria. In the absence of γ/δ T cells granuloma formation is reduced and bacterial growth is increased[56]. It was shown that this is likely to be caused

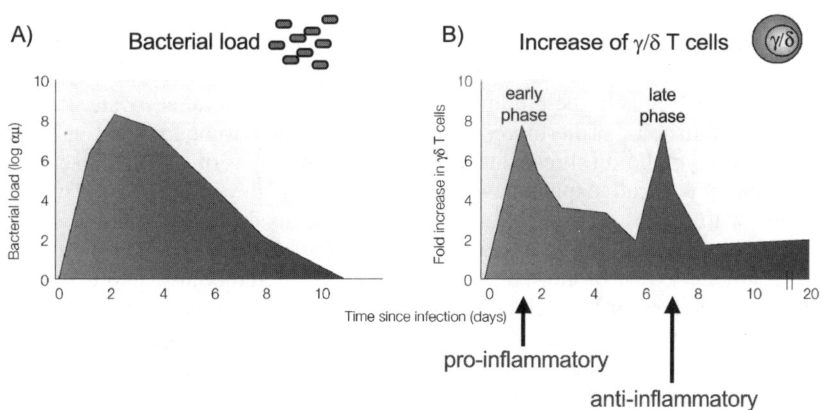

Figure 4 γ/δ T cells consist of distinct subsets which carry out different functions depending on the stage of the immune response (according to ref. 4). **A:** Bacterial clearance after infection of mice with listeria. **B:** The corresponding number of γ/δ T cells during the immune response which consists of two peaks. The peak during the early phase is likely to be caused by proinflammatory γ/δ T cells which help to clear the bacteria, whereas the second peak, around day 7, is probably due to anti-inflammatory γ/δ T cells which help to terminate the immune response

by the decreased secretion of IFN-γ. The second wave, around day 7, is likely to be characterized by anti-inflammatory γ/δ T cells which down-modulate the inflammatory response at the termination of an immune response to infection. This is supported by γ/δ-deficient mice which developed an exaggerated inflammatory response which was characterized by liver necrosis[57,58].

Two distinct waves of γ/δ T cells were also observed in several mouse models of virus and parasite infection[4,59–63]. Thus, it is possible that an early and late γ/δ T-cell response is present in many infections. An important question is if these two waves consist of two completely distinct γ/δ T-cell subsets or of γ/δ T cells which switch from a proinflammatory to an anti-inflammatory state. Analysis of the TCR repertoire suggests that the two waves consist of distinct γ/δ T cells. In some mouse models these waves were associated with γ/δ T cells which express different Vδ and Vγ chains. For example in murine influenza the first wave is dominated by V$\gamma4^+$ γ/δ T cells[63], whereas the second wave consists of V$\gamma1^+$ γ/δ T cells[62]. The same finding was observed in schistosome-induced liver granulomas where V$\delta4^+$ γ/δ T cells were followed by V$\delta6^+$ γ/δ T cells[60]. In murine studies with coxsackievirus B3-induced myocarditis selective depletion of V$\gamma1^+$ γ/δ T cells resulted in an exacerbation of myocarditis, whereas depletion of V$\gamma4^+$ subsets suppressed myocarditis. Furthermore, V$\gamma1^+$ cells biased the CD4 T cells to a Th2 cell response whereas V$\gamma4$ cells resulted in a Th1 response[64,65]. Thus, the specialized functions of γ/δ T cells coincide with the expression of distinctive γ/δ TCR[66,67], and there is evidence that these different subsets are recruited based on their various chemokine receptor expression[68,69].

THE ROLE OF γ/δ T CELLS IN CROHN'S DISEASE AND ULCERATIVE COLITIS

Several studies support the notion that γ/δ T cells play a key role in the pathogenesis of IBD. Immunohistochemical studies[70,71] reported an increased number of γ/δ T cells in the inflamed mucosa, although contradictory studies[72–74] were also published. Furthermore, γ/δ T cells were found to be frequent in T-cell areas around lymphoid follicles and epithelioid granulomas of Crohn's disease[75], and clonal γ/δ T-cell expansions were described in the inflamed mucosa of patients with Crohn's disease[76]. In addition, analysis of peripheral blood lymphocytes revealed an increased percentage of γ/δ T cells expressing the V$\delta1$ gene segment[72,77,78]. In normal subjects V$\delta2$ is preferentially expressed by peripheral γ/δ T cells[79], whereas intestinal γ/δ T cells express mainly V$\delta1$[9,80]. V$\delta1$ is also the dominant V region in the inflamed mucosa of patients with IBD[70,71,78]. Thus, circulating V$\delta1$-expressing γ/δ T cells might be derived from colonic γ/δ T cells leaving the inflamed gut.

In order to discover if γ/δ T cells are involved in IBD we analysed the TCR δ repertoire of γ/δ T cells in the intestine and peripheral blood of normal subjects[9,10] and patients with IBD[81]. In healthy adults we found an oligoclonal TCR δ repertoire which was almost unchanged along the entire colon, and the TCR δ repertoire of the peripheral blood was distinct from that in the intestine. These findings were irrespective of the Vδ region analysed. We do not know which antigens are recognized by these γ/δ T cells, but it is possible that the oligoclonal repertoire is shaped by stress-induced self antigens such as MICA which are constitutively expressed in the non-inflamed intestine.

Our initial hypothesis was to find clonally expanded γ/δ T cells in the inflamed intestine of subjects with IBD which are not present in the non-inflamed colon. This would support the notion that autoreactive γ/δ T cells might damage the mucosa. However, we rarely identified γ/δ T cells exclusively expanded in the inflamed mucosa, and identical TCR δ repertoires were present in inflamed and non-inflamed mucosa of patients with Crohn's disease (CD)[81]. Furthermore, the TCR δ repertoire of the peripheral blood was distinct from that in the colon, indicating that circulating γ/δ T cells are not derived from the inflamed gut.

Interestingly, in several patients with ulcerative colitis we observed a striking loss of several dominant γ/δ T cells within the highly inflamed colon[81]. Dominant γ/δ T cells which were present in non-inflamed and slightly inflamed colon were absent in highly inflamed colon. However, this was not found in the patients with CD and not in all patients with ulcerative colitis (UC). Nevertheless, in a subset of patients there might be a loss of protective γ/δ T cells within the inflamed colon which might result in an impaired down-regulation of the intestinal inflammation. Thus, it is likely that γ/δ T cells are not primarily causing the intestinal inflammation. Instead there might be a lack of immune activation or recruitment of these cells[82]. A regulatory role for γ/δ T cells was also suggested in patients with active pulmonary tuberculosis. The progression of the disease was associated with an increasing absence or loss of *Mycobacterium*-reactive γ/δ T cells[83,84]. The hypothesis that γ/δ T cells have an important role in mucosal healing is further supported by murine models of colitis in which a delayed tissue repair or increased mortality was observed in γ/δ-deficient mice[41,48,85].

CONCLUSION

Collectively, these findings suggest that γ/δ T cells consist of functionally specialized subsets which are often segregated by the tissue distribution and stage of the immune response. Furthermore, those specialized functions coincide with the expression of distinctive γ/δ TCR[66,67,86,87]. Thus, different γ/δ T-cell subsets are likely to be activated by distinct groups of antigens. Stress-induced self antigens such as MICA/B or CD1 were shown to be important; however, additional self antigens, which are expressed at different time points during the immune response, are likely to be identified.

Acknowledgement

This work was funded by grants from the Deutsche Forschungsgemeinschaft DFG (HO 1521/3-1 and 3-2).

References

1. Mak TW, Ferrick DA. The γ/δ T-cell bridge: linking innate and acquired immunity. Nat Med. 1998;4:764–5.

2. Hayday A, Tigelaar R. Immunoregulation in the tissues by γ/δ T cells. Nat Rev Immunol. 2003;3:233–42.

3. Havran WL, Chien YH, Allison JP. Recognition of self antigens by skin-derived T cells with invariant γ/δ antigen receptors. Science. 1991;252:1430–2.

4. Carding SR, Egan PJ. γ/δ T cells: functional plasticity and heterogeneity. Nat Rev Immunol. 2002;2:336–45.

5. Groh V, Steinle A, Bauer S, Spies T. Recognition of stress-induced MHC molecules by intestinal epithelial γ/δ T cells. Science. 1998;279:1737–40.

6. Spies T. Induction of T cell alertness by bacterial colonization of intestinal epithelium. Proc Natl Acad Sci USA. 2002;99:2584–6.

7. Pardoll DM. Immunology – stress, NK receptors, and immune surveillance. Science. 2001;294:534–6.

8. Chowers Y, Holtmeier W, Harwood J, Morzycka-Wroblewska E, Kagnoff MF. The Vδ1 T cell receptor repertoire in human small intestine and colon. J Exp Med. 1994;180:183–90.

9. Holtmeier W, Chowers Y, Lumeng A, Morzycka-Wroblewska E, Kagnoff MF. The δ T cell receptor repertoire in human colon and peripheral blood is oligoclonal irrespective of V region usage. J Clin Invest. 1995;96:1108–17.

10. Holtmeier W, Witthöft T, Hennemann A, Winter HS, Kagnoff MF. The TCR-δ repertoire in human intestine undergoes characteristic changes during fetal to adult development. J Immunol. 1997;158:5632–41.

11. Holtmeier W, Käller J, Geisel W et al. Development and compartmentalization of the porcine TCR δ repertoire at mucosal and extraintestinal sites: the pig as a model for analyzing the effects of age and microbial factors. J Immunol. 2002;169:1993–2002.

12. Holtmeier W, Pfänder M, Hennemann A et al. The TCR δ repertoire in normal human skin is restricted and distinct from the TCR δ repertoire in the peripheral blood. J Invest Dermatol. 2001;116:275–80.

13. Groh V, Bahram S, Bauer S et al. Cell stress-regulated human major histocompatibility complex class I gene expressed in gastrointestinal epithelium. Proc Natl Acad Sci USA. 1996; 93:12445–50.

14. Bauer S, Groh V, Wu J et al. Activation of NK cells and T cells by NKG2D, a receptor for stress-inducible MICA. Science. 1999;285:727–9.

15. Roberts AI, Lee L, Schwarz E et al. NKG2D receptors induced by IL-15 costimulate CD28-negative effector CTL in the tissue microenvironment. J Immunol. 2001;167:5527–30.

16. Ohteki T. Critical role for IL-15 in innate immunity. Curr Mol Med. 2002;2:371–80.

17. Garcia VE, Jullien D, Song M et al. IL-15 enhances the response of human gamma delta T cells to nonpeptide microbial antigens. J Immunol. 1998;160:4322–9.

18. Liu Z, Geboes K, Colpaert S et al. IL-15 is highly expressed in inflammatory bowel disease and regulates local T cell-dependent cytokine production. J Immunol. 2000;164:3608–15.

19. Groh V, Rhinehart R, Secrist H et al. Broad tumor-associated expression and recognition by tumor-derived γ/δ T cells of MICA and MICB. Proc Natl Acad Sci USA. 1999;96:6879–84.

20. Das H, Groh V, Kuijl C et al. MICA engagement by human Vγ2Vδ2 T cells enhances their antigen-dependent effector function. Immunity. 2001;15:83–93.

21. Wu J, Groh V, Spies T. T cell antigen receptor engagement and specificity in the recognition of stress-inducible MHC class I-related chains by human epithelial γ/δ T cells. J Immunol. 2002;169:1236–40.

22. Vetter CS, Groh V, Straten PT et al. Expression of stress-induced MHC class I related chain molecules on human melanoma. J Invest Dermatol. 2002;118:600–5.

23. Ferrarini M, Ferrero E, Dagna L, Poggi A, Zocchi MR. Human γ/δ T cells: a nonredundant system in the immune-surveillance against cancer. Trends Immunol. 2002;23:14–18.

24. Girardi M, Oppenheim DE, Steele CR et al. Regulation of cutaneous malignancy by γ/δ T cells. Science. 2001;294:605–9.

25. Groh V, Wu J, Yee C, Spies T. Tumour-derived soluble MIC ligands impair expression of NKG2D and T-cell activation. Nature. 2002;419:734–8.

26. Tieng V, Le Bouguenec C, du ML et al. Binding of *Escherichia coli* adhesin AfaE to CD55 triggers cell-surface expression of the MHC class I-related molecule MICA. Proc Natl Acad Sci USA. 2002;99:2977–82.

27. Darfeuille-Michaud A, Neut C, Barnich N et al. Presence of adherent *Escherichia coli* strains in ileal mucosa of patients with Crohn's disease. Gastroenterology. 1998;115:1405–13.

28. Masseret E, Boudeau J, Colombel JF et al. Genetically related *Escherichia coli* strains associated with Crohn's disease. Gut. 2001;48:320–5.

29. Stephens HAF. MICA and MICB genes: can the enigma of their polymorphism be resolved? Trends Immunol. 2001;22:378–85.

30. Orchard TR, Dhar A, Simmons JD et al. MHC class I chain-like gene A (MICA) and its associations with inflammatory bowel disease and peripheral arthropathy. Clin Exp Immunol. 2001;126:437–40.

31. Takeda K, Kaisho T, Akira S. Toll-like receptors. Annu Rev Immunol. 2003;21:335–76.

32. Leslie DS, Vincent MS, Spada FM et al. CD1-mediated γ/δ T cell maturation of dendritic cells. J Exp Med. 2002;196:1575–84.

33. Vincent MS, Leslie DS, Gumperz JE et al. CD1-dependent dendritic cell instruction. Nat Immunol. 2002;3:1163–8.

34. Ismaili J, Olislagers V, Poupot R, Fournie JJ, Goldman M. Human γ/δ T cells induce dendritic cell maturation. Clin Immunol. 2002;103:296–302.

35. Jameson J, Witherden D, Havran WL. T-cell effector mechanisms: γ/δ and CD1d-restricted subsets. Curr Opin Immunol. 2003;15:349–53.

36. Spada FM, Grant EP, Peters PJ et al. Self-recognition of CD1 by γ/δ T cells: Implications for innate immunity. J Exp Med. 2000;191:937–48.

37. Beckman EM, Porcelli SA, Morita CT et al. Recognition of a lipid antigen by CD1-restricted α/β+ T cells. Nature. 1994;372:691–4.

38. Matsuda JL, Kronenberg M. Presentation of self and microbial lipids by CD1 molecules. Curr Opin Immunol. 2001;13:19–25.

39. Boismenu R, Havran WL. Modulation of epithelial cell growth by intraepithelial γ/δ T cells. Science. 1994;266:1253–5.

40. Havran WL. A role for epithelial γ/δ T cells in tissue repair. Immunol Res. 2000;21:63–9.

41. Chen YP, Chou K, Fuchs E, Havran WL, Boismenu R. Protection of the intestinal mucosa by intraepithelial γ/δ T cells. Proc Natl Acad Sci USA. 2002;99:14338–43.

42. Fahrer AM, Konigshofer Y, Kerr EM et al. Attributes of γ/δ intraepithelial lymphocytes as suggested by their transcriptional profile. Proc Natl Acad Sci USA. 2001;98:10261–6.

43. Salvati VM, Bajaj-Elliott M, Poulsom R et al. Keratinocyte growth factor and coeliac disease. Gut. 2001;49:176–81.

44. Jameson J, Ugarte K, Chen N et al. A role for skin γ/δ T cells in wound repair. Science. 2002;296:747–9.

45. Workalemahu G, Foerster M, Kroegel C, Braun RK. Human γ/δ-T lymphocytes express and synthesize connective tissue growth factor: effect of IL-15 and TGF-β1 and comparison with α/β-T lymphocytes. J Immunol. 2003;170:153–7.

46. Hsieh B, Schrenzel MD, Mulvania T et al. *In vivo* cytokine production in murine listeriosis. Evidence for immunoregulation by γ/δ+ T cells. J Immunol. 1996;156:232–7.

47. Lagler H, Willheim M, Traunmuller F et al. Cellular profile of cytokine production in a patient with visceral leishmaniasis: γ/δ+ T cells express both type 1 cytokines and interleukin-10. Scand J Immunol. 2003;57:291–5.

48. Hoffmann JC, Peters K, Henschke S et al. Role of T lymphocytes in rat 2,4,6-trinitrobenzene sulphonic acid (TNBS) induced colitis: increased mortality after γ/δ T cell depletion and no effect of α/β T cell depletion. Gut. 2001;48:489–95.

49. Guan H, Zu G, Slater M, Elmets C, Xu H. γ/δ T cells regulate the development of hapten-specific CD8+ effector T cells in contact hypersensitivity responses. J Invest Dermatol. 2002;119:137–42.

50. Girardi M, Lewis J, Glusac E et al. Resident skin-specific γ/δ T cells provide local, nonredundant regulation of cutaneous inflammation. J Exp Med. 2002;195:855–67.

51. Lahn M, Kanehio A, Takeda K et al. Negative regulation of airway responsiveness that is dependent on γ/δ T cells and independent of α/β T cells. Nat Med. 1999;5:1150–6.

52. Skeen MJ, Rix EP, Freeman MM, Ziegler HK. Exaggerated proinflammatory and Th1 responses in the absence of γ/δ T cells after infection with *Listeria monocytogenes*. Infect Immun. 2001;69:7213–23.

53. Egan PJ, Carding SR. Downmodulation of the inflammatory response to bacterial infection by γ/δ T cells cytotoxic for activated macrophages. J Exp Med. 2000;191:2145–58.

54. Carding SR, Egan PJ. The importance of γ/δ T cells in the resolution of pathogen-induced inflammatory immune responses. Immunol Rev. 2000;173:98–108.

55. Belles C, Kuhl AK, Donoghue AJ et al. Bias in the γ/δ T cell response to *Listeria monocytogenes*. Vδ6.3+ cells are a major component of the γ/δ T cell response to *Listeria monocytogenes*. J Immunol. 1996;156:4280–9.
56. Ladel CH, Blum C, Kaufmann SH. Control of natural killer cell-mediated innate resistance against the intracellular pathogen *Listeria monocytogenes* by γ/δ T lymphocytes. Infect Immun. 1996;64:1744–9.
57. Mombaerts P, Arnoldi J, Russ F, Tonegawa S, Kaufmann SH. Different roles of α/β and γ/δ T cells in immunity against an intracellular bacterial pathogen. Nature. 1993;365:53–6.
58. Fu YX, Roark CE, Kelly K et al. Immune protection and control of inflammatory tissue necrosis by γ/δ T cells. J Immunol. 1994;153:3101–15.
59. Carding SR, Allan W, McMickle A, Doherty PC. Activation of cytokine genes in T cells during primary and secondary murine influenza pneumonia. J Exp Med. 1993;177:475–82.
60. Sandor M, Sperling AI, Cook GA et al. Two waves of γ/δ T cells expressing different Vδ genes are recruited into schistosome-induced liver granulomas. J Immunol. 1995;155:275–84.
61. Hou S, Katz JM, Doherty PC, Carding SR. Extent of γ/δ T cell involvement in the pneumonia caused by Sendai virus. Cell Immunol. 1992;143:183–93.
62. Augustin A, Kubo RT, Sim GK. Resident pulmonary lymphocytes expressing the γ/δ T-cell receptor. Nature. 1989;340:239–41.
63. Carding SR, Allan W, Kyes S et al. Late dominance of the inflammatory process in murine influenza by γ/δ+ T cells. J Exp Med. 1990;172:1225–31.
64. Huber SA, Graveline D, Born WK, O'Brien RL. Cytokine production by Vγ(+)-T-cell subsets is an important factor determining CD4(+)-Th-cell phenotype and susceptibility of BALB/c mice to coxsackievirus B3-induced myocarditis. J Virol. 2001;75:5860–9.
65. Huber SA, Graveline D, Newell MK, Born WK, O'Brien RL. Vγ1(+) T cells suppress and Vγ4(+) T cells promote susceptibility to coxsackievirus B3-induced myocarditis in mice. J Immunol. 2000;165:4174–81.
66. O'Brien RL, Lahn M, Born WK, Huber SA. T cell receptor and function cosegregate in γ/δ T cell subsets. Chem Immunol. 2001;79:1–28.
67. Lahn M, Kanehiro A, Takeda K et al. MHC class I-dependent Vγ4(+) pulmonary T cells regulate α/β T cell-independent airway responsiveness. Proc Natl Acad Sci USA. 2002;99:8850–5.
68. Boismenu R, Feng L, Xia YY, Chang JC, Havran WL. Chemokine expression by intraepithelial γ/δ T cells. Implications for the recruitment of inflammatory cells to damaged epithelia. J Immunol. 1996;157:985–92.
69. Kunkel EJ, Butcher EC. Chemokines and the tissue-specific migration of lymphocytes. Immunity. 2002;16:1–4.
70. McVay LD, Li B, Biancaniello R et al. Changes in human mucosal γ/δ T cell repertoire and function associated with the disease process in inflammatory bowel disease. Mol Med. 1997;3:183–203.
71. Yeung MMW, Melgar S, Baranov V et al. Characterisation of mucosal lymphoid aggregates in ulcerative colitis: immune cell phenotype and TCR-γ/δ expression. Gut. 2000;47:215–27.
72. Bucht A, Soderstrom K, Esin S et al. Analysis of γ/δ V region usage in normal and diseased human intestinal biopsies and peripheral blood by polymerase chain reaction (PCR) and flow cytometry. Clin Exp Immunol. 1995;99:57–64.
73. Cuvelier CA, De Wever N, Mielants H et al. Expression of T cell receptors α/β and γ/δ in the ileal mucosa of patients with Crohn's disease and with spondylarthropathy. Clin Exp Immunol. 1992;90:275–9.
74. Trejdosiewicz LK, Calabrese A, Smart CJ et al. γ/δ T cell receptor-positive cells of the human gastrointestinal mucosa: occurrence and V region gene expression in *Helicobacter pylori*-associated gastritis, coeliac disease and inflammatory bowel disease. Clin Exp Immunol. 1991;84:440–4.
75. Fukushima K, Masuda T, Ohtani H et al. Immunohistochemical characterization, distribution, and ultrastructure of lymphocytes bearing T-cell receptor γ/δ in inflammatory bowel disease. Gastroenterology. 1991;101:670–8.
76. Landau SB, Probert CS, Stevens CA, Balk SP, Blumberg RS. Over-utilization of the Jδ3 gene-segment in Crohn's disease. J Clin Lab Immunol. 1996;48:33–44.
77. Giacomelli R, Parzanese I, Frieri G et al. Increase of circulating γ/δ T lymphocytes in the peripheral blood of patients affected by active inflammatory bowel disease. Clin Exp Immunol. 1994;98:83–8.

78. Soderstrom K, Bucht A, Halapi E et al. Increased frequency of abnormal γ/δ T cells in blood of patients with inflammatory bowel diseases. J Immunol. 1996;156:2331–9.

79. Borst J, Wicherink A, van Dongen JJ et al. Non-random expression of T cell receptor γ and δ variable gene segments in functional T lymphocyte clones from human peripheral blood. Eur J Immunol. 1989;19:1559–68.

80. Deusch K, Luling F, Reich K et al. A major fraction of human intraepithelial lymphocytes simultaneously expresses the γ/δ T cell receptor, the CD8 accessory molecule and preferentially uses the Vδ1 gene segment. Eur J Immunol. 1991;21:1053–9.

81. Holtmeier W, Hennemann A, May E, Duchmann R, Caspary WF. T cell receptor δ repertoire in inflamed and noninflamed colon of patients with IBD analyzed by CDR3 spectratyping. Am J Physiol Gastrointest Liver Physiol. 2002;282:G1024–34.

82. Bradley LM. Migration and T-lymphocyte effector function. Curr Opin Immunol. 2003; 15:343–8.

83. Szereday L, Baliko Z, Szekeres-Bartho J. γ/δ T cell subsets in patients with active *Mycobacterium tuberculosis* infection and tuberculin anergy. Clin Exp Immunol. 2003;131:287–91.

84. Li B, Rossman MD, Imir T et al. Disease-specific changes in γ/δ T cell repertoire and function in patients with pulmonary tuberculosis. J Immunol. 1996;157:4222–9.

85. Kuhl AA, Loddenkemper C, Westermann J, Hoffmann JC. Role of γ/δ T cells in inflammatory bowel disease. Pathobiology. 2002;70:150–5.

86. Mukasa A, Born WK, O'Brien RL. Inflammation alone evokes the response of a TCR-invariant mouse γ/δ T cell subset. J Immunol. 1999;162:4910–13.

87. O'Brien RL, Yin X, Huber SA, Ikuta K, Born WK. Depletion of a γ/δ T cell subset can increase host resistance to a bacterial infection. J Immunol. 2000;165:6472–9.

3
NOD2 (CARD 15) gene mutation and defensin expression

J. WEHKAMP, K. FELLERMANN and E. F. STANGE

INTRODUCTION

Despite active research for many decades the aetiology of Crohn's disease is still enigmatic. Most of the research has focused on a potential dysregulation of specific mucosal immunology. These investigations have elegantly described the mucosal cellular populations and cytokine profiles associated with inflammatory bowel disease but have not succeeded in finding the aetiological culprit. In this chapter we will outline a novel concept of how epidemiological, pathophysiological, genetic, molecular, clinical and pharmacological sets of data may be synthesized into a unifying hypothesis compatible with many features of this disease.

Several years ago we became interested in the innate mucosal system of antibiotic peptides contributing to the defensive array of substances and structures opposed to the invasion of luminal bacteria and other potential invaders. This system of antibiotic peptides is apparently synthesized and secreted by the intestinal mucosa as part of innate immunity, but has received little attention. In this chapter we will outline some recent findings regarding innate immunity which might be crucial for the pathophysiology of inflammatory bowel diseases.

DEFENSINS: GENETICS, EXPRESSION AND REGULATION

Probably the most important peptide family of endogenous antibiotics is the still-growing number of defensins[1-3]; they comprise a class of cationic antimicrobial peptides with a molecular weight of 3–5 kDa conserved throughout phylogeny. All defensins have been mapped to chromosome 8 in humans[4-6]. Six α-defensins and four β-defensins have so far been identified in humans. The α-defensins comprise human neutrophil peptide 1–4, abundant in granulocytes, and human defensin 5 and 6 synthesized in Paneth cells[7]. The β-defensins are of epithelial origin and abundant in skin, intestine and lung. The concept of a certain defensin exclusively formed by specialized tissues or cells needs revision, as inflammation induces epithelial expression of human neutrophil peptides[7] and β-defensins in monocytes and lymphocytes[8]. Defensins can be divided into constitutive forms, e.g. HBD-1 with its widespread stable distribution[9], and inducible peptides such as HBD-2[10]. The mechanisms of activation are currently under investigation. A cytokine-driven induction, e.g. by IL-1β and TNF-α, has been shown, besides a direct response to bacterial components such as lipopolysaccharides and lipoproteins. Possible signalling pathways involve Toll-like receptors, especially TLR2 and 4, eventually leading to NFκB-mediated activation of transcription. NOD2/CARD15 as an intracellular LPS receptor induces NFκB[11], which in turn is known to trigger HBD-2 transcription. Interestingly, this NFκB response is impaired in the NOD2 insertion mutation associated with Crohn's disease[12,13], suggesting a diminished innate response to bacterial components. Human defensin 5 is released as a propeptide from Paneth cells and activated by trypsinogen in the lumen of the intestinal crypts[14]. The functional significance in bacterial infection has recently been shown in HD-5 transgenic mice, which are protected from lethal *Salmonella* infection[15]. On the other hand, matrilysin-deficient mice fail to process defensins efficiently, and exhibit higher bacterial counts[16].

DEFENSINS AND INFLAMMATORY BOWEL DISEASES (IBD)

Some defensins appear to be induced in both Crohn's disease and ulcerative colitis. Human neutrophil peptides 1–3, as well as lysozyme, are expressed in surface enterocytes of mucosa with active IBD but surprisingly not in controls [7]. HD-5 is stored in a precursor form in normal Paneth cells and is expressed by metaplastic colonic Paneth cells[17]. Notably, both α-defensins HD-5 and HD-6 are induced in the colonic mucosa of IBD patients[17–19]. The alterations in β-defensins are more intriguing because there is a conspicuous difference between Crohn's disease and ulcerative colitis. It has been suggested that HBD-1 is constitutively expressed in the intestinal epithelium[20], and qualitative investigations showed constitutive expression in normal tissue and IBD mucosa[21]. With the quantitative approach a decrease of HBD-1 was found in inflamed mucosa of both Crohn's disease and ulcerative colitis[22]. However, it remains to be shown that such a decrease actually translates into a diminished mucosal antibacterial activity.

The inducible HBD-2 which has been described originally in skin[10] is also expressed in the colon during inflammation[20], particularly in ulcerative colitis[21]. It has now been shown by three different independent studies[21–23] that HBD-2 is highly induced in inflamed mucosa of ulcerative colitis patients. As compared to ulcerative colitis this induction is missing in Crohn's disease[22,23]. Most likely there is a lack of β-defensin induction in Crohn's disease contributing to a defective antimicrobial barrier or, alternatively, there is an excessive induction in ulcerative colitis.

The third defensin studied was HBD-3, which was reported by Harder et al. as a novel inducible β-defensin in skin[24]. Another group described HBD-3 based on genomic analysis[25]. Our recent study first described HBD-3 in the human colon. Although HBD-3 was also slightly induced in inflamed Crohn's mucosa, its expression was preferentially enhanced in inflamed and non-inflamed ulcerative colitis[22]. A deficiency in the antimicrobial defence systems of defensins may be a reasonable and plausible explanation for the break of the antibacterial barrier function in IBD.

In conclusion, the decrease of HBD-1 in both IBD, and the lack of induction of both inducible β-defensins HBD-2 and HBD-3 in Crohn's disease, suggest a deficient mucosal barrier function. This may in part be compensated by the induction of the α-defensins. A lack in the innate defence system of antimicrobial peptides may lead to a permanent but slow bacterial invasion triggering the inflammatory process, but further direct studies on antimicrobial peptide activity in IBD mucosa are required to validate this hypothesis.

NOD2, A PETIDOGLYCAN RECEPTOR AND DEFENSIN EXPRESSION

Although the aetiology of Crohn's disease is still enigmatic, the recent finding in about a third of Crohn's disease patients of a loss of function mutation in the putative intracellular peptidoglycan receptor NOD2 represents a major advance[11,12]. The pathophysiology of NOD2 in Crohn's disease was proposed to

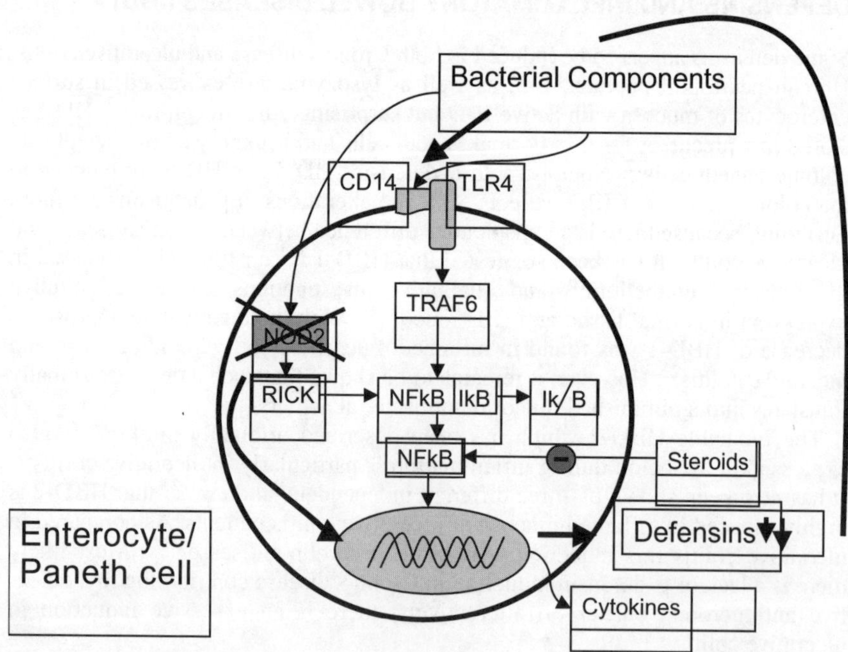

Figure 1 The putative pathomechanism of the NOD2 mutations in Crohn's disease. NOD2 is also expressed in epithelial cells and a loss of function mutation may lead to disturbed Paneth cell defensin expression as well as diminished barrier

link to immunological dysregulation in monocytes. Alternatively, intestinal epithelial cells[26,27] and Paneth cells[28], which have also been demonstrated to express this putative receptor, might be compromised in their antibacterial response. It has been demonstrated that NOD2-mutated epithelial cells display a disturbed response against *Salmonella*[29], supporting the hypothesis of a defensin deficiency. Unpublished data from our laboratory show that mutation in the NOD2 gene leads to a disturbed expression of antimicrobial Paneth cell defensins. This disturbed Paneth cell defensin expression might explain the ileal preference in NOD2-mutated Crohn's disease patients.

CONCLUDING REMARKS

Seventy years after Crohn's description of the disease named after him it becomes apparent that Crohn's disease is not a disease but a syndrome. It is not surprising that the diverse facets of genetic predisposition, where only a minority of patients display a defective NOD2 gene, modified by environmental factors such as childhood hygiene and others, may lead to very different forms of disease with respect to localization, natural course and therapeutic response. Although in no way perfect, the present hypothesis appears to be plausible for the reasons presented above, but particularly since the multitude of defensins, other antibiotic peptides and related transcription factors or transporters leaves enough room for clinical diversity. The link between mutations of the NOD2 gene in Crohn's disease patients related to a diminished defensin expression gives further evidence for our hypothesis that Crohn's disease may be a defensin deficiency syndrome[30].

Acknowledgements

Helpful discussions and joint investigations with JM Schröder and J Harder are gratefully acknowledged. The work was generously supported by the Robert Bosch Foundation, Stuttgart, Germany.

References

1. Fellermann K, Stange EF. Defensin – innate immunity at the epithelial fontier. Eur J Gastroenterol Hepatol. 2001;13:771–6.
2. Cunliffe RN, Mahida YR. Antimicrobial peptides in innate intestinal host defence. Gut. 2000;47:16–17.
3. Lehrer RI, Ganz T. Defensins of vertebrate animals. Curr Opin Immunol. 2002;14:96–102.
4. Harder J, Siebert R, Zhang Y et al. Mapping of the gene encoding human beta-defensin-2 (DEFB2) to chromosome region 8p22-p23.1. Genomics. 1997;46:472–5.
5. Liu L, Zhao C, Heng HH, Ganz T. The human beta-defensin-1 and alpha-defensins are encoded by adjacent genes: two peptide families with differing disulfide topology share a common ancestry. Genomics. 1997;43:316–20.
6. Liu L, Wang L, Jia HP et al. Structure and mapping of the human beta-defensin HBD-2 gene and its expression at sites of inflammation. Gene. 1998;222:237–44.
7. Cunliffe RN, Kamal M, Rose FR, James PD, Mahida YR. Expression of antimicrobial neutrophil defensins in epithelial cells of active inflammatory bowel disease mucosa. J Clin Pathol. 2002;55:298–304.
8. Duits LA, Ravensbergen B, Rademaker M, Hiemstra PS, Nibbering PH. Expression of beta-defensin 1 and 2 mRNA by human monocytes, macrophages and dendritic cells. Immunology. 2002;106:517–25.

9. Zhao C, Wang I, Lehrer RI. Widespread expression of beta-defensin hBD-1 in human secretory glands and epithelial cells. FEBS Lett. 1996;396:319–22.

10. Harder J, Bartels J, Christophers E, Schröder JM. A peptide antibiotic from human skin [letter; see comments]. Nature. 1997;387:861.

11. Ogura Y, Bonen DK, Inohara N et al. A frameshift mutation in NOD2 associated with susceptibility to Crohn's diease. Nature. 2001;411:603–6.

12. Hugot J-P, Chamaillard C, Zouali H et al. Association of NOD2 leucine-rich repeat variants with susceptibility to Crohn's disease. Nature. 2001;411:599–603.

13. Ogura Y, Inohara N, Benito A, Chen FF, Yamaoka S, Nunez G. Nod2, a Nod1/Apaf-1 family member that is restricted to monocytes and activates NF-kappaB. J Biol Chem. 2001;276:4812–18.

14. Ghosh D, Porter E, Shen B et al. Paneth cell trypsin is the processing enzyme for human defensin-5. Nat Immunol. 2002;3:583–90.

15. Salzman NH, Ghosh D, Huttner KM, Paterson Y, Bevins CL. Protection against enteric salmonellosis in transgenic mice expressing a human intestinal defensin. Nature. 2003;422:522–6.

16. Wilson CL, Ouellette AJ, Satchell DP et al. Regulation of intestinal α-defensin activation by the metalloproteinase matrilysin in innate host defense. Science. 1999;286:113–17.

17. Cunliffe RN, Rose FRAJ, Keyte J, Abberley L, Chan WC, Mahida YR. Human defensin 5 is stored in precursor form in normal Paneth cells and is expressed by some villous epithelial cells and by metaplastic Paneth cells in the colon in inflammatory bowel disease. Gut. 2001;48:176–85.

18. Lawrance IC, Fiocchi C, Chakravarti S. Ulcerative colitis and Crohn's disease: distinctive gene expression profiles and novel susceptibility candidate genes. Hum Mol Genet. 2001;10:445–56.

19. Wehkamp J, Schwind B, Herrlinger KR et al. Innate immunity and colonic inflammation: enhanced expression of epithelial alpha-defensins. Dig Dis Sci. 2002;47:1349–55.

20. O'Neil DA, Porter EM, Elewaut D et al. Expression and regulation of the human β-defensins hBD-1 and hBD-2 in intestinal epithelium. J Immunol. 1999;163:6718–24.

21. Wehkamp J, Fellermann K, Herrlinger KR et al. Human beta-defensin 2 but not beta-defensin 1 is expressed preferentially in colonic mucosa of inflammatory bowel disease. Eur J Gastroenterol Hepatol. 2002;14:745–52.

22. Wehkamp J, Harder J, Weichenthal M et al. Inducible and constitutive beta-defensins are differentially expressed in Crohn's disease and ulcerative colitis. Inflamm Bowel Dis. 2003;91:215–23.

23. Fahlgren A, Hammarstrom S, Danielsson A, Hammarstrom ML. Increased expression of antimicrobial peptides and lysozyme in colonic epithelial cells of patients with ulcerative colitis. Clin Exp Immunol. 2003;131:90–101.

24. Harder J, Bartels J, Christophers E, Schröder JM. Isolation and characterization of human β-defensin-3, a novel human inducible peptide antibiotic. J Biol Chem. 2001;276:5707–13.

25. Garcia JR, Jaumann F, Schulz S et al. Identification of a novel, multifunctional beta-defensin (human beta-defensin 3) with specific antimicrobial activity. Its interaction with plasma membranes of *Xenopus* oocytes and the induction of macrophage chemoattraction. Cell Tissue Res. 2001;306:257–64.

26. Berrebi D, Maudinas R, Hugot JP et al. Card15 gene overexpression in mononuclear and epithelial cells of the inflamed Crohn's disease colon. Gut. 2003;52:840–6.

27. Rosenstiel P, Fantini M, Brautigam K et al. TNF-alpha and IFN-gamma regulate the expression of the NOD2 (CARD15) gene in human intestinal epithelial cells. Gastroenterology. 2003;124:1001–9.

28. Lala S, Ogura Y, Osborne C et al. Crohn's disease and the NOD2 gene: a role for Paneth cells. Gastroenterology. 2003;125:47–57.

29. Hisamatsu T, Suzuki M, Reinecker HC, Nadeau WJ, McCormick BA, Podolsky DK. CARD15/NOD2 functions as an antibacterial factor in human intestinal epithelial cells. Gastroenterology. 2003;124:993–1000.

30. Fellermann K, Wehkamp J, Herrlinger KR, Stange EF. Crohn's disease: a defensin deficiency syndrome? Eur J Gastroenterol Hepatol. 2003;15:627–34.

Section II
Handling of luminal antigens II:
Role of dendritic cells

4
Dendritic cells and epithelial cells crosstalk at mucosal surfaces

M. RIMOLDI, M. CHIEPPA, M. VULCANO, P. ALLAVENA and M. RESCIGNO

INTRODUCTION

Entry of pathogens across the intestinal mucosa occurs mainly through specialized epithelial cells, called M cells, which are located in Peyer's patches (PP)[1]; however, we have recently described a new mechanism for bacterial entry which is mediated by dendritic cells (DC)[2]. DC are distributed as immature cells in non-lymphoid organs and in the blood where they perform a sentinel function for incoming pathogens[3-8]. Immature DC are characterized by the capacity to take up antigens and to phagocytose macroparticles[9,10]. During infection or inflammation, DC are mobilized in and out of peripheral tissues[11,12] and activated DC are targeted to secondary lymphoid organs[13,14]. Here, DC have the unique function, among antigen-presenting cells, to activate naive T cells. Thus DC play an important role in the induction of immune responses.

As often occurs, understanding the mechanisms underlying the physiology of the organism allows the unveiling of the uncontrolled steps which lead to some pathological condition, and vice-versa. In this regard the comparison of how microorganisms are handled by DC in healthy or diseased environments can shed some light on the development of uncontrolled inflammatory states to non-dangerous commensal microorganisms. We have described that, during infection, lamina propria DC are able to open the tight junctions (TJ) between adjacent epithelial cells and to capture bacteria directly across the mucosal epithelium. The epithelial barrier is preserved because DC express TJ proteins whose level is regulated by bacteria or bacterial products, and establish TJ-like structures with neighbouring epithelial cells[2]. Interestingly, lamina propria DC can discriminate between pathogenic and non-pathogenic bacteria. When the intestine is infected with non-pathogenic bacteria, DC do not receive any migratory signal and stay *in situ*, whereas infection with pathogenic bacteria induces a large migration of DC from the mucosa, presumably to the mesenteric node[2]. Thus, DC play an active role of bacterial handling across mucosal surfaces; but how can DC sense the presence of bacteria from the apical side of the mucosal epithelium and discriminate between pathogenic and commensal bacteria? We know from previous studies that bacteria, regardless of their pathogenicity[15], easily activate DC from the spleen or from the bone marrow. This results in secretion of proinflammatory and anti-inflammatory cytokines, and in the up-regulation of those molecules which are necessary for their antigen-presenting function and for cell migration[16,17]. This suggests that DC by themselves are unable to discriminate between pathogenic and non-pathogenic bacteria. Thus, what is the role of epithelial cells that are the first cells encountering bacteria in the intestinal lumen? Can they perform a control action on DC function according to the type of microorganism encountered? In this study we analysed the role of epithelial cell-derived factors in mediating DC–epithelial cell crosstalk in terms of DC recruitment and activation. We used an *in vitro* co-culture model that we set up in our laboratory. Epithelial cells were tested for their capacity to release chemokines such as IL-8 and MIP-3α and to activate DC after encounter with *Salmonella typhimurium*. Epithelial cells or epithelial cells/DC co-cultures were incubated with several *Salmonella* strains deficient in different pathways of pathogenicity and invasiveness.

METHODS

Cells and reagents

DC are derived from peripheral blood monocytes according to a slightly modified protocol[18]. Briefly, monocytes are purified by positive selection with anti-CD14 antibodies coupled to magnetic beads (Miltenyi). CD14$^+$ cells are incubated for 6 days in complete medium containing GM-CSF (50 ng/ml, Peprotech) and IL-4 (20 ng/ml, Endogen) in order to obtain immature DC.

Bacterial strains

Bacillus subtilis is an aerobe commonly found in soil, water sources or associated to plants whose genome has been completely sequenced[19]. Lactic acid bacteria (LAB), including *Lactobacillus plantarum*, are present in the intestine of most animals. *Salmonella typhimurium* is a typical pathogen entering the host across mucosal surfaces[20]. The types of mutations carried by the attenuated *Salmonella* strains that have been used are: msbB (lipid A); purE; AroA; surA; invA (SPI I deficient); ssaV (SPI II deficient); htrA; ompCompF; and ompR. These strains are impaired either in invasiveness (as SPI I deficient), in their capacity to survive inside the phagosome (as SPI II), in growth (as purE) or in general toxicity (as msbB).

Cells are incubated with live bacteria for 1 h and then bacteria are killed by addition of antibiotics (including gentamicin, 100 μg/ml, and tetracycline, 10 μg/ml).

Cytokine assay and cell phenotype

The ability of DC to produce proinflammatory and anti-inflammatory cytokines (IL-10, IL-12, IL-8, IL-6) has been tested by ELISA in culture supernatants 24 h after bacterial incubation (R&D system). Cells have been analysed for acquisition of maturation markers (CD83, CD80, DC-Lamp, HLA-DR) by cytofluorimetry (FACScalibur, Becton Dickinson).

Dendritic cells/epithelial cells co-culture

Generation of an epithelial monolayer (equal for situations a and b)

In brief, Caco-2 cells are seeded in the upper chamber of a transwell filter (Costar 3 μm diameter of pores) for 5–7 days until a trans-epithelial resistance of 300 Ohm $\cdot$ cm^2 is achieved.

Situation a (Figure 1a). Epithelial cell monolayers are incubated with bacteria from the apical surface (upper chamber). One hour after incubation the bacteria are washed out and the medium is changed to one containing antibiotics (gentamicin 100 μg/ml, and tetracycline 10 μg/ml). Culture supernatants are collected at different time points from the lower chamber (facing the basolateral membrane) and are used to activate DC. DC are incubated for 24 h in culture supernatant and are then analysed phenotypically for expression of activation markers (surface activation markers: CD83, CD80, HLA-DR). Distinction of cytokines released by epithelial cells or dendritic cells is performed by analysing culture supernatants before and after DC incubation. Culture supernatants are collected at different time points from the lower chamber and analysed for the presence of cytokines (IL-10, IL-12, IL-6, IL-8), respectively.

Situation b (Figure 1b). Filters are turned upside-down and DC are seeded on the filter facing the basolateral membrane of epithelial cells for 4 h to allow the cells to attach to the filter. Filters are then again turned upside-down into the 24-well plate. The transwells are either left untreated for a suitable amount of time (5 h) before treatment with bacteria to allow the 'conditioning' of DC by epithelial cells, or are treated directly with bacteria (ratio of 10 bacteria to one EC) from the apical surface (upper chamber). One hour after incubation the bacteria are washed out and the medium is changed to one containing antibiotics (gentamicin 100 μg/ml, and tetracycline 10 μg/ml). DC and culture supernatants are collected at different time points and analysed as in situation *a*.

Analysis of the ability of DC to creep between epithelial cells

The ability of DC to intercalate between EC and open tight junction proteins has been analysed by laser confocal microscopy after staining of filters for DC (CD11c+) or tight junction markers (occludin) as already described[2].

RESULTS AND DISCUSSION

DC–epithelial cell interaction was studied by using an *in-vitro* system established in our laboratory. This system is particularly suitable to dissect out the contribution of epithelial cell-derived factors or bacterial products in the activation

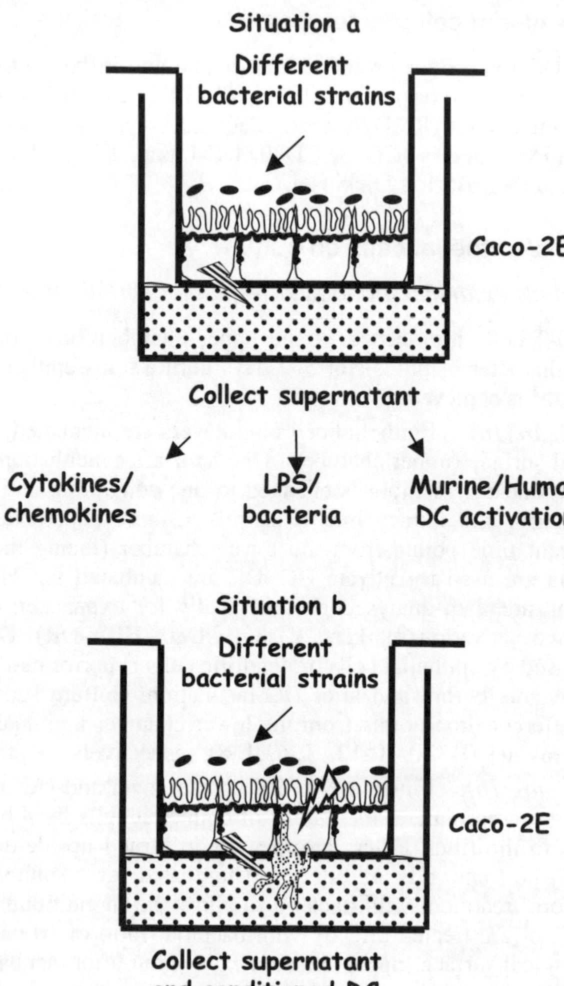

Figure 1 Graphical description of experimental models. In situation *a* the DC are incubated with supernatants of epithelial cells previously treated with bacteria; in situation *b* the interaction of DC with epithelial cells and bacteria is studied directly, across a monolayer of epithelial cells. *Situation* a: Epithelial cell monolayers are incubated with bacteria from the apical surface (upper chamber). One hour after incubation the bacteria are washed out and the medium is changed to one containing antibiotics (gentamicin 100 µg/ml, and tetracyclin 10 µg/ml). Culture supernatants are collected at different time points from the lower chamber (facing the basolateral membrane) and are used to activate DC. DC are incubated for 24 h in culture supernatant and are analysed phenotypically for expression of activation markers. *Situation* b: Filters are turned upside-down and DC are seeded on the filter facing the basolateral membrane of epithelial cells for 4 h to allow the cells to attach to the filter. Filters are then again turned upside-down into the 24-well plate. The transwells are either left untreated for a suitable amount of time (5 h) before treatment with bacteria, to allow the 'conditioning' of DC by epithelial cells, or are treated directly with bacteria (ratio of 10 bacteria to one EC) from the apical surface (upper chamber). DC and culture supernatants are collected at different time points from the lower chamber and analysed either functionally (surface activation markers) or for the presence of cytokines, respectively

of DC. It allows simplifying the mucosal barrier to just three players: DC, epithelial cells and bacteria in a spatial distribution similar to that found *in vivo*. Thus it can help to identify possible interactions and factors responsible for the ability or inability of DC to 'sense' different bacterial strains. Two possible scenarios are considered (Figure 1). In situation *a* the DC are incubated with supernatants of epithelial cells previously treated with bacteria; in situation *b* the interaction of DC with epithelial cells and bacteria is studied directly, across a monolayer of epithelial cells.

We observed that incubation of invasive salmonellae, but not of non-invasive bacteria, from the apical side of epithelial cell monolayers in the absence of DC (situation *a*) induced the release of proinflammatory cytokines, such as IL-8 (Table 1). As we could not detect any bacteria from the lower chamber of the epithelial monolayer this suggests that the observed effect is due either to bacteria staying intracellularly or to bacterial products translocated across the monolayer to basolateral membrane receptors. Interestingly, incubation of DC with culture supernatant of epithelial cells treated with invasive bacteria, but not with non-invasive bacteria, induced DC activation, as attested by an increased number of cells expressing high levels of activation markers, CD83 and DC-LAMP (Table 1). Activation of DC could be due simply to bacterial products that have crossed the epithelial cell monolayer; however, when we incubated murine DC that can respond to bacteria or bacterial products together with the same epithelial cell supernatants, some cell activation was observed (Figure 2, top graph). This correlated with the detection of traces of bacterial lipopolysaccharide (LPS). Indeed, when we incubated murine DC derived from C3H/HeJ mice that are mutated in the Toll-like receptor 4 gene, and cannot respond to LPS, DC

Table 1 Analysis of cell culture supernatants of epithelial cells activated with different bacterial strains in terms of IL-8 production and dendritic cells activating properties. The percentage of CD83[hi] and DC-LAMP[hi] cells is shown as an indicator of activated DC

Bacterial strains[a]	IL-8 (ng/ml)	Percentage CD83[hi] cells	Percentage DC-LAMP[hi] cells	MIP-3α (ng/ml)	Invasive
C5 WT	2.27	61.6	70.9	1.02	Yes
SL1344 WT	1.55	82.5	50.6	0.96	Yes
htrA	1.13	70.8	77	1.08	Yes
ssaV (SPI-II)	1.31	91.8	96	1.13	Yes
ompCompF	0.72	89.5	73.5	0.658	Yes
msbB	0.07	33.9	29.4	0.46	No
SurA	0.56	30.6	30.3	1.03	No
InvA (SPI-I)	0.16	47.6	52	0.88	No
DH5α	0	32	33.4	0.08	No
B. subtilis	0	N.D.	N.D.	1.2	No
untreated	0	27.2	28	0.04	—
LPS	—	85.8	98.8	—	—
iDC	—	10.8	12.2	—	—

[a] Bacterial strains: invasive: (a) *Salmonella*: C5 WT; SL1344 WT; htrA; SPI-II (ssaV); ompC-ompF; non-invasive: (a) *Salmonella*: msbB (lipid A mutant); SurA; SPI-I (InvA⁻); (b) *E. coli*: DH5α; (c) *B. subtilis*.

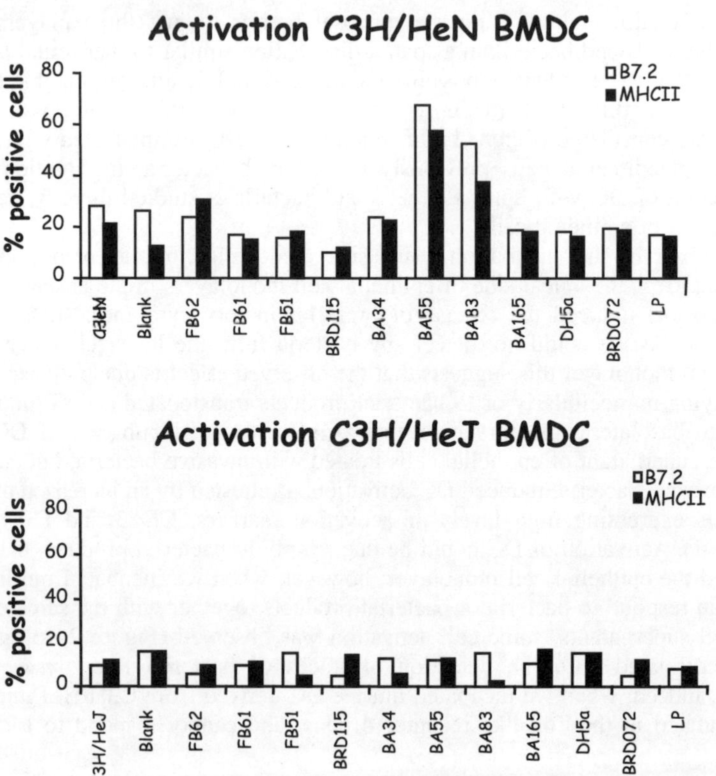

Figure 2   LPS is responsible for murine DC activation after incubation with epithelial cells/bacteria derived co-culture supernatants. *Salmonella* (invasive: FB62: WT; BA55: htrA; BA83: SPI-II (ssaV); BA 165: ompC-ompF; FB51: purE; or non-invasive: FB61: msbB; BRD115: SurA; BA34: SPI-I (InvA); *E. coli* (non-invasive: DH5a) or *Lacobacillus plantarum* (LP: commensal) were seeded from the apical side of epithelial cell monolayers, for 1 h in medium without antibiotics and then washed out. Cells were left for 18 additional hours in medium containing gentamicin (100 μg/ml) and tetracycline (10 μg/ml). Culture supernatants were used to activate wild-type bone marrow-derived DC (from C3H/HeN mice, top graph) or TLR4 mutated DC (from C3H/HeJ mice, lower graph). Expression of activation markers MHC II and B7.2 is shown. DC are partially activated only with supernatants of epithelial cells treated with invasive bacteria

activation was abrogated (Figure 2, lowest graph). This indicates that human DC activation that occurs only after incubation with supernatants of epithelial cells infected with invasive bacteria is due to a combination of factors, including bacterial products and epithelial cell-derived molecules. LPS was detected in the lower chamber of epithelial cell/bacteria co-cultures only when invasive bacteria were seeded from the apical side. LPS is the major bacterial component able to induce DC translocation across a monolayer of epithelial cells (Figure 3), probably by up-regulating the expression of tight junction proteins (not shown). LPS alone can induce the translocation of DC (Figure 3), and commensal bacteria

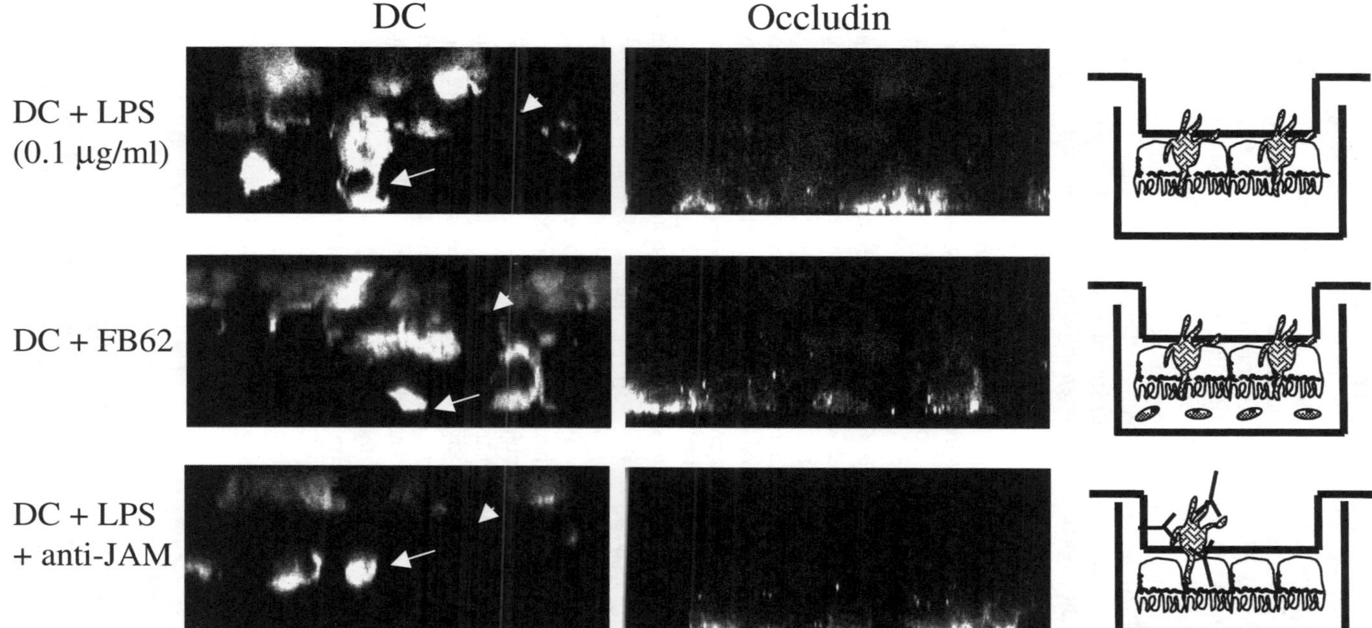

Figure 3 Anti-JAM antibodies block LPS-induced DC translocation. *Salmonella* (invasive: FB62: WT) or LPS (0.1 µg/ml) induce DC migration across a monolayer of epithelial cells all the way to the apical face. Preincubation of DC with anti-JAM 1 antibody (10 µg/ml), for 30 min before addition to the epithelial monolayer from the basolateral membrane, blocks DC migration. Transwell filters were fixed 2 h after addition of bacteria and were processed for laser confocal microscopy analysis. Left photographs: CD11c staining of DC; right photographs, occludin staining of epithelial tight junctions. White arrowheads show the location of the filter (dark black). White arrows indicate the position of DC migrated across the filters: note that preincubation of DC with anti-JAM 1 antibody does not block DC migration across the filter, but inhibits their ability to open the tight junctions and reach the apical surface

such as *Lactobacillus plantarum* lacking LPS are unable to recruit DC into the apical side (not shown). Tight junction proteins expressed by DC are necessary to allow DC translocation. Preincubation of DC with antibodies directed to the extracellular portion of the tight junction protein Junctional adhesion protein (JAM) 1 with anti-JAM1 antibodies inhibits the ability of DC to open adjacent epithelial cell junctions (Figure 3). Interestingly, both invasive and non-invasive salmonellae, as long as they express flagellin, induce the release of MIP-3α, a chemokine responsible for the recruitment of immature DC (Table 1). This is consistent with a recent report showing that flagellated salmonellae can induce the release of MIP-3α by epithelial cells[21]. This suggests that the presence of flagellated bacteria induces the recruitment of immature DC regardless of their invasiveness or pathogenicity. *Bacillus subtilis*, a flagellated soil bacterium, is also able to induce MIP-3α release by epithelial cells (Table 1). By contrast, only invasive bacteria induce DC activation. If, however, we switch to situation *b* in which DC are coincubated with epithelial cells and can sense the bacteria directly across the monolayer, they are activated both by invasive and non-invasive bacteria (not shown), even by commensal bacteria such as *Lactobacillus plantarum*, due to their capacity to cross the monolayer (not shown). This suggests that during infection two situations are generated. In the first one the invasive bacteria transduce activation signals to epithelial cells that release inflammatory chemokines such as IL-8 and activating factors for DC. As a consequence, DC that have not encountered the bacteria will also be activated. By contrast, in the second situation, non-invasive bacteria that are not 'sensed' by epithelial cells will not induce bystander DC activation. In both cases, with invasive or non-invasive salmonellae, because they do express flagellin, they will recruit immature DC. Thus, in the second situation, non-invasive bacteria will induce the activation only of those DC that creep between epithelial cells and contact them directly from the luminal side. Whether this activation then results in a different capability to polarize T cells remains to be established. The signals that induce DC migration across the monolayer after infection with non-invasive salmonellae also remain to be elucidated.

In conclusion, we have demonstrated that, during a bacterial infection, DC respond differently if they receive signals from invasive or non-invasive bacteria. In particular, invasive bacteria induce a broad DC activation due to a combination of epithelial cell-derived and bacteria-derived factors, whereas non-invasive bacteria induce activation only of those DC that they have contacted directly. If non-invasive or commensal bacteria, by inducing an immunosuppressive effect on epithelial cells, as recently suggested[22], also modulate DC function remains to be established. Hence, epithelial cells are not simply a barrier to bacteria entering via the oral route, they also actively influence the activating properties of bystander DC.

Acknowledgements

This work was supported by grants from the Italian Association for Cancer Research (AIRC) and from the Ministero della Salute (Ricerca finalizzata). We thank Dr Gordon Dougan and Liljana Petrovska for providing the *Salmonella typhimurium*-mutated strains.

References

1. Neutra MR. M cells in antigen sampling in mucosal tissues. Curr Top Microbiol Immunol. 1999;236:17–32.
2. Rescigno M, Urbano M, Valzasina B et al. Dendritic cells express tight junction proteins and penetrate gut epithelial monolayers to sample bacteria. Nat Immunol. 2001;2:361–7.
3. Palucka K, Banchereau J. How dendritic cells and microbes interact to elicit or subvert protective immune responses. Curr Opin Immunol. 2002;14:420–31.
4. Banchereau J, Briere F, Caux C et al. Immunobiology of dendritic cells. Annu Rev Immunol. 2000;18:767–811.
5. Rescigno M. Dendritic cells and the complexity of microbial infection. Trends Microbiol. 2002;10:425.
6. Pulendran B, Palucka K, Banchereau J. Sensing pathogens and tuning immune responses. Science. 2001;293:253–6.
7. Reis e Sousa C. Dendritic cells as sensors of infection. Immunity. 2001;14:495–8.
8. Wick MJ. The role of dendritic cells in the immune response to *Salmonella*. Immunol Lett. 2003;85:99–102.
9. Inaba K, Inaba M, Naito M, Steinman RM. Dendritic cell progenitors phagocytose particulates, including bacillus Calmette–Guerin organisms, and sensitize mice to mycobacterial antigens *in vivo*. J Exp Med. 1993;178:479–88.
10. Reis e Sousa C, Austyn JM. Phagocytosis of antigens by Langerhans cells. Adv Exp Med Biol. 1993;329:199–204.
11. De Smedt T, Pajak B, Muraille E et al. Regulation of dendritic cell numbers and maturation by lipopolysaccharide *in vivo*. J Exp Med. 1996;184:1413–24.
12. Robert C, Fuhlbrigge RC, Kieffer JD et al. Interaction of dendritic cells with skin endothelium: a new perspective on immunosurveillance. J Exp Med. 1999;189:627–36.
13. Saeki H, Moore AM, Brown MJ, Hwang ST. Cutting edge: secondary lymphoid-tissue chemokine (SLC) and CC chemokine receptor 7 (CCR7) participate in the emigration pathway of mature dendritic cells from the skin to regional lymph nodes. J Immunol. 1999;162:2472–5.
14. Sozzani S, Allavena P, D'Amico G et al. Differential regulation of chemokine receptors during dendritic cell maturation: a model for their trafficking properties. J Immunol. 1998;161:1083–6.
15. Rescigno M, Urbano M, Rittig M et al. Interaction of dendritic cells with bacteria. In: Thomson MLA, editor. Dendritic Cell. Biology and Clinical Applications, 2nd edn. San Diego: Academic Press; 2001:473–86.
16. Rescigno M, Citterio S, Théry C et al. Bacteria-induced neo-biosynthesis, stabilization, and surface expression of functional class I molecules in mouse dendritic cells. Proc Natl Acad Sci USA. 1998;95:5229–34.
17. Rescigno M, Granucci F, Ricciardi-Castagnoli P. Molecular events of bacterial-induced maturation of dendritic cells [In process citation]. J Clin Immunol. 2000;20:161–6.
18. Sallusto F, Lanzavecchia A. Efficient presentation of soluble antigen by cultured human dendritic cells is maintained by granulocyte/macrophage colony-stimulating factor plus interleukin 4 and downregulated by tumor necrosis factor alpha. J Exp Med. 1994;179:1109–18.
19. Kunst F, Ogasawara N, Moszer I et al. The complete genome sequence of the gram-positive bacterium *Bacillus subtilis*. Nature. 1997;390:249–56.
20. Mastroeni P, Menager N. Development of acquired immunity to *Salmonella*. J Med Microbiol. 2003;52:453–9.
21. Sierro F, Dubois B, Coste A, Kaiserlian D, Kraehenbuhl JP, Sirard JC. Flagellin stimulation of intestinal epithelial cells triggers CCL20-mediated migration of dendritic cells. Proc Natl Acad Sci USA. 2001;98:13722–7.
22. Neish AS, Gewirtz AT, Zeng H et al. Prokaryotic regulation of epithelial responses by inhibition of IkappaB-alpha ubiquitination. Science. 2000;289:1560–3.

5
Effect of CpG oligonucleotides in animal models of inflammatory bowel disease

F. OBERMEIER, U. G. STRAUCH, N. DUNGER, N. GRUNWALD,
H. C. RATH, H. HERFARTH, J. SCHÖLMERICH and W. FALK

INTRODUCTION

There is abundant evidence that the resident intestinal flora plays a critical role in the initiation and perpetuation of chronic intestinal inflammation, as demonstrated in numerous genetic mouse and rat models of spontaneous colitis which fail to develop disease under germ-free conditions[1–7]. On the other hand there are several observations suggesting that an 'over-clean' environment, especially in early childhood, increases the risk of inflammatory bowel disease (IBD)[8,9].

Recently the importance of bacterial DNA as an activating product of the vertebrate immune system was recognized[10]. As shown by Krieg et al., CpG sequence motifs composed of unmethylated CpG dinucleotides are the immunostimulatory component of bacterial DNA[11]. CpG motifs occur stochastically in bacterial DNA (5%) and are rare in vertebrate DNA (1.5%)[12]. Additionally, the cytosines in vertebrate DNA are mostly methylated, in contrast to bacterial DNA. Based on these differences the vertebrate immune system has developed mechanisms to specifically recognize bacterial DNA. Recent findings indicate that Toll-like receptor (TLR) 9 is critical for the recognition of CpG motifs of bacterial DNA[13].

So far known oligodeoxynucleotides (ODN) containing CpG motifs are able to directly activate murine macrophages, natural killer cells, B lymphocytes, and dendritic cells, resulting in the differentiation and activation of T lymphocytes. Interestingly, the specific immune stimulatory properties of bacterial DNA lead to a strong Th$_1$ response with elevated production of IFN-γ, IL-12, TNF, and IL-6 that shows a pattern similar to the exaggerated immune response described for IBD. Therefore, and with regard to the possible contribution of bacteria in the pathomechanism of colitis, we hypothesized that the interaction between bacterial DNA and the intestinal immune system is a critical factor within the pathogenesis of IBD.

Previously we were able to demonstrate a proinflammatory effect of CpG-ODN treatment during DSS-induced colitis, most evident in the chronic phase of the disease[14]. In line with that is a report from Katakura et al., who found a colitis-exacerbating effect of a CpG motif containing plasmid in TNBS colitis[15]. In contrast Rachmilewitz et al.[16] demonstrated a protective role of bacterial DNA and CpG-ODN treatment in experimental models of colitis. These – at first glance contradictory – results will be analysed and discussed in the following section.

'THERAPEUTIC' APPROACHES: APPLICATION OF CpG MOTIF CONTAINING DNA AFTER THE ONSET OF ACUTE OR CHRONIC EXPERIMENTAL COLITIS

To determine whether CpG motifs of bacterial DNA have the potential to modulate intestinal inflammation we tested the effect of a systemic CpG-ODN therapy both in acute and chronic DSS-induced colitis. In acute colitis treatment started with the onset of clinical symptoms of colitis on day 3 of DSS feeding, and was continued with daily applications throughout day 7, when DSS feeding was terminated and animals were sacrificed. An aggravation of colitis by CpG-ODN treatment was clearly indicated by an increased loss of body weight (day 7: CpG-ODN vs. control GpG-ODN: -4.6 ± 0.3 g vs. -2.9 ± 0.3 g) and an augmented inflammatory infiltration and epithelial damage as illustrated by the histological score which was increased by $30.0 \pm 5.3\%$ ($p = 0.019$) compared to controls (Figure 1).

Along with that finding, IFN-γ, IL-6 and IL-12 production in colonic tissue and mesenterial lymph node cells increased significantly. In previous studies we had shown that IL-12 induced IFN-γ aggravated acute DSS-induced colitis[17]. Thus, the colitis-accelerating effects of CpG-ODN administration during acute colitis might be explained by their Th$_1$-favouring, proinflammatory properties.

Even more pronounced was the CpG-ODN-induced exacerbation of intestinal inflammation during the chronic phase of DSS colitis[14]. A 5-day treatment with CpG-ODN resulted in a dose-dependent increase of the histological score by 56% compared to GpG-ODN-treated controls. IFN-γ and TNF expression, which were previously shown to have a pathophysiological role in this model of chronic colitis[18], both increased significantly (150–200-fold) in colonic tissue. Coadministration of neutralizing IFN-γ antibodies blocked the proinflammatory effects of CpG-ODN treatment in chronic DSS-induced colitis, indicating that IFN-γ mediates the effects of CpG-ODN in this setting.

The colitis-exacerbating potential of CpG-ODN treatment was further confirmed in the SCID-transfer model of colitis when treatment was started together with the onset of clinical signs of colitis at week 3 after transfer. This was illustrated by an accelerated weight loss in CpG-ODN-treated animals compared to control GpG-ODN-treated mice (Figure 2). Again IFN-γ secretion was significantly elevated in CpG-ODN-treated animals compared to controls (CpG-ODN: 5560 ± 404 pg/ml vs. control GpG-ODN: 1841 ± 582 pg/ml).

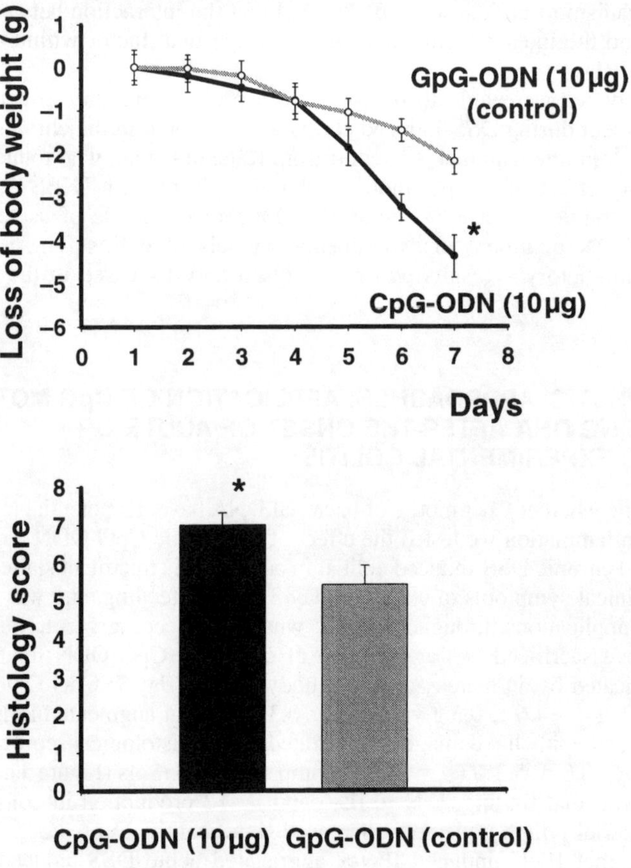

Figure 1 CpG-ODN treatment from day 3 to day 7 of DSS administration aggravates acute DSS-induced colitis

Together with the data from Katakura et al.[15], which indicate an increase of intestinal inflammation in TNBS-induced colitis in mice when exposed to CpG-motif containing plasmid DNA after the onset of disease, there is convincing evidence for a proinflammatory effect of exogenous CpG-ODN exposition after the establishment of experimental colitis. Moreover, these data suggest that DNA might be an important bacterial constituent contributing to the well-established pacemaker function of the intestinal flora in the development and perpetuation of chronic colitis[7]. Our preliminary data, which show that CpG-ODN-blocking (inhibitory) ODNs containing adenoviral motifs ameliorate chronic colitis in the DSS model further strengthen this hypothesis.

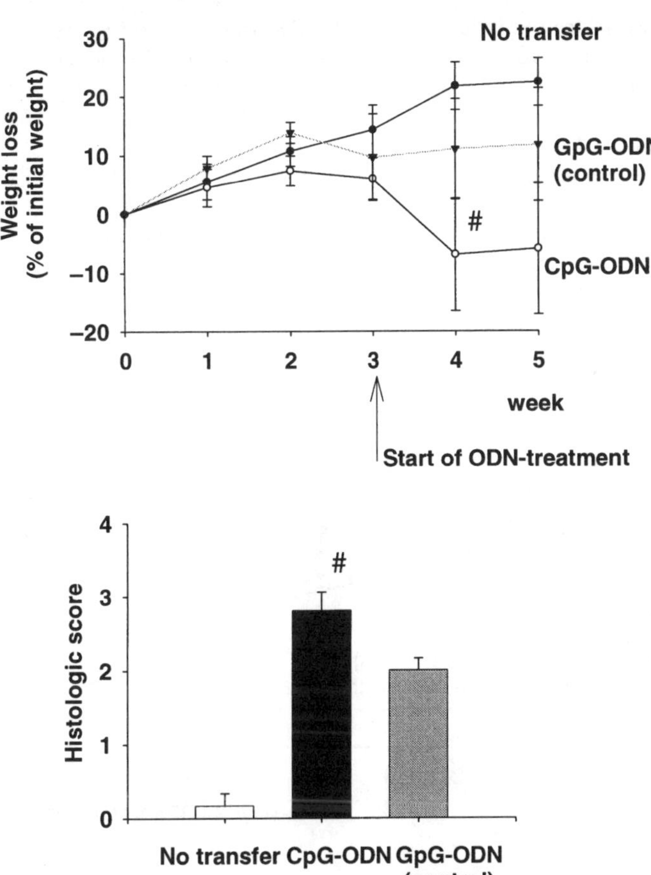

Figure 2   CpG-ODN treatment beginning at week 3 (twice weekly, 10 μg) aggravates inflammation in the SCID transfer of colitis. (# One mouse out of five died between weeks 4 and 5)

PROPHYLACTIC APPROACHES: APPLICATION OF CpG MOTIF CONTAINING DNA BEFORE THE ONSET OF EXPERIMENTAL COLITIS

Pretreatment schedules revealed that CpG-ODNs are protective when applied before the onset of colitis. Rachmilewitz et al.[16] demonstrated an amelioration of intestinal inflammation in acute DSS-induced colitis as well as in hapten-induced colitis (both TNBS and DNBS) and in spontaneous colitis which develops in IL-10-deficient mice. In this work CpG-ODN treatment was performed in all models before the induction/manifestation of colitis. This is in line with our observations, which clearly indicated a protective effect of CpG-ODN pretreatment over 5 days before the induction of acute DSS-induced colitis. As demonstrated in Figure 3, mice were significantly protected from DSS-induced weight loss ($p < 0.0001$) and the histological score was significantly and dose-dependently reduced (CpG-ODN 10 µg: 3.6 ± 0.2 and CpG-ODN 2 µg: 4.3 ± 0.6 vs. control 6.6 ± 0.2) (Figure 3).

The reduced disease activity was accompanied by a significant 85% decrease of IFN-γ and IL-6 mRNA levels and a 55% reduction of TNF mRNA expression in the colonic tissue at the end of DSS application, whereas mRNA expression levels of the anti-inflammatory cytokine IL-10 were found to be elevated 4-fold compared to controls.

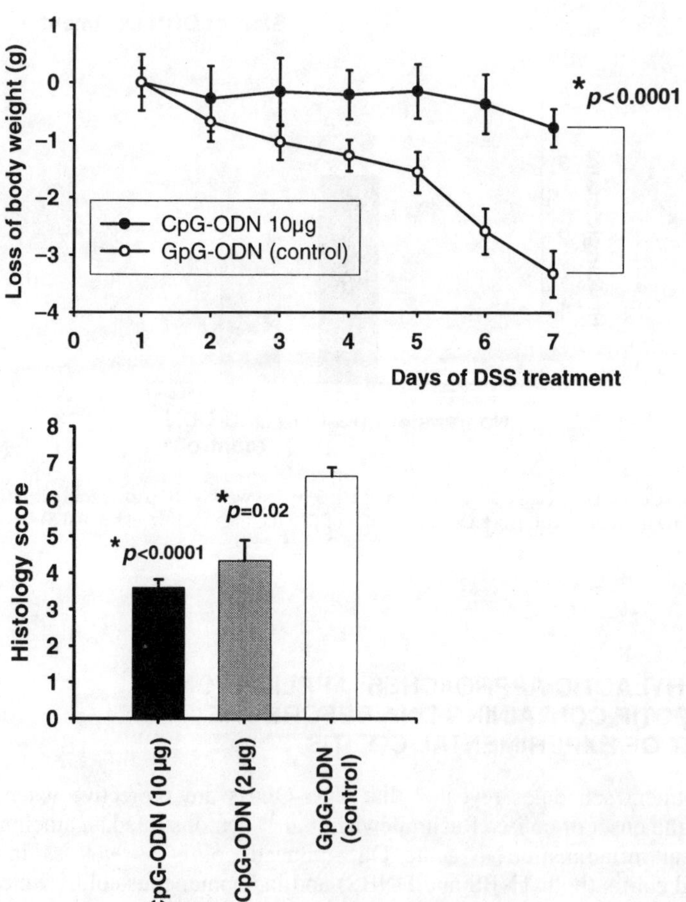

Figure 3 CpG-DNA pretreatment over 5 days (10 µg per day) before DSS feeding reduces the severity of acute DSS-induced colitis

PROPHYLACTIC CpG-ODN APPLICATION: POSSIBLE UNDERLYING MECHANISMS

As the changes in cytokine patterns induced by CpG-ODN pretreatment implicated a modulation towards a regulatory response, we decided to further characterize the role of T cells in this process by using the SCID transfer model of colitis.

We found that animals receiving $CD4^+CD62L^+$ T cells from CpG-ODN-treated donor mice were highly protected, and developed only mild or no intestinal inflammation (Figure 4).

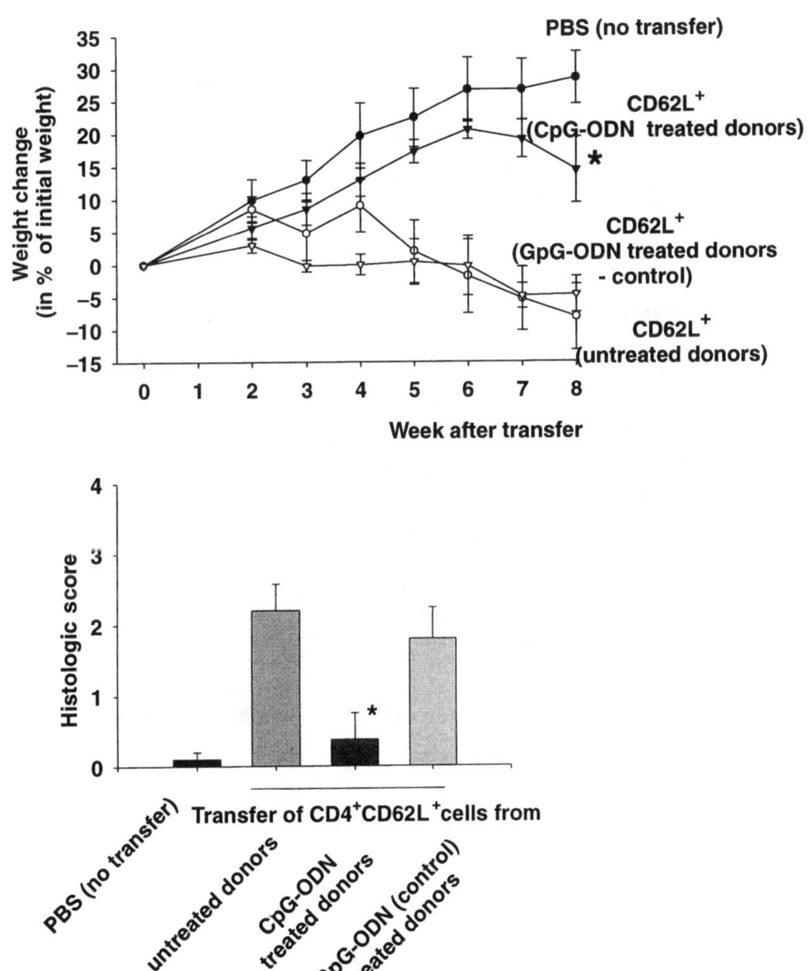

Figure 4 CpG-ODN treatment (10 µg/day over 5 days) of donor mice protects SCID recipients from the development of colitis

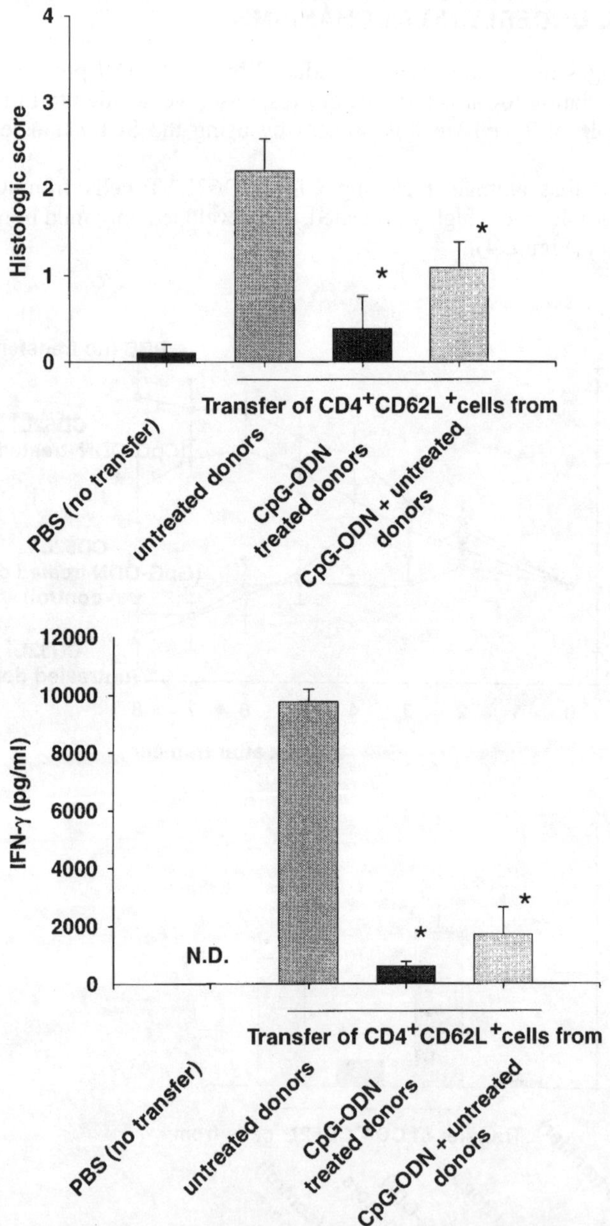

Figure 5 CD4$^+$CD62L$^+$ cells from CpG-ODN-treated donors develop regulatory potential indicated by the suppression of colitis development and IFN-γ production in SCID recipients transferred with both CD4$^+$CD62L$^+$ cells from untreated and CpG-ODN-treated donors. N.D. = not detected

This prophylactic effect was accompanied by low IFN-γ secretion from draining mesenterial lymph-node cells, comparable to those from mice used as negative control which were not transferred at all.

To further analyse whether the $CD4^+CD62L^+$ T cells just lose their colitis-inducing potential upon CpG-ODN treatment of donor animals, or whether they even develop regulatory qualities, we performed a co-transfer experiment. In this experiment animals were transferred either with cells from untreated donors or from CpG-ODN-treated donor mice or both. Recipients co-transferred with cells from CpG-ODN-treated and untreated donors were also significantly protected, and IFN-γ production was inhibited.

These results demonstrate that CpG-ODN treatment of donor mice did not only reduce the colitis-inducing potential of the transferred $CD4^+CD62L^+$ cells, but even induced colitis-suppressive qualities. We therefore suggest that the prophylactic application of CpG-ODN protected against development of colitis via induction of regulatory T cells.

CONCLUSIONS

In summary, CpG-ODN treatment proved to be a two-sided sword in experimental colitis, having both a disease-aggravating and -improving potential, depending on the time point of administration. Therefore, possible therapeutic use in IBD should be carefully evaluated. Due to the proinflammatory effects of CpG-ODN after the onset of colitis, as shown by us and others[14,15], therapeutic approaches using CpG-ODN during active disease – as recently suggested[16,19] – might have deleterious consequences.

However, the fact that pre-exposure to bacterial DNA was protective, possibly via the induction of regulatory T cells, is of special interest with regard to results from epidemiological studies which suggest that the incidence of IBD positively correlates with the increase of hygienic standards in developed countries[8,9]. Therefore, it is tempting to speculate that the reduced exposure to microbial components (such as bacterial DNA) contributes to an increased risk to develop a deregulated intestinal immune response – eventually leading to inflammatory bowel diseases in genetically susceptible hosts.

References

1. Brimnes J, Reimann J, Nissen M, Claesson M. Enteric bacterial antigens activate CD4(+) T cells from scid mice with inflammatory bowel disease. Eur J Immunol. 2001;31:23–31.
2. Dianda L, Hanby AM, Wright NA, Sebesteny A, Hayday AC, Owen MJ. T cell receptor-alpha beta-deficient mice fail to develop colitis in the absence of a microbial environment. Am J Pathol. 1997;150:91–7.
3. Madsen KL, Malfair D, Gray D, Doyle JS, Jewell LD, Fedorak RN. Interleukin-10 gene-deficient mice develop a primary intestinal permeability defect in response to enteric microflora. Inflamm Bowel Dis. 1999;5:262–70.
4. Schultz M, Tonkonogy SL, Sellon RK et al. IL-2-deficient mice raised under germfree conditions develop delayed mild focal intestinal inflammation. Am J Physiol. 1999;276:G1461–72.
5. Veltkamp C, Tonkonogy SL, De Jong YP et al. Continuous stimulation by normal luminal bacteria is essential for the development and perpetuation of colitis in Tg(epsilon26) mice. Gastroenterology. 2001;120:900–13.

6. Sartor RB. Review article: Role of the enteric microflora in the pathogenesis of intestinal inflammation and arthritis. Aliment Pharmacol Ther. 1997;11:17–22.
7. Sartor RB. The influence of normal microbial flora on the development of chronic mucosal inflammation. Res Immunol. 1997;148:567–76.
8. Duggan AE, Usmani I, Neal KR, Logan RF. Appendicectomy, childhood hygiene, *Helicobacter pylori* status, and risk of inflammatory bowel disease: a case control study. Gut. 1998;43:494–8.
9. Gent AE, Hellier MD, Grace RH, Swarbrick ET, Coggon D. Inflammatory bowel disease and domestic hygiene in infancy. Lancet. 1994;343:766–7.
10. Krieg AM. Now I know my CpGs. Trends Microbiol. 2001;9:249–52.
11. Krieg AM, Yi AK, Matson S et al. CpG motifs in bacterial DNA trigger direct B-cell activation. Nature. 1995;374:546–9.
12. Burge C, Campbell AM, Karlin S. Over- and under-representation of short oligonucleotides in DNA sequences. Proc Natl Acad Sci USA. 1992;89:1358–62.
13. Hemmi II, Takeuchi O, Kawai T et al. A Toll-like receptor recognizes bacterial DNA. Nature. 2000;408:740–5.
14. Obermeier F, Dunger N, Deml L, Herfarth H, Schölmerich J, Falk W. CpG motifs of bacterial DNA exacerbate colitis of dextran sulfate sodium-treated mice. Eur J Immunol. 2002;32: 2084–92.
15. Katakura K, Sato Y, Sato N et al. CpG motifs in plasmid DNA exacerbate inflammation in experimental colitis. Gastroenterology. 2001;120(Suppl. 1):A518.
16. Rachmilewitz D, Karmeli F, Takabayashi K et al. Immunostimulatory DNA ameliorates experimental and spontaneous murine colitis. Gastroenterology. 2002;122:1428–41.
17. Hans W, Scholmerich J, Gross V, Falk W. Interleukin-12 induced interferon-gamma increases inflammation in acute dextran sulfate sodium induced colitis in mice. Eur Cytokine Netw. 2000;11:67–74.
18. Obermeier F, Kojouharoff G, Hans W, Schölmerich J, Gross V, Falk W. Interferon-gamma (IFN-gamma)- and tumour necrosis factor (TNF)-induced nitric oxide as toxic effector molecule in chronic dextran sulphate sodium (DSS)-induced colitis in mice. Clin Exp Immunol. 1999;116:238–45.
19. Bradbury J. New treatment for inflammatory bowel disease could soon enter clinical trials. Lancet. 2002;359:1583.

6
Organ-specific pathology of the small intestine mediated by hsp60 CD8$^+$ T cells: proteasomal antigen processing is different in the small intestine and colon

U. STEINHOFF and U. KUCKELKORN

INTRODUCTION

CD8$^+$ T cells exert their effector function mainly by the cytotoxic damage of target cells expressing MHC class I molecules and a relevant antigenic peptide, as well as by the production of proinflammatory cytokines such as IFN-γ and TNF-α. As almost all cells express MHC class I molecules, activation of CD8$^+$ T cells bears a great potential for tissue damage. Although their importance in autoimmune diseases such as type 1 diabetes, multiple sclerosis, thyroiditis and rheumatoid arthritis is not yet well recognized, the number of reports describing the involvement of CD8$^+$ T cells in experimental and clinical autoimmune diseases is continuously growing. Thus CD8$^+$ T cells emerge as important contributors as well as targets for therapeutic intervention in murine and human autoimmune diseases[1].

T cell-mediated autoimmune disorders are often restricted to specific organs despite the ubiquitous expression of a self-antigen[2]. In a model of CD8$^+$ T cell-mediated pathology of the small intestine we propose tissue-specific antigen processing by proteasomes as a potential mechanism to control organ-specific CD8$^+$ T-cell responses. Further, we demonstrate that, in contrast to the colon, the small intestine is a preferable target tissue of hsp60-crossreactive CD8$^+$ T cells.

AUTOIMMUNE INTESTINAL INFLAMMATION BY hsp60-SPECIFIC CD8$^+$ T CELLS

The intestinal immune system is continuously stimulated with antigens derived from the food, the microbial flora or invading pathogenic bacteria. To discriminate between noxious and normal constituents of the intestine the mucosal immune system requires tight regulation to avoid pathological immune responses. However, the undefined antigen specificity of intestinal lymphocytes has hampered the understanding of mechanisms leading to T cell-mediated protection or pathology of the intestine.

We have established mycobacterial hsp60-specific CD8$^+$ T cells that crossreact with the murine homologue. Peptides of either mycobacterial (AA499–508: SALQNAASIA) or murine hsp60 origin (AA162–171: KDIGNIISDA) were recognized in a H-2D^b-restricted fashion[3]. The hsp60-specific T cells expressed the TCR Vβ8.1 and Vα8 chains, exhibited cytolytic activity that was mainly Fas-mediated, and secreted large amounts of the proinflammatory cytokines IFN-γ and TNF-α upon antigenic stimulation. Analysis of surface marker expression revealed the phenotype of activated T cells (high expression of CD69) with no obvious homing receptors for the intestine, as demonstrated by the barely detectable expression of the integrin α4 chain and no detectable expression of the integrin α$_{IEL}$ and L-selectin[4].

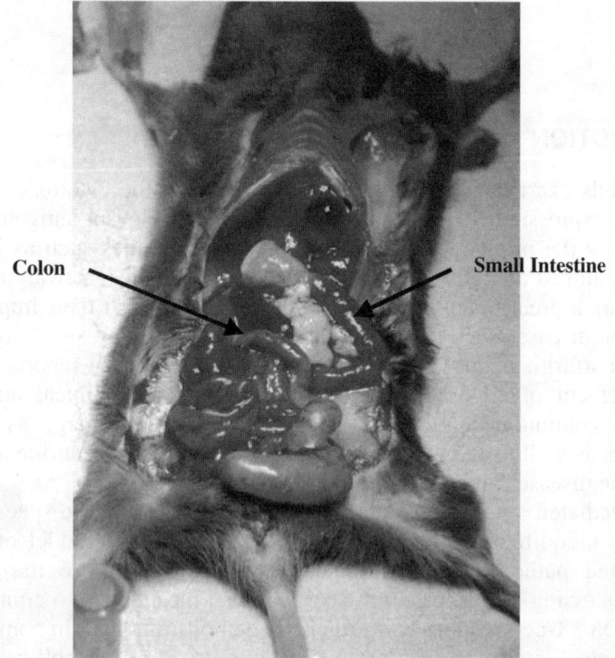

Figure 1　hsp60-specific CD8$^+$ T cells cause inflammation of the small intestine. β TCR$^{-/-}$ mice were reconstituted (i.v.) with 5×10^6 hsp60-specific CD8$^+$ T cells and monitored for pathology 24 days after reconstitution. Arrows indicate inflammation of the small intestine but normal colon

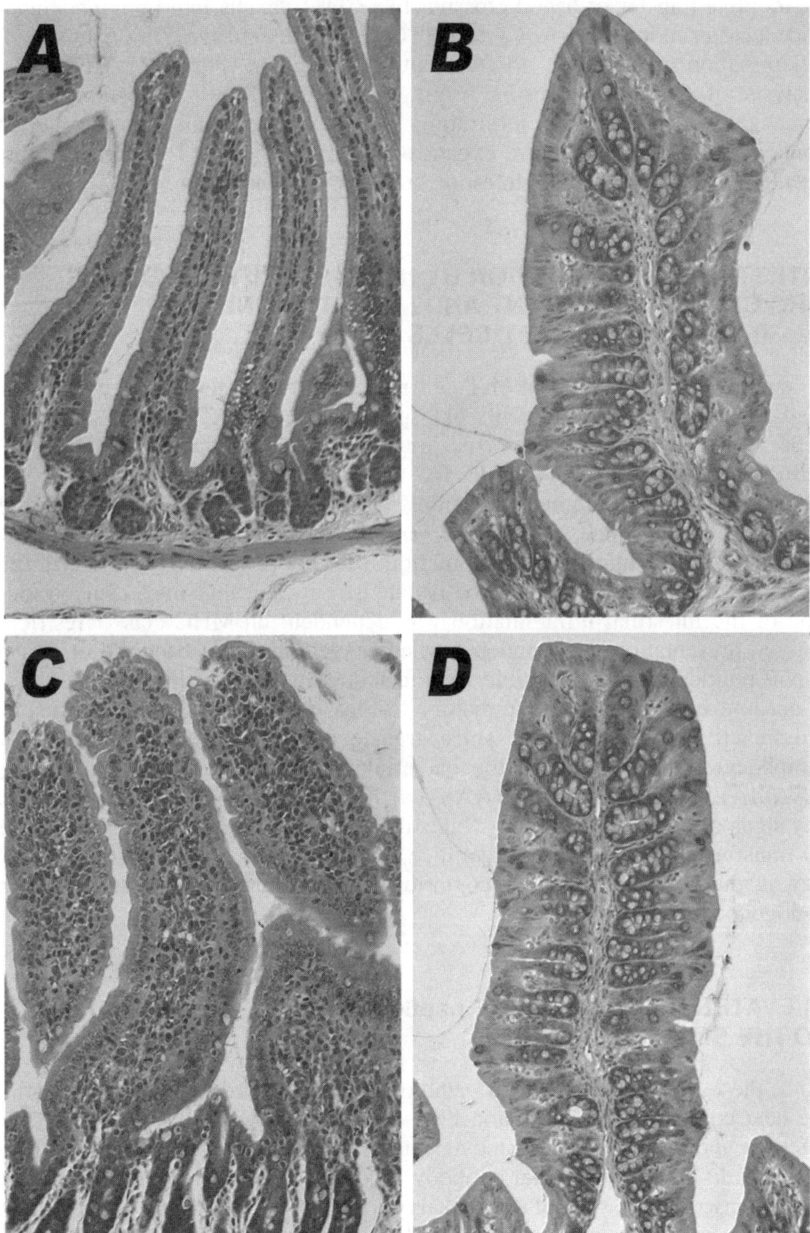

Figure 2 CD8$^+$ T cell-mediated inflammation of the small intestine due to tissue-specific proteasomal processing of hsp60. The upper panel shows haematoxylin–eosin-stained cross-sections of a naive small intestine (**A**) and colon (**B**), and the lower panel represents the same organs 16 days after transfer of hsp60-specific CD8$^+$ T cells. Massive expansion of these autoreactive CD8$^+$ T lymphocytes causing inflammation and tissue destruction is observed in the small intestine (**C**) but not in the colon (**D**)

Adoptive transfer of hsp60 crossreactive CD8$^+$ T cells into immunodeficient mice lacking endogenous α/β T cells (TCR$\beta^{-/-}$ mice) resulted in organ-specific inflammation of the small intestine but not the colon (Figure 1). Histological analysis of the small intestine from control and T cell-reconstituted mice revealed large numbers of infiltrating T cells in the lamina propria and the epithelium, indicating massive expansion of hsp60-specific T cells with subsequent pathology in the small intestine but not the colon (Figure 2).

INTESTINAL INFLAMMATION BY hsp60-SPECIFIC T CELLS IS MHC CLASS I DEPENDENT AND MEDIATED ONLY BY hsp60-CROSSREACTIVE T CELLS

To determine the mechanism of T cell-mediated intestinal pathology we examined the activation requirements of hsp60-crossreactive T cells. Therefore, T cells were adoptively transferred into double mutant mice (TCR$\beta^{-/-}$ × $\beta2m^{-/-}$) lacking endogenous α/β T cells and MHC class I molecules and the development of inflammatory lesions was observed. In contrast to single mutant TCR$\beta^{-/-}$ mice, double deficient TCR$\beta^{-/-}$ × $\beta2m^{-/-}$ animals developed no signs of intestinal inflammation after adoptive transfer. Accordingly, no hsp60-specific T cells could be isolated from their intestines. Since induction of the intestinal inflammation was dependent on MHC class I restricted antigen presentation, we wondered whether recognition of bacterial or murine hsp60 peptides was responsible for the induction of intestinal inflammation. It became obvious that inflammatory lesions were only mediated by hsp60-crossreactive CD8$^+$ T cells since transfer of non-crossreactive CD8$^+$ T lymphocytes that react with the bacterial hsp60 epitope (AA$_{499-508}$ SALQNAASIA) but not the murine (AA$_{162-171}$ KDIGNIIDDA) hsp60 did not induce any signs of intestinal pathology. Intestinal inflammation could also be induced by transfer of T cells in germfree mice, supporting the finding that the pathology is due to autoimmune recognition of self-hsp60 independently of the endogenous flora[4].

ELEVATED EXPRESSION OF hsp60 IN THE COLON COMPARED TO THE SMALL INTESTINE

Since the hsp60 T cell-mediated pathology was restricted to the small intestine, we next compared the expression levels of the endogenous hsp60 in the small intestine and the colon before and after transfer of T cells. Western-blot analysis performed with a monoclonal antibody specific for the murine hsp60 revealed: (a) increased expression of the eukaryotic hsp60 in the small intestine after T cell reconstitution and (b) significantly higher levels of endogenous hsp60 in the colon and not the small intestine (Figure 3). This finding showed an apparent discrepancy to the tissue-specific, autoimmune pathology of the small intestine. How can these findings be reconciled? The most feasible explanation was that the efficiency of processing and presentation of the hsp60 T cell epitope differs between the small intestine and the colon.

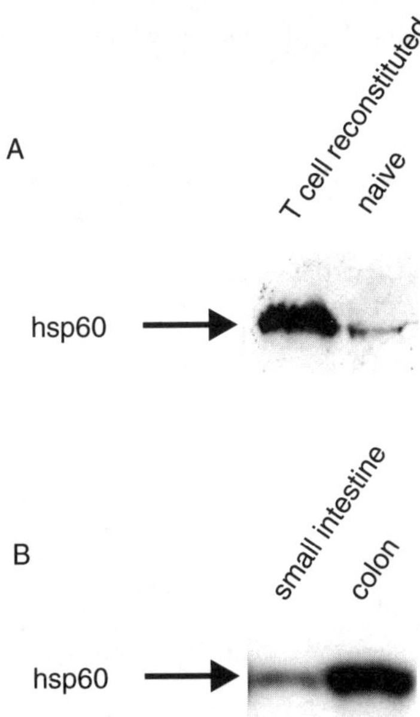

Figure 3   Expression of hsp60 in the small intestine and colon. **A**: Expression levels of eukaryotic hsp60 in the small intestine before and after T cell reconstitution was evaluated by Western blot analysis using a mAb specific for eukaryotic hsp60. **B**: Comparison of endogenous hsp60 expression between the colon and small intestine of naive mice. Equivalent amounts of proteins, as determined by UV absorbance (280 nm), were loaded

MHC CLASS I ANTIGEN PROCESSING BY PROTEASOMES

MHC class I molecules usually bind peptides of 8–10 amino acids for display to the T cells. These peptides are antigenic side-products originating from the turnover of intracellular proteins, mainly ubiquitin-tagged proteins[5]. Most of these peptides are generated by 26S proteasomes, the major proteolytic enzyme machinery of a cell[6–8]. Although other proteases with selective cleavage specificity might also contribute to the MHC class I peptide pool, this seems to apply only for a limited subset of peptides, and cannot substitute for proteasome function[9].

The active sites of the 26S proteasomes are located within the 20S core complex that is composed of four stacked rings with seven subunits each. The outer rings contain the α subunits ($\alpha1$–$\alpha7$) which shape the gates of substrate entry and product release. The two inner rings harbour the β subunits ($\beta1$–$\beta7$) of which three β subunits, $\beta1$, $\beta5$ and $\beta2$ are catalytically active[10,11]. Stimulation with IFN-γ results in an exchange of these constitutive β subunits by the inducible i$\beta1$ (LMP2), i$\beta5$ (LMP7), and i$\beta2$ (MECL-1) subunits leading to the formation of immunoproteasomes[12–14]. Further, cytokine-induced subunit exchange occurs during proteasome assembly, and profoundly alters the cleavage specificity of 20S proteasomes[15].

In order to investigate whether tissue-restricted inflammation of the small intestine is directly influenced by organ-specific processing of MHC class I ligands, the subunit composition of 20S proteasomes was analysed and compared with their ability to generate T-cell epitopes which are involved in the induction of intestinal pathology.

SUBUNIT COMPOSITION OF 20S PROTEASOMES DIFFERS BETWEEN THE SMALL INTESTINE AND THE COLON

The composition of the 20S proteasomes from various organs was analysed by two-dimensional gel electrophoresis (2-DE) and proteins were identified by

Immunosubunit expression

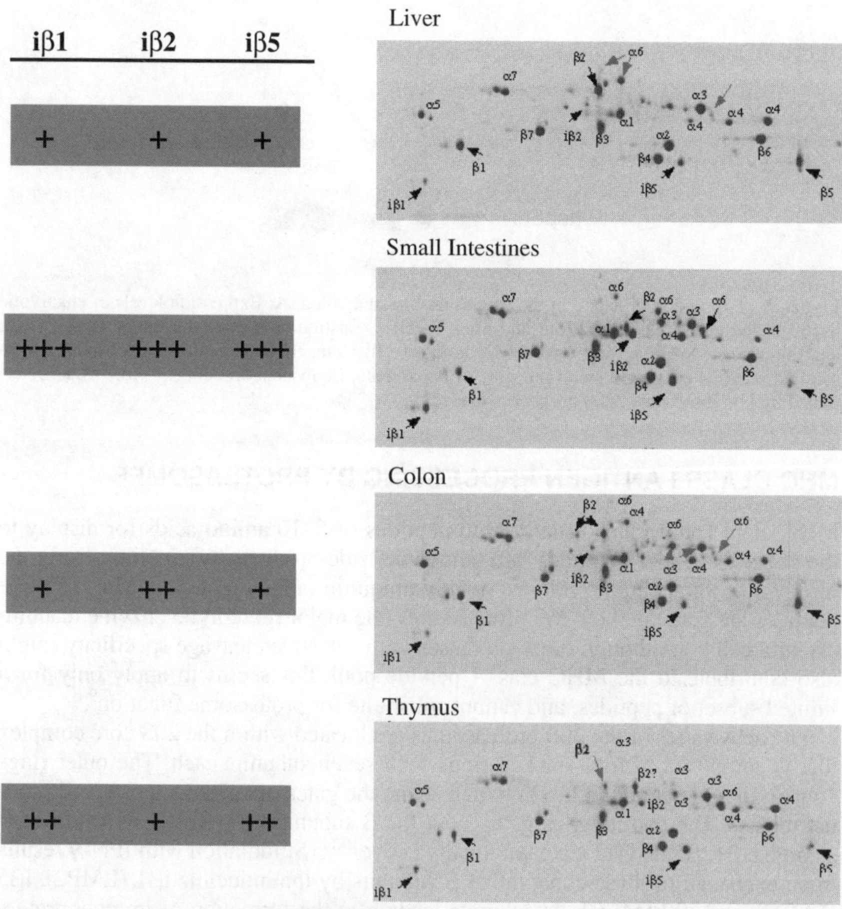

Figure 4 The subunit composition of 20S proteasomes varies between different organs. Purified 20S proteasomes were analysed by 2-DE, and MS identified spots of the thymus, small intestine and colon were compared with proteasome subunits of the liver. The α and β subunits of the small intestine, colon and thymus were related to the liver (standard proteasome) and differences were marked by black arrows. The relative expression of the immunosubunits iβ1, iβ2 and iβ5 of organ-isolated proteasomes is schematically indicated at the left side

mass spectroscopy (MALDI-MS). We found marked differences between the small intestine and the colon, including both α and β subunits of the 20S proteasome (Figure 4). A detailed MALDI-MS analysis of the 20S proteasome subunits from the small intestine and the colon revealed that the $\alpha4$ and $\alpha6$ subunits were identified in three spots each with similar molecular mass (M_r) but different isoelectric points (pI). This finding suggests posttranslational modifications as the cause for this polymorphism. The small intestine and the colon differed in the expression ratio of both α subunits. The $\alpha4$ and $\alpha6$ subunits are known to interact with the proteasomal regulatory complexes PA700 and PA28 and other proteins of cellular and viral origin, suggesting that the $\alpha4$ and $\alpha6$ subunits modulate the proteasomal activity by controlling substrate entry into the catalytic activity[16–18]. Polymorphisms in the subunit composition of 20S proteasomes may be due to tissue-specific functional modifications, including differential transcription and posttranslational modification, as discussed previously[19–21].

Further, proteasomes of the small intestine and the colon also revealed characteristic differences in the composition of β subunits. The immunoproteasome

Table 1 Subunit differences of the 20S proteasomes isolated from the small intestine and the colon

	Gene	Spot	Small intestine	Colon
α Subunits				
α1 (Jota)	PSMA 6	α1	+	+
α2 (C3)	PSMA 2	α2	+	+
α3 (C9)	PSMA 4	α3.1/α3.2	+	+
α4 (C6)	PSMA 7	α4.1 α4.2 α4.3	α4.1 > α4.3 > α4.2	α4.1 = α4.2 = α4.3
α5 (Zeta)	PSMA 5	α5	+	+
α6 (C2)	PSMA 1	α6.1 α6.2 α6.3	α6.3 > α6.2 > α6.1	α6.1 > α6.2 > α6.3
α7 (C8)	PSMA 3	α7	+	+
β Subunits				
β1 (delta)	PSMB 6	β1	+	++
iβ1 (LMP2)	PSMB 9	iβ1	++	(+)
		β2	−	++
β2 (Z)	PSMB 7	β2.2	++	(+)
		iβ2	−	+
iβ2 (MECL1)	PSMB 10	iβ2	++	(+)
β3 (C10)	PSMB 3	β3	+	+
β4 (C7)	PSMB 2	β4	+	+
β5 (MB1)	PSMB 5	β5	(+)	++
iβ5 (LMP7)	PSMB 8	iβ5	++	(+)
β6 (C5)	PSMB 1	β6	+	+
β7 (N3)	PSMB 4	β7	+	+

MS identified α and β subunits of the 20S proteasomes isolated from the small intestine and colon are compared and evaluated as follows: + comparable amounts; (+) traces; − not detectable; + normal intensity; ++ increased intensity. β2 and iβ2 were detected in two isoforms, differing in their IP (anionic and cathodic, respectively). The basic isoforms of β2 and iβ2 were strongly expressed in the small intestine and only marginally in the colon and thymus.

subunits iβ1, iβ2 and iβ5 were predominantly found in the small intestine, whereas large amounts of the constitutive proteasome subunits β1, β2 and β5 were detected in the proteasomes of the colon[22]. Data are summarized in Table 1. It remained to be analysed whether these structural differences have functional consequences with respect to the generation of T-cell epitopes.

PROTEASOMES OF THE SMALL INTESTINE AND THE COLON GENERATE DIFFERENT T-CELL EPITOPES

To examine the functional impact of organ-specific proteasome subunit composition, the generation of distinct cleavage fragments of a 30mer polypeptide substrate of the murine hsp60 by 20S proteasomes derived from various tissues was compared. Therefore, organ-purified 20S proteasomes were normalized according to their protein amount, and the purity of proteasomal preparations was assessed by native PAGE following the overlay of fluorogenic substrates, which excludes the copurification of contaminating proteases[23]. Sequence information of cleavage products was obtained by tandem MS. The main cleavage products of the murine hsp60 from tissue derived proteasomes are summarized in Figure 5. Although there were few qualitative differences in cleavage products, some tissues varied markedly in the quantity of peptides generated. The quantitative assignment of peptides demonstrated that the majority of fragments were most efficiently produced by tissues expressing high levels of immunosubunits, i.e. the small intestine and thymus. Interestingly, despite the fact that the small intestine and the thymus express comparable levels of immunoproteasomes, they differed significantly in their cleavage site preferences. As proteasomes of the small intestine and the thymus differed mainly in their α-subunit composition, these data indicate that modifications in the α subunits may also influence the processing characteristics of proteasomes by regulating substrate entry into the catalytic cavity.

With respect to the localized inflammation mediated by hsp60-specific T cells, we analysed the ability of 20S proteasomes from various tissues to generate epitopes of a murine hsp60 polypeptide substrate. Although it is assumed that *in vivo* most of the antigens are processed by the 26S proteasomes, it has been demonstrated for many tumour and viral antigens that *in-vitro* processing of polypeptide substrates containing MHC class I epitopes by 20S proteasomes closely resembles the situation in living cells[24]. The relative abundance of T-cell epitopes produced by organ-derived 20S proteasomes is summarized in Figure 6. The mu hsp60 T-cell epitope KDIGNIISD and the NH_2-terminally elongated fragments which could serve as precursors were generated significantly more efficiently by proteasomes of the small intestine compared to the colon.

RECOGNITION OF *IN-VITRO*-GENERATED EPITOPES BY hsp60-SPECIFIC CD8[+] T CELLS CORRELATES WITH THE INTESTINAL PATHOLOGY OF T CELL-RECONSTITUTED MICE

We wondered whether *in-vitro*-generated epitopes were of functionally relevant amounts and quality. Therefore, recognition of hsp60 digests was determined in

cleavage products   organs

Position: 1 … 5 … 10 … 15 … 20 … 25 … 30	SI	C	L	SP	T
V A T I S A N G D K D I G N I I S D A M K K V G R K G V I T					
V A T I S	0.7	0.2	0.5	0.5	**1.0**
V A T I S A	**1.0**	0.3	**1.0**	0.5	**0.9**
V A T I S A N G D	**0.8**	0.2	0.5	0.6	1.0
S A N G D K D I G N I I S D	1.0	0.1	0.1	0.2	0.5
N G D K D I G N I I S D A M K K V G R K G V I T	1.0	0.3	**0.8**	0.4	**0.9**
K D I G N I I S D	1.0	0.1	0.2	0.1	0.5
K V G R K G V I T	0.7	0.6	0.2	**1.0**	**0.9**
V G R K G V I T	**1.0**	**0.8**	0.1	0.1	0.1
K G V I T	0.6	**1.0**	0.1	0.1	0.1

Figure 5 Generation of organ-specific peptide fragments by 20S proteasomes. The murine hsp60 substrate (VATISANGDKDIGNIISDAMKKV-GRKGVIT) was digested by isolated 20S proteasomes from various organs (SI, small intestine; C, colon; L, liver; SP, spleen and T, thymus). Peptide sequences were analysed by MS, maximal signal intensities of individual peptides were arbitrarily defined as 1.0. (A) Main cleavage products of the murine hsp60 substrate are listed, and the relative amounts generated by individual organs are shown to the right

Murine hsp60 Substrate

V A T I S A N G D K D I G N I I S D A M K K V G R K G V I

(5–18)

(10–18)

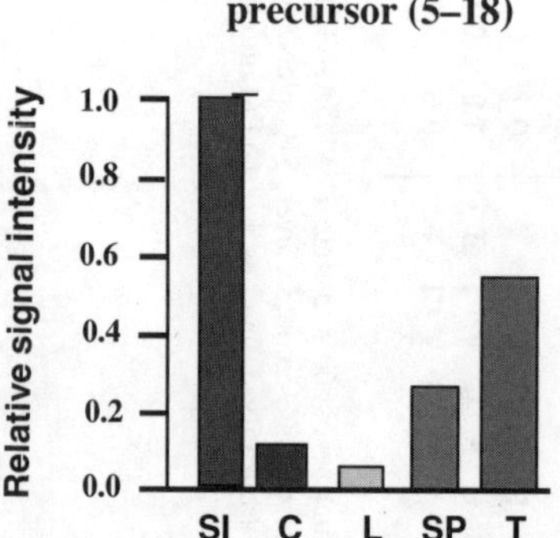

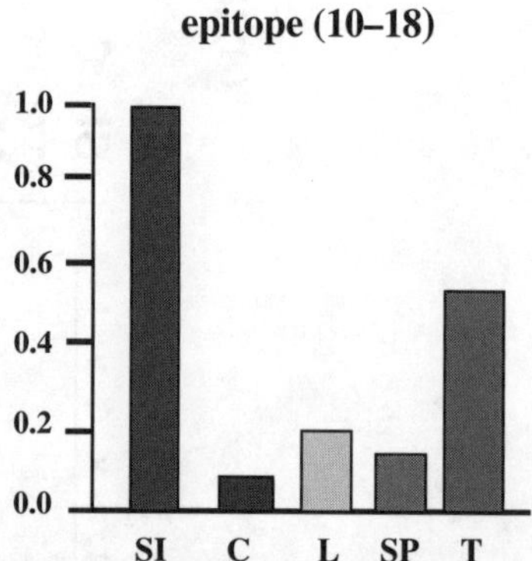

Figure 6 Generation of the hsp60 precursor and T cell epitope by 20S proteasomes. Relative amounts of a potential precursor (5–18) and the T cell epitope (10–18) of the mu hsp60. Peptide sequences were analysed by MS, maximal signal intensities of individual peptides were arbitrarily defined as 1.0. Data from three experiments, means ± SD are shown

a ^{51}Cr release assay with the hsp60-specific CD8[+] T cell clones. Studies with overlapping peptides revealed that the epitopes KDIGNIISDA and KDIGNIISD of the murine hsp60 were recognized[3] by T cells at physiological concentrations of 10^{-10} M. Target cells pulsed with cleavage products derived from 20S proteasomes of the small intestine but not from the colon or other organs were lysed by hsp60-specific T cells. Addition of the specific proteasome inhibitor MG 132 to the *in-vitro* digests blocked the generation of T-cell epitopes, indicating that cleavage of the hsp60 substrate is strictly proteasome-dependent (Figure 7). Specific recognition of the murine hsp60 T-cell epitope in the small intestine but not the colon is in accordance with the pathology observed in hsp60 T cell-reconstituted β TCR[−/−] mice.

SUMMARY

We here show that recognition of a ubiquitously expressed self-antigen by CD8[+] T cells leads to organ-specific pathology of the small intestine and not the colon due to differential, tissue-specific processing of the self-antigen by proteasomes. We further could demonstrate that 20S proteasomes are sufficient to generate the CD8[+] T-cell epitopes of the murine hsp60 and that 20S proteasomes derived from different organs produce distinct peptide patterns due to

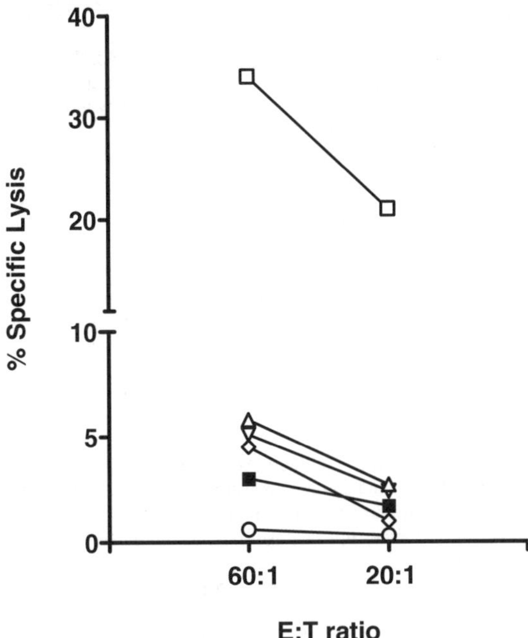

Figure 7 hsp60-specific T cells recognize peptides generated by 20S proteasomes from the small intestine. Cytolytic activity of a crossreactive hsp60-specific T cell clone was measured in a ^{51}Cr-release assay on EL-4 cells loaded with equal amounts of digests (20 μl) of hsp60 performed by 20S proteasomes from the small intestine (□), the liver (△), the colon (◇), the thymus (▽) or left untreated (○). EL-4 cells were loaded with digests performed by small intestinal 20S proteasomes in the presence of 3 μM proteasome inhibitor MG132 (■)

their organ-characteristic subunit composition. Further, generation of large quantities of self-epitopes in selected tissues may correlate with organ-specific autoimmunity. Thus we propose that, in addition to peripheral immune regulatory mechanisms, tissue-specific antigen processing by proteasomes represents an important mechanism to control the activity of CD8[+] T cells.

The reason why the polar forms of constitutive proteasomes and immunoproteasomes are predominantly found in the colon and small intestine, respectively, still remains speculative. One could hypothesize that in the very specialized immune system of the gut, which is confronted with a multitude of harmless as well as pathogenic antigens, efficient processing in the small intestine is necessary for the induction of CD8[+] T cells exerting protective or regulatory functions, i.e. establishment of oral tolerance. However, in order to avoid uncontrolled and adverse CD8[+] T-cell responses in the colon, which contains myriads of bacteria and bacterial products, the proteasomal activity should be limited to ensure the cellular protein turnover but otherwise to avoid stimulation of T cells.

References

1. Liblau RS, Wong FS, Mars LT, Santamaria P. Autoreactive CD8 T cells in organ-specific autoimmunity: emerging targets for therapeutic intervention. Immunity. 2002;17:1–6.
2. Matsumoto I, Staub A, Benoist C, Mathis D. Arthritis provoked by linked T and B cell recognition of a glycolytic enzyme. Science. 1999;286:1732–5.
3. Zugel U, Schoel B, Yamamoto S, Hengel H, Morein B, Kaufmann SH. Crossrecognition by CD8 T cell receptor alpha beta cytotoxic T lymphocytes of peptides in the self and the mycobacterial hsp60 which share intermediate sequence homology. Eur J Immunol. 1995;25:451–8.
4. Steinhoff U, Brinkmann V, Klemm U et al. Autoimmune intestinal pathology induced by hsp60-specific CD8 T cells. Immunity. 1999;11:349–58.
5. Grant EP, Michalek MT, Goldberg AL, Rock KL. Rate of antigen degradation by the ubiquitin–proteasome pathway influences MHC class I presentation. J Immunol. 1995;55:3750–8.
6. Cerundolo V, Benhan A, Braud V et al. The proteasome-specific inhibitor lactacystin blocks presentation of cytotoxic T lymphocyte epitopes in human and murine cells. Eur J Immunol. 1997;27:336–41.
7. Rock KL, Gramm C, Rothstein L et al. Inhibitors of the proteasome block the degradation of most cell proteins and the generation of peptides presented on MHC class I molecules. Cell. 1994;78:761–71.
8. Michalek MT, Grant EP, Gramm G, Goldberg AL, Rock KL. A Role for the ubiquitin-dependent pathway in MHC-class I restricted antigen presentation. Nature. 1993;363:552–554.
9. Schwarz K, de Giuli R, Schmidtke G et al. The selective proteasome inhibitors lactacystin and epoxomicin can be used to either up- or down-regulate antigen presentation at nontoxic doses. J Immunol. 2000;164:6147–57.
10. Groll M, Ditzel L, Lowe J et al. Structure of 20S proteasome from yeast at 2.4 Å resolution. Nature. 1997;386:463–71.
11. Ditzel L, Stock D, Lowe J. Structural investigation of proteasome inhibition. Biol Chem. 1997;378:239–47.
12. Akiyama K, Kagawa S, Tamura T et al. Replacement of proteasome subunits X and Y by LMP7 and LMP2 induced by interferon-gamma for acquirement of the functional diversity responsible for antigen processing. FEBS Lett. 1994;343:85–8.
13. Fruh K, Gossen M, Wang K, Bujard H, Peterson PA, Yang Y. Displacement of housekeeping proteasome subunits by MHC-encoded LMPs: a newly discovered mechanism for modulating the multicatalytic proteinase complex. EMBO J. 1994;13:3236–44.
14. Nandi D, Jiang H, Monaco JJ. Identification of MECL-1 (LMP-10) as the third IFN-gamma-inducible proteasome subunit. J Immunol. 1996;156:2361–4.
15. Boes B, Hengel H, Ruppert T, Multhaup G, Koszinowski UH, Kloetzel PM. Interferon gamma stimulation modulates the proteolytic activity and cleavage site preference of 20S mouse proteasomes. J Exp Med. 1994;179:901–9.
16. Kania MA, Demartino GN, Baumeister W, Goldberg AL. The proteasome subunit, C2, contains an important site for binding of the PA28 (11S) activator. Eur J Biochem. 1996;236:510–16.
17. Zhang Z, Torii N, Furusaka A, Malayaman N, Hu Z, Liang TJ. Structural and functional characterization of interaction between hepatitis B virus X protein and the proteasome complex. J Biol Chem. 2000;275:15157–65.
18. Groll M, Bajorek M, Kohler A et al. A gated channel into the proteasome core particle. Nat Struct Biol. 2000;7:1062–7.
19. Seelig A, Boes B, Kloetzel PM. Characterization of mouse proteasome subunit MC3 and identification of proteasome subtypes with different cleavage characteristics. Proteasome subunits, proteasome subpopulations. Enzyme Protein. 1993;47:330–42.
20. Arribas J, Arizti P, Castano JG. Antibodies against the C2 COOH-terminal region discriminate the active and latent forms of the multicatalytic proteinase complex. J Biol Chem. 1994;269:12858–64.
21. Covi JA, Belote JM, Mykles DL. Subunit compositions and catalytic properties of proteasomes from developmental temperature-sensitive mutants of *Drosophila melanogaster*. Arch Biochem Biophys. 1999;368:85–97.
22. Kuckelkorn U, Ruppert T, Strehl B et al. Link between organ-specific antigen processing by 20S proteasomes and CD8(+) T cell-mediated autoimmunity. J Exp Med. 2002;195:983–90.

23. Kuckelkorn U, Frentzel S, Kraft R, Kostka S, Groettrup M, Kloetzel PM. Incorporation of major histocompatibility complex-encoded subunits LMP2 and LMP7 changes the quality of the 20S proteasome polypeptide processing products independent of interferon-gamma. Eur J Immunol. 1995;25:2605–11.
24. Kloetzel PM. Antigen processing by the proteasome. Nat Rev Mol Cell Biol. 2001;2:179–87.

7

Interaction between T cells and dendritic cells in the development and control of colitis

H. H. UHLIG, C. MOTTET, B. SINGH, V. MALMSTROM and F. POWRIE

INTRODUCTION

Studies of chronic intestinal inflammation in mice have provided insight the pathogenesis of human Crohn's disease or ulcerative colitis[1]. A well-studied model of inflammatory bowel disease (IBD) is the T cell adoptive transfer model. In this system the transfer of predominantly naive $CD4^+CD45RB^{high}$ T cells into immunodeficient SCID or RAG-knockout mice leads to wasting disease and colon immunopathology[2,3]. Histological aspects of the immuno-pathology are infiltration of the colonic lamina propria (LP) by lymphocytes, granulocytes, monocytes, macrophages and dendritic cells (DC)[4–6]. Th1-associated proinflammatory cytokines including IL-12p40, IFN-γ and TNF-α are present in the colonic mucosa and drive the pathogenesis of IBD[4].

The T-cell transfer model has allowed the identification and characterization of a population of naturally occurring regulatory T (T_R) cells. Early studies showed that these cells were contained within the $CD4^+CD45RB^{low}$ population. More recently T_R activity was found to enrich within the $CD25^+$ subset of $CD45RB^{low}$ cells. T_R cells prevent the immune activation caused by transfer of $CD4^+CD45RB^{high}$ T cells through active regulation involving cytokines such as IL-10 and TGF-β[7,8].

There is a large body of evidence showing that the development of intestinal inflammation in various model systems of murine chronic colitis is dependent on the presence of the intestinal flora[1]. Thus, in the T-cell transfer system, colitis does not develop after adoptive transfer of $CD4^+CD45RB^{high}$ T cells into immuno-deficient recipient mice with a reduced bacterial load, or housed under germfree conditions, and antibiotic treatment of colitic mice can ameliorate disease[9–11].

Consistent with this, CD4$^+$ T cells that are responsive against intestinal commensal bacteria can be isolated from T cell-reconstituted SCID mice, and these cells are likely to be involved in the pathogenicity of the disease[12].

To understand how the bacterial flora drives the pathogenic T-cell response, the influence and functional activity of key antigen-presenting cells (APC) in the mucosa, as well as in the secondary lymphoid organs, needs to be dissected. In the T-cell transfer model DC and macrophages are the dominant professional APC since SCID and RAG-knockout mice lack B-cell populations. DC that are characterized by the expression of the CD11c integrin are the dominant population with regard to the activation of naive T-cell populations[13] and are therefore likely to be involved in the initiation of the disease. In contrast a variety of myeloid cells, including DC and macrophages, may contribute to the maintenance of the disease. Furthermore, during intestinal inflammation other cell types, such as epithelial cells, may also present MHC-II restricted antigens to CD4$^+$ T cells[14]. Here we discuss the role of intestinal CD11c$^+$ DC in the initiation and maintenance of colitis, with particular focus on the T-cell transfer model.

DC ACCUMULATE IN THE MUCOSA AND THE MESENTERIC LYMPH NODE (MLN) DURING INTESTINAL INFLAMMATION

The characterization of intestinal DC has been predominantly restricted to those in the LP and the organized lymphoid tissue of the small intestine and the draining MLN[15–18]. Knowledge concerning these cells in the colon is much more limited. Under non-inflammatory conditions DC are scattered throughout the colonic mucosa and are present within small clusters of leucocytic cells[6,19,20]. It is likely that the enteric flora provides inflammatory signals that lead to the activation of some of these cells, enabling them to migrate towards the secondary lymphoid organs and to activate naive T cells with specificity for intestinal antigens[21]. However, the migration of intestinal DC is not completely dependent on the encounter of intestinal bacteria, since similar DC populations are present in the MLN of germfree animals[22]. In colitis, DC accumulate in the MLN and also in the colon, where they form cell aggregates[6,19,20] (Figure 1).

CD134L$^+$ DC ARE INVOLVED IN THE DEVELOPMENT OF INTESTINAL INFLAMMATION

CD134L is a TNF family member molecule that is expressed on DC after activation via CD40[23,24]. CD134L on DC interacts with its receptor CD134 that is expressed on T cells, providing costimulatory signals to activated T cells[25].

Analysis of CD134L expression on DC in the T-cell transfer model revealed that 20–30% of DC in the MLN of colitic mice were positive, whereas less than 5% were positive in normal lymphocyte-replete mice. In contrast to the MLN, few DC were positive in the inflamed colon, suggesting a higher frequency of activated DC in the former. CD134L$^+$ DC play an important role in the pathogenesis of colitis, since administration of an anti-CD134L monoclonal antibody

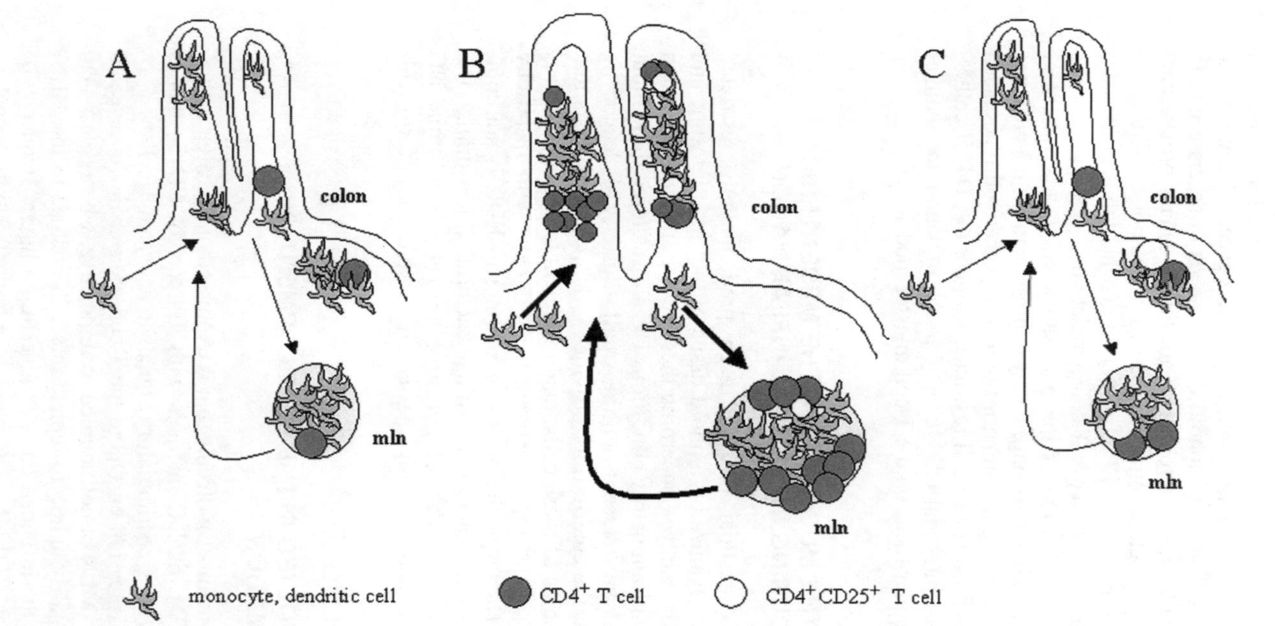

Figure 1 Model of T cell–DC interactions in the T cell transfer model of colitis. **A**: Under non-inflammatory conditions bone marrow-derived monocytes and DC/DC precursor cells enter the colon via the blood. They distribute in a scattered pattern throughout the colon LP and accumulate in small leucocytic clusters in the colon. After antigen encounter the cells travel towards the draining lymph node. If potentially pathogenic CD4$^+$CD45RB^{high} T cells are transferred at this stage, these T cells accumulate in secondary lymphoid organs such as in the mesenteric lymph node, as well as in the CD11c$^+$ cell-enriched intestinal leucocytic clusters, proliferate and redistribute towards the LP effector site. **B**: During established colitis, effector T cells that are derived from the CD4$^+$CD45RB^{high} progeny, as well as DC, form large clusters in the LP as well as in the MLN. In both sites the effector T cells proliferate. When CD4$^+$CD25$^+$ regulatory T cells are adoptively transferred into colitic mice at this time point, these cells accumulate in the inflamed mucosa as well as in the draining lymph nodes, preferentially at the interface between pathogenic effector cells and clusters of CD11c$^+$ cells. Under inflammatory conditions, CD4$^+$CD25$^+$ T$_R$ cells have the potential to proliferate at both sites. **C**: CD4$^+$CD25$^+$ regulatory T cells can reduce the proliferation of T cells in the LP and resolve the inflammatory infiltrate that includes effector T cells and CD11c$^+$ APC. After the resolution of colitis, which might involve the activity of the immunosuppressive cytokines IL-10 or TGF-β, the progeny of the regulatory T cells are preferentially located in remaining leucocytic clusters as well as in the MLN

(mAb) prevented the development of disease in immunodeficient mice transfused with CD4$^+$CD45RB^{high} T cells. The anti-CD134L mAb (OX89) used in these experiments has been shown to block CD134–CD134L interactions *in vitro*, although it cannot be ruled out that *in vivo* the antibody modulates CD134L expression or delivers signals to CD134L$^+$ DC[6].

Several studies suggest that CD134L–CD134 interactions are involved in the maintenance of the T-cell response as opposed to its initial priming[26]. A similar mechanism may also be operational in the T-cell transfer model where the blockade of CD134–CD134L interactions may not impede the initial T-cell priming but prevent the amplification of the T-cell response. Consistent with this, administration of anti-CD134L antibody did not affect T-cell accumulation in the spleen, but did prevent the chronic pathogenic intestinal T-cell response. These results are compatible with the view that CD134L$^+$CD11c$^+$ DC are functionally required for the maintenance of the T-cell response towards bacteria, and that after encountering bacterial antigens in the MLN, bacteria-reactive T cells home to the intestine where they re-encounter antigen and mediate their pathogenic effector function.

The adoptive transfer of CD4$^+$CD25$^+$ T$_R$ cells together with potentially pathogenic CD4$^+$CD45RB^{high} T cells inhibited the T-cell and DC accumulation in the intestinal mucosa, as well as the draining lymph nodes. In addition to inhibiting the accumulation of DC, the presence of CD4$^+$CD25$^+$ T$_R$ cells inhibited the frequency of those that express CD134L, indicating that (whether primarily or as a bystander reaction via the suppression of other inflammatory and chemoattractant stimuli) T$_R$ cells modulate the activation status of DC preventing the maintenance of the intestinal Th1 response.

Taken together, these results suggest that CD134L$^+$ DC may play a key factor in the development of intestinal inflammation and that targeting of activated CD134L$^+$ DC populations can control intestinal inflammation.

CD40 STIMULATION INDUCES T-CELL-INDEPENDENT INTESTINAL INFLAMMATION

CD40–CD40L (CD154) interactions play a crucial role in the initiation and maintenance of T-cell-mediated intestinal inflammation since the blockade of CD40–CD40L interactions inhibits the development of colitis in the T-cell transfer model as well as in other T-cell-mediated mouse models of IBD[27–30]. CD40$^+$ APC were found in the inflamed intestinal tissue of T cell-reconstituted mice, but also in human IBD patients[29,31,32]. After antigen encounter, activated CD4$^+$CD40L$^+$ T cells could stimulate CD40$^+$ APC via the CD40L–CD40 pathway, leading to further activation of APC and T cells and initiating a positive feedback loop of immune activation[33].

To investigate the functional consequence of CD40-mediated signals on DC and macrophage activation and effector function, B- and T-cell-deficient mice were injected with an anti-CD40 stimulatory mAb; a signal mimicking activated T cells. We found that systemic CD40 stimulation led not only to systemic DC activation and accumulation in secondary lymphoid organs, but also to local intestinal inflammation in immunodeficient SCID or RAG-1$^{-/-}$ mice (H. Uhlig and F. Powrie, unpublished results). The development of the T-cell-independent colon pathology is associated with an accumulation and activation of $CD40^+CD11c^+$ DC, and was dependent on an immune cascade involving TNF-α, IL-12p40, and IFN-γ secretion. These *in-vivo* experiments provide evidence that activated DC and macrophages may not only influence the activation and maintenance of a T cell response, but can exhibit potent effector functions and are capable of inducing IBD-like lesions.

POTENTIAL OF CD4$^+$CD25$^+$ T$_R$ CELLS TO REVERSE WASTING DISEASE AND COLITIS

It is now well established that $CD4^+CD25^+$ T$_R$ cells can prevent the development of intestinal immunopathology[7,34,35]. However, the ability of $CD4^+CD25^+$ T$_R$ cells to influence established colitis and to regulate ongoing T-cell responses would be a functional prerequisite for the use of these cells in a therapeutic setting. To investigate whether T$_R$ cells can ameliorate established colitis we injected immunodeficient mice with clinical signs of colitis including piloerection, hunching, anal inflammation, diarrhoea and weight loss with $CD4^+CD25^+$ or $CD4^+CD45RB^{low}CD25^-$ T cells[19]. Mice receiving 10^6 $CD4^+CD25^+$ T cells recovered from wasting disease and colitis, as indicated by a resolution of the histological signs of intestinal inflammation including a significantly reduced epithelial cell hyperplasia, a reduction of the $CD4^+$ T-cell infiltrate and the reappearance of goblet cells. Isolated clusters of leucocytes in the LP remained. The therapeutic effects seen after the adoptive transfer of $CD4^+CD25^+$ cells were not found after transfer of 10^6 $CD4^+CD45RB^{low}CD25^-$ T cells into colitic mice.

To track the $CD4^+CD25^+$ T$_R$ cell progeny *in vivo*, when these cells are injected into colitic recipients, we used a congenic system allowing the differentiation of the progeny of effector and T$_R$ cells. Colitis was induced by transfer of $CD4^+CD45RB^{high}$ cells from wild-type mice, and colitic mice were then injected with $CD4^+CD25^+$ T cells from mice expressing a congenic marker protein. We could show that 2 weeks after injection of the $CD4^+CD25^+$ T$_R$ cells the progeny were present in low frequency (1–5% of total $CD4^+$ T cells) in spleen, MLN and colon. Ten weeks after the secondary transfer of T$_R$ cells the frequency of T$_R$ cells increased to 41% in the MLN and 18% in the LP. This suggests that $CD4^+CD25^+$ T cells may act in the draining MLN as well as in the inflamed colon.

The increased frequency of T$_R$ cells that is associated with the resolution of colitis may be a consequence either of the expansion of the T$_R$ population *in vivo*, or the reduction of pathogenic effector cells, or both. To examine the influence of $CD4^+CD25^+$ T cells on the effector T cell proliferation, and to identify whether $CD4^+CD25^+$ progeny proliferate *in vivo*, we examined the histological expression of the proliferation marker Ki67. The transfer of $CD4^+CD25^+$ T cells reduced the frequency of proliferating effector T cells in both the MLN and the LP. Furthermore, $CD4^+CD25^+$ T$_R$ cells strongly proliferate in MLN and colon under inflammatory conditions, which would indicate that, in contrast to *in-vitro* data, $CD25^+$ T$_R$ cells have proliferative and immunoregulatory capacity *in vivo*.

These data show that the $CD4^+CD25^+$ T_R cells accumulate and expand not only in the MLN, but also in the inflamed colon where they are able to influence the proliferation of the pathogenic T-cell population. Our findings support the hypothesis that T_R cell expansion is driven by the inflammation that is regulated, providing a feedback mechanism for the control of chronic inflammation[7].

$CD4^+CD25^+$ T CELLS ARE IN CONTACT WITH $CD11c^+$ CELLS AND EFFECTOR $CD4^+$ T CELLS *IN VIVO*

The finding that effector as well as regulatory T-cell populations proliferate in the inflamed colon suggests the presence of appropriate antigen presentation and costimulation in the inflamed but not the non-inflamed mucosa. To determine the localization of $CD4^+CD25^+$ T cells in relation to $CD11c^+$ cells and the progeny of $CD4^+CD45RB^{high}$ T cells, the histological distribution of these cells in MLN and colon LP was analysed. The $CD4^+CD25^+$ T cell progeny were found to be in direct contact with the $CD4^+CD45RB^{high}$ progeny, as well as with $CD11c^+$ cells, predominantly located between clusters of $CD11c^+$ cells and the $CD4^+CD45RB^{high}$ T cell progeny (Figure 1). The direct physical contact of $CD4^+CD25^+$ cells with $CD11c^+$ cells was a consistent pattern.

Whereas it has been shown that interactions between pathogenic T cells and $CD11c^+$ cells within MLN and colon are important for the initiation of colitis in this IBD model[6,36], the observed location of T_R cells at the interface of APC and effector T cells also supports a role for the $CD11c^+$ cells in T_R activation and/or migration. The functional activity of T_R cells requires a specific quality and strength of costimulation by APC[37]. In return, T_R cells may influence the activation state of the APC itself, which might thus interfere with their ability to activate effector T-cell responses[38]. Furthermore, the ability of T_R cells to resolve established colitis may also involve direct T_R–T effector interactions, as suggested by *in-vitro* experiments[37,39].

OUTLOOK

Our data concerning the interplay between DC activation and $CD4^+$ T cell effector and $CD4^+CD25^+$ T_R function support the hypothesis that strategies to target activated DC may be beneficial for the treatment of IBD, and suggest that some of the suppressive activities of T_R cells *in vivo* may be mediated via effects on DC. The finding that T_R activity *in vivo* can reverse established inflammation, leading to cure of colitis, indicates that cell therapy with T_R cells might aid therapeutic strategies using their potential of inflammation-dependent homing, expansion and immunosuppression.

Acknowledgements

F.P. is supported by the Wellcome Trust; H.U. and V.M. were funded by EU grant QLGI-1999-00050; H.U. is supported by the Deutsche Forschungsgemeinschaft;

C.M received funding by the Swiss National Science Foundation; and B.S. by the MRC.

References

1. Strober W, Fuss IJ, Blumberg RS. The immunology of mucosal models of inflammation. Annu Rev Immunol. 2002;20:495–549.
2. Powrie F, Leach MW, Mauze S, Barcomb Caddle L, Coffman RL. Phenotypically distinct subsets of CD4$^+$ T cells induce or protect from chronic intestinal inflammation in C. B-17 *scid* mice. Int Immunol. 1993;5:1461–71.
3. Morrissey PJ, Charrier K, Braddy S, Liggitt D, Watson JD. CD4+ T cells that express high levels of CD45RB induce wasting disease when transferred into congenic severe combined immunodeficient mice. Disease development is prevented by cotransfer of purified CD4+ T cells. J Exp Med. 1993;178:237–44.
4. Powrie F, Leach MW, Mauze S, Menon S, Barcomb Caddle L, Coffman RL. Inhibition of Th1 responses prevents inflammatory bowel disease in *scid* mice reconstituted with CD45RB^{hi} CD4$^+$ T cells. Immunity. 1994;1:553–62.
5. Leach MW, Bean AG, Mauze S, Coffman RL, Powrie F. Inflammatory bowel disease in C.B-17 scid mice reconstituted with the CD45RBhigh subset of CD4+ T cells. Am J Pathol. 1996;148:1503–15.
6. Malmstrom V, Shipton D, Singh B et al. CD134L expression on dendritic cells in the mesenteric lymph nodes drives colitis in T cell-restored SCID mice. J Immunol. 2001;166:6972–81.
7. Maloy KJ, Powrie F. Regulatory T cells in the control of immune pathology. Nat Immunol. 2001;2:816–22.
8. Read S, Malmstrom V, Powrie F. Cytotoxic T lymphocyte-associated antigen 4 plays an essential role in the function of CD25(+)CD4(+) regulatory cells that control intestinal inflammation. J Exp Med. 2000;192:295–302.
9. Aranda R, Sydora BC, McAllister PL et al. Analysis of intestinal lymphocytes in mouse colitis mediated by transfer of CD4+, CD45RBhigh T cells to SCID recipients. J Immunol. 1997;158:3464–73.
10. Powrie F. T cells in inflammatory bowel disease: protective and pathogenic roles. Immunity. 1995;3:171–4.
11. Morrissey PJ, Charrier K. Induction of wasting disease in SCID mice by the transfer of normal CD4$^+$/CD45RBhi T cells and the regulation of this autoreactivity by CD4+/CD45RBlo T cells. Res Immunol. 1994;145:357–62.
12. Brimnes J, Reimann J, Nissen M, Claesson M. Enteric bacterial antigens activate CD4(+) T cells from scid mice with inflammatory bowel disease. Eur J Immunol. 2001;31:23–31.
13. Itano AA, Jenkins MK. Antigen presentation to naive CD4 T cells in the lymph node. Nat Immunol. 2003;4:733–9.
14. Hershberg RM, Framson PE, Cho DH et al. Intestinal epithelial cells use two distinct pathways for HLA class II antigen processing. J Clin Invest. 1997;100:204–15.
15. Mowat AM. Anatomical basis of tolerance and immunity to intestinal antigens. Nat Rev Immunol. 2003;3:331–41.
16. Henri S, Vremec D, Kamath A et al. The dendritic cell populations of mouse lymph nodes. J Immunol. 2001;167:741–8.
17. Iwasaki A, Kelsall BL. Unique functions of CD11b$^+$, CD8 alpha$^+$, and double-negative Peyer's patch dendritic cells. J Immunol. 2001;166:4884–90.
18. Iwasaki A, Kelsall BL. Localization of distinct Peyer's patch dendritic cell subsets and their recruitment by chemokines macrophage inflammatory protein (MIP)-3alpha, MIP-3beta, and secondary lymphoid organ chemokine. J Exp Med. 2000;191:1381–94.
19. Mottet C, Uhlig HH, Powrie F. Cutting edge: cure of colitis by CD4$^+$CD25$^+$ regulatory T cells. J Immunol. 2003;170:3939–43.
20. Krajina T, Leithauser F, Moller P, Trobonjaca Z, Reimann J. Colonic lamina propria dendritic cells in mice with CD4$^+$ T cell-induced colitis. Eur J Immunol. 2003;33:1073–83.
21. Neutra MR, Pringault E, Kraehenbuhl JP. Antigen sampling across epithelial barriers and induction of mucosal immune responses. Annu Rev Immunol. 1996;14:275–300.
22. Huang FP, Platt N, Wykes M et al. A discrete subpopulation of dendritic cells transports apoptotic intestinal epithelial cells to T cell areas of mesenteric lymph nodes. J Exp Med. 2000;191:435–44.

23. Straw AD, MacDonald AS, Denkers EY, Pearce EJ. CD154 plays a central role in regulating dendritic cell activation during infections that induce Th1 or Th2 responses. J Immunol. 2003;170:727–34.

24. Ohshima Y, Tanaka Y, Tozawa H, Takahashi Y, Maliszewski C, Delespesse G. Expression and function of OX40 ligand on human dendritic cells. J Immunol. 1997;159:3838–48.

25. Lane P. Role of OX40 signals in coordinating CD4 T cell selection, migration, and cytokine differentiation in T helper (Th)1 and Th2 cells. J Exp Med. 2000;191:201–6.

26. Weinberg AD, Vella AT, Croft M. OX-40: life beyond the effector T cell stage. Semin Immunol. 1998;10:471–80.

27. De Jong YP, Comiskey M, Kalled SL et al. Chronic murine colitis is dependent on the CD154/CD40 pathway and can be attenuated by anti-CD154 administration. Gastroenterology. 2000;119:715–23.

28. Cong Y, Weaver CT, Lazenby A, Elson CO. Colitis induced by enteric bacterial antigen-specific CD4+ T cells requires CD40-CD40 ligand interactions for a sustained increase in mucosal IL-12. J Immunol. 2000;165:2173–82.

29. Liu Z, Geboes K, Colpaert S et al. Prevention of experimental colitis in SCID mice reconstituted with CD45RBhigh CD4$^+$ T cells by blocking the CD40-CD154 interactions. J Immunol. 2000;164:6005–14.

30. Kelsall BL, Stuber E, Neurath M, Strober W. Interleukin-12 production by dendritic cells. The role of CD40-CD40L interactions in Th1 T-cell responses. Ann NY Acad Sci. 1996;795:116–26.

31. Liu Z, Colpaert S, D'Haens GR et al. Hyperexpression of CD40 ligand (CD154) in inflammatory bowel disease and its contribution to pathogenic cytokine production. J Immunol. 1999;163:4049–57.

32. Polese L, Angriman I, Cecchetto A et al. The role of CD40 in ulcerative colitis: histochemical analysis and clinical correlation. Eur J Gastroenterol Hepatol. 2002;14:237–41.

33. van Kooten C, Banchereau J. CD40-CD40 ligand. J Leukoc Biol. 2000;67:2–17.

34. Sakaguchi S, Sakaguchi N, Shimizu J et al. Immunologic tolerance maintained by CD25$^+$ CD4$^+$ regulatory T cells: their common role in controlling autoimmunity, tumor immunity, and transplantation tolerance. Immunol Rev. 2001;182:18–32.

35. Shevach EM. CD4$^+$ CD25$^+$ suppressor T cells: more questions than answers. Nat Rev Immunol. 2002;2:389–400.

36. Leithauser F, Trobonjaca Z, Moller P, Reimann J. Clustering of colonic lamina propria CD4(+) T cells to subepithelial dendritic cell aggregates precedes the development of colitis in a murine adoptive transfer model. Lab Invest. 2001;81:1339–49.

37. Ermann J, Szanya V, Ford GS, Paragas V, Fathman CG, Lejon K. CD4(+)CD25(+) T cells facilitate the induction of T cell anergy. J Immunol. 2001;167:4271–5.

38. Cederbom L, Hall H, Ivars F. CD4$^+$CD25$^+$ regulatory T cells down-regulate co-stimulatory molecules on antigen-presenting cells. Eur J Immunol. 2000;30:1538–43.

39. Piccirillo CA, Shevach EM. Cutting edge: control of CD8+ T cell activation by CD4$^+$CD25$^+$ immunoregulatory cells. J Immunol. 2001;167:1137–40.

8
A model of the mechanism underlying chronic inflammatory bowel disease

W. MÜLLER

The mechanisms underlying the development of chronic inflammatory bowel disease are not understood, and the disease is probably due to many different mechanisms. While treatment of the disease has to focus on already-established (active) disease, the use of experimental animals allows us to better understand the start of the disease, and may lead to new therapies, once the underlying mechanisms for the establishment of the inflammation are understood. Here I discuss two key elements for a mechanistic model for the induction and maintenance of inflammatory bowel disease.

The first aspect is based on the recent finding that mutations in the nod-2 gene of humans result in a higher incidence of chronic inflammatory bowel disease. Cells in the intestine are probably able to sense the presence of the various microorganisms in the gut lumen. A balance is established between the microflora and the activation status of the intestine (Figure 1, left side). The composition of the microorganism in the gut may require a particular awareness of the cells in the gut. This awareness is correlated to signals to the various pathogen-recognizing molecules (PAMs) expressed on the cell surface, as well as in the cell. Nod-2 is one such molecule present in the cell, and recognizes products of both Gram-positive and Gram-negative bacteria. The recognition of such products leads to an increased expression of nod-2 signal-driven genes. The expression of such genes, or some of such genes, leads to an activation state which is appropriate to avoid chronic inflammation. In the absence of nod-2 the activation state of the cells in the gut is not correctly set, resulting in an imbalance between the microflora and the activation state of the cells in the intestine, and chronic inflammation is induced when too many of the pathogenic microorganisms are present in the gut lumen. Defining the target genes of nod-2 may allow identification of genes setting the correct threshold, and thus may allow bypassing of the nod-2 gene by direct activation of the target gene. Alternatively, other PAMs may be triggered artificially by synthetic compounds to increase the

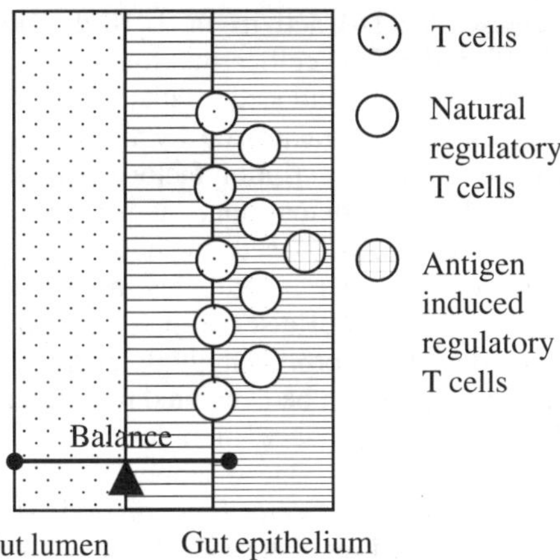

Figure 1 Model of the mechanism underlying chronic inflammatory bowel disease. *Left side*: cells of the intestine and the composition of the microflora develop a balance, which prevents the development of inflammation. The balance can be disturbed by alteration of the microflora or by alteration of signals required to determine awareness of the cells in the gut. *Right side*: in IL-10-deficient mice, antigen-induced regulatory T cells may be absent or non-functional, leading to imbalance in the gut and finally resulting in the development of chronic inflammatory bowel disease

activation state of the cells in the gut, and in this way altering the balance may prevent onset of disease. This idea of compensating the nod-2 deficiency by triggering alternative PAMs is highly speculative at present, and needs to be tested in the correct animal model in order to prove whether the initial idea is correct. The problem in this approach would be that treatment would have to start prior to the onset of the disease. This balance model may also provide a clue to the activity of probiotic microorganisms. The use of probiotic organisms may alter the balance between the flora and the cells in the intestine by lowering the overall activation status and thereby decreasing the chance of inflammation. In order to verify the balance model we need ways to determine the activation state of the cells in the intestine, and then follow the changes in the activation state after altering the microflora of the gut.

The second aspect concerns the role of interleukin-10 for the development of chronic inflammatory bowel disease. Interleukin-10 is an anti-inflammatory cytokine expressed by many different cell types. It can act on various cell types in order to prevent inflammation. In interleukin-10-deficient mice chronic inflammation is induced when interleukin-10-deficient mice are maintained in an environment rich in microorganisms. The type of inflammation may vary, depending on the microorganisms present in the microflora and on the genetic background of the interleukin-10-deficient mutant. In the mutant the disease which develops is a Th1-dominated CD4 cell-driven immune reaction. In the absence of IL-10 high levels of IL-12 are produced in the mutant, and many of the pathological changes can be explained not only as a consequence of loss of IL-10 production but also as the consequence of high levels of IL-12 production.

The source of the IL-12 in the mutant is not known, but it may well be produced by macrophages upon activation in the absence of IL-10. Removing IL-12 from the system decreases the Th1 activity in IL-10-deficient mice. What could be the key role of IL-10 in the CD4 cell compartment? It has been shown in cell transfer experiments that naturally induced regulatory T cells are able to prevent inflammation. These cells are characterized by the cell surface expression of CD25 and by expression of the transcription factor foxp3. It has been shown that such cells are present in IL-10-deficient mice, and that IL-10 is not required for the *in-vitro* activity of these cells. Based on these findings the population of natural induced regulatory T cells is probably not initially involved in the development of inflammatory bowel disease in IL-10-deficient mice. A second CD4 cell type has been described, producing high levels of IL-10, the TR-1 cells (Figure 1; right side). Such cells can be generated *in vitro* in the presence of high levels of IL-10. They in turn produce high levels of IL-10, and also have suppressive activity. These antigen-induced suppressor T cells may be dependent in their generation and/or for their effector function on IL-10. It may well be that the lack of such antigen-induced regulatory CD4 T cells may be the main reason for the development of inflammatory bowel disease in IL-10-deficient mice. This idea is compatible with the differences seen in phenotypes of mice with deficiencies in foxp3, namely early onset of the inflammation, and in mice deficient for IL-10, namely late onset of inflammation and restricted to certain locations.

In order to better understand the role of IL-10 in the development of inflammatory bowel disease we generated conditional mouse mutants deficient for either the IL-10 gene or the IL-10-binding receptor chain. Using these conditional mouse mutants will allow us to specifically inactivate the genes in various cell types or at a given time-point. We will be able to identify the biologically relevant IL-10-producing and IL-10-responsive cells. At the Falk-133 Symposium in Berlin our results of the T cell-specific, IL-10-deficient mouse mutant were presented.

9
Consequences of the modulation of luminal bacterial antigens for the intestinal immune response

R. DUCHMANN

INTRODUCTION

Bacteria from the normal flora provide a major and permanent immune stimulus and activate the intestinal immune system through receptors of both the innate and the antigen-specific immune system. As the first two chapters focusing on innate immunity and dendritic cells have described, basic research has success-fully dissected this complex and fascinating field using extensive efforts and new technologies. Together with the increasing understanding of the effector func-tions of the induced inflammatory and regulatory T-cell populations addressed in the following two chapters, detailed explorations of the genetic, immune and microbial factors that govern the life-long crosstalk between host and intestinal flora are already providing new insights into general aspects of human immunol-ogy, immune regulation and IBD pathogenesis. The plethora of immune mole-cules of the innate immune system (e.g. extracellular receptors of the TLR family, intracellular receptors of the NOD family) and the acquired immune sys-tem (e.g. antigen-specific receptors, accessory molecules and soluble mediators) known to be involved in the generation and regulation of intestinal inflammation constitute an extremely valuable repertoire for therapeutic targets. These targets can be hit by more conventional approaches or by defined modulation of luminal antigens. The latter opens its own universe of opportunities for therapeutic manipulation of host immune responses. Of these, reducing the number of 'inflammatory antigens' by antibiotics, increasing the number of 'non-inflamma-tory antigens' by probiotics, and different approaches to influence the intestinal immune response by using bacterial vectors will be discussed below in more detail.

REDUCTION OF 'INFLAMMATORY ANTIGENS' AND INCREASE OF 'NON-INFLAMMATORY ANTIGENS'

Since the intestinal flora provides the major immune stimulus leading to chronic intestinal inflammation in IBD, modulation of luminal bacteria to prevent or to treat intestinal inflammation is increasingly regarded as a promising therapeutic option. Among these, antibiotic and probiotic agents are established modulators of the intestinal flora; the former through eradication or reduction, the latter through establishment or increase of luminal bacteria. Despite the proven clinical effectiveness of both approaches their relevant mechanisms of action remain largely unknown.

Antibiotics

Antibiotics are an effective treatment for active Crohn's disease and pouchitis, but not for ulcerative colitis[1]. Why that is the case, is not sufficiently clear. We also do not know exactly whether, or to what extent, the positive effect of antibiotics in the relevant clinical trials was mediated via their antibiotic effect or via direct immunological effects. Clearly, at least certain antibiotics, including those frequently used for IBD treatment, have their own immunological effects, as demonstrated by the reduction of serum IL-6 and TNF-α in LPS-treated mice by fluoroquinolones[2], effects on cytokine production by human monocytes[3-6] and general outcome measures of cell-mediated immunity[7,8].

Probiotics

Clinical studies clearly demonstrate that probiotics are effective for remission maintenance in ulcerative colitis and pouchitis[9]. The mechanisms that contribute to the beneficial clinical effects, be it direct effects (bacteria – immune), indirect effects (e.g. bacteria – bacteria – immune; metabolic – intestinal barrier – immune) or other, are still unclear.

With regard to their immunological effects an increasing body of literature is beginning to dissect the differential and complex immunological interplay of the host immune system and pathogenic and probiotic bacteria. Clearly both types of bacteria interact with host epithelial cells and immune cells through a large variety of mechanisms. Highlighting effects on the level of human intestinal epithelial cells it was elegantly shown that some non-pathogenic bacteria can prevent inflammatory immune responses by inhibiting the ubiquitination of IκB-α. The subsequent increase of IκB-α prevents the release of the transcription factor NFκB, its nuclear translocation and the subsequent induction of inflammatory genes, which is typically seen in response to pathogenic bacteria[10]. Differential immune effects are observed not only between pathogens and probiotic bacteria but also between different probiotic species. *In-vitro* studies comparing the immunological effects of Gram-positive vs. Gram-negative probiotic bacteria on epithelial cell lines[11], human intestinal mucosal explants[12,13] and peripheral blood mononuclear cells[14] showed differential effects on a variety of cytokines, including IL-8, TNF-α, IL-10 and IL-12 production. Clearly, LPS present in the cell wall of Gram-negative but not Gram-positive bacteria is expected to account at least for some of the difference. Interestingly, however, the level of complexity

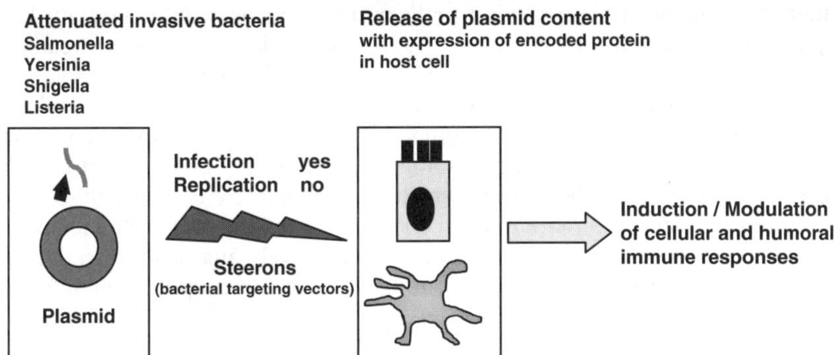

Figure 1 Bacteria used as vectors can release plasmid encoded antigens in the host. This strategy is currently investigated for use in oral vaccination. Within the appropriate immunological context, which can be modified by the experimental system, such regulated antigen expression might also be useful for treatment of autoimmune and chronic inflammatory diseases

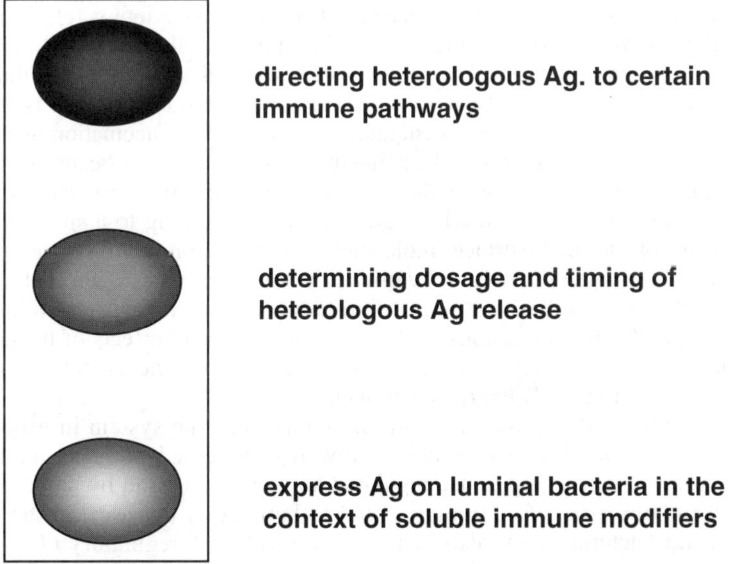

Figure 2 Several variables can be modified in order to generate an immunological context in which antigen release in the host by bacterial vectors induces regulatory mechanisms

is even greater, since studies in humans and mice clearly demonstrate that bacteria which differ only on the level of the bacterial strain also generate greatly divergent immune responses[12,14–19]. Thus, in order to understand what is really going on in the host after exposure to probiotic bacteria, well-controlled clinical studies that are accompanied by careful investigation of induced cellular and humoral immune responses[20], and inform us regarding the functional consequences within the relevant populations of immune cells, are certainly needed.

Identification of critical bacteria or bacterial antigens would certainly be a major step forward to set up more specific probiotic or antibiotic treatment strategies. New types of molecular analyses with high reliability and resolving power for the study of complex bacterial samples are already available, and facilitate the investigation of complex effects on the composition of the intestinal flora. Together with immunological studies they could detect bacteria or certain dominant bacterial antigens which play a major role in IBD pathogenesis. In addition to allowing a more rational choice of antibiotic and probiotic agents, these relevant antigens could be used to very selectively augment protective and regulatory immune responses by presenting them in the correct immunological context.

MODULATION OF THE INTESTINAL IMMUNE RESPONSE BY USING BACTERIAL VECTORS

Attenuated derivatives of invasive bacteria, such as *Salmonella, Shigella, Yersinia* and *Listeria*, can specifically infect antigen-presenting cells and epithelial cells, including enterocytes. Within the cell their plasmid content is released, and encoded proteins are expressed leading to the induction of specific cellular and humoral immune responses. The mutant strain then dies, since genes that are essential for its survival have been deleted. Mutant bacteria expressing heterologous antigens are extensively investigated for use in oral vaccination against a variety of infectious diseases and malignant tumours[21–28]. The beauty of using these mutant bacteria for the induction of antigen-specific responses is that multiple approaches can be used to optimize them according to a specific goal. Expression of defined surface molecules (steerons) on carrier strains, for example, might guide the bacterial carrier to distinct cell types[21]. Promotors can be selected from an increasing set for fine-tuning of antigen expression levels[24] and the type of immune response[26]. Furthermore, adjuvant effects of the carrier bacterium itself are likely to influence the type of immune response elicited against the recombinantly expressed antigen.

Thus, bacteria which interfere with the innate immune system in ways that promote regulatory immune responses towards expressed antigens might be advantageous when trying to use regulated antigen expression by recombinant bacteria for treatment of autoimmune and inflammatory diseases. In the same way certain bacteria might also increase the level of T regulatory (T_R) cells. Thus, it was recently shown that T_R cells expand after stimulation via Toll-like receptors (TLR)[29] and subsequently augment their regulatory capacity. Here, as in other instances, immunological context is important, since activation of TLR on antigen-presenting cells (APC) disinhibits T_R cells and supports inflammatory responses through production of interleukin (IL)-6 and other substances[30].

In a landmark study Steidler and colleagues introduced genetically manipulated bacteria into the treatment of chronic intestinal inflammation. They demonstrated that intragastric administration of *Lactococcus lactis* secreting IL-10 had beneficial effects in two mouse models of IBD[31]. IL-10 has multiple actions and was shown to facilitate the generation of Tr1 cells. In the C3H/HeJBir mouse,

Cong and colleagues showed that repeated culture of CD4[+] T cells in the presence of caecal bacterial antigens, antigen-presenting cells and IL-10 generated Tr1 cells. These bacterial-reactive Tr1 cells prevented colitis upon cotransfer with pathogenic Bir CD4[+] Th1 cells in SCID mice[32]. Generation of Tr1 cells might also be inducible *in vivo* through combined expression of bacterial antigen and IL-10 in orally delivered recombinant bacteria.

References

1. Sands BE. Therapy of inflammatory bowel disease. Gastroenterology. 2000;118(Suppl. 1): S68–82.
2. Khan AA, Slifer TR, Araujo FG, Suzuki Y, Remington JS. Protection against lipopolysaccharide-induced death by fluoroquinolones. Antimicrob Agents Chemother. 2000;44:3169–73.
3. Khan AA, Slifer TR, Remington JS. Effect of trovafloxacin on production of cytokines by human monocytes. Antimicrob Agents Chemother. 1998;42:1713–17.
4. Khan AA, Slifer TR, Araujo FG, Remington JS. Effect of clarithromycin and azithromycin on production of cytokines by human monocytes. Int J Antimicrob Agents. 1999;11:121–32.
5. Khan AA, Slifer TR, Araujo FG, Remington JS. Effect of quinupristin/dalfopristin on production of cytokines by human monocytes. J Infect Dis. 2000;182:356–8.
6. Yoshimura T, Kurita C, Usami E et al. Immunomodulatory action of levofloxacin on cytokine production by human peripheral blood mononuclear cells. Chemotherapy. 1996;42:459–64.
7. Rockwell S, Irvin CG, Neaderland MH. Inhibition of delayed hypersensitivity by metronidazole and misonidazole. Int J Radiat Oncol Biol Phys. 1983;9:701–6.
8. Rockwell S, Neaderland MH. Suppression of cell-mediated immunity by misonidazole. Int J Radiat Biol Relat Stud Phys Chem Med. 1982;42:185–9.
9. Hart AL, Stagg AJ, Kamm MA. Use of probiotics in the treatment of inflammatory bowel disease. J Clin Gastroenterol. 2003;36:111–19.
10. Neish A, Gewirtz A, Zeng H et al. Prokaryotic regulation of epithelial responses by inhibition of IκB-alpha ubiquitination. Science. 2000;289:1560–3.
11. Lammers KM, Helwig U, Swennen E et al. Effect of probiotic strains on interleukin 8 production by HT29/19A cells. Am J Gastroenterol. 2002;97:1182–6.
12. Borruel N, Casellas F, Antolin M et al. Effects of nonpathogenic bacteria on cytokine secretion by human intestinal mucosa. Am J Gastroenterol. 2003;98:865–70.
13. Borruel N, Carol M, Casellas F et al. Increased mucosal tumour necrosis factor alpha production in Crohn's disease can be downregulated *ex vivo* by probiotic bacteria. Gut. 2002;51:659–64.
14. Hessle C, Andersson B, Wold AE. Gram-positive bacteria are potent inducers of monocytic interleukin-12 (IL-12) while gram-negative bacteria preferentially stimulate IL-10 production. Infect Immun. 2000;68:3581–6.
15. Hosoi T, Hirose R, Saegusa S, Ametani A, Kiuchi K, Kaminogawa S. Cytokine responses of human intestinal epithelial-like Caco-2 cells to the nonpathogenic bacterium *Bacillus subtilis* (natto). Int J Food Microbiol. 2003;82:255–64.
16. Haller D, Bode C, Hammes WP, Pfeifer AM, Schiffrin EJ, Blum S. Non-pathogenic bacteria elicit a differential cytokine response by intestinal epithelial cell/leucocyte co-cultures. Gut. 2000;47:79–87.
17. Ibnou-Zekri N, Blum S, Schiffrin EJ, Von Der Weid T. Divergent patterns of colonization and immune response elicited from two intestinal *Lactobacillus* strains that display similar properties *in vitro*. Infect Immun. 2003;71:428–36.
18. Christensen HR, Frokiaer H, Pestka JJ. Lactobacilli differentially modulate expression of cytokines and maturation surface markers in murine dendritic cells. J Immunol. 2002;168:171–8.
19. Maassen CB, van Holten JC, Balk F et al. Orally administered *Lactobacillus* strains differentially affect the direction and efficacy of the immune response. Vet Q. 1998;20(Suppl. 3):S81–3.
20. Cukrowska B, LodInova-Zadnikova R, Enders C, Sonnenborn U, Schulze J, Tlaskalova-Hogenova H. Specific proliferative and antibody responses of premature infants to intestinal colonization with nonpathogenic probiotic *E. coli* strain Nissle 1917. Scand J Immunol. 2002;55:204–9.

21. Autenrieth IB, Schmidt MA. Bacterial interplay at intestinal mucosal surfaces: implications for vaccine development. Trends Microbiol. 2000;8:457–64.
22. Dietrich G, Gentschev I, Hess J, Ulmer JB, Kaufmann SH, Goebel W. Delivery of DNA vaccines by attenuated intracellular bacteria. Immunol Today. 1999;20:251–3.
23. Bumann D, Metzger WG, Mansouri E et al. Safety and immunogenicity of live recombinant *Salmonella enterica* serovar Typhi Ty21a expressing urease A and B from *Helicobacter pylori* in human volunteers. Vaccine. 2001;20:845–52.
24. Bumann D. Regulated antigen expression in live recombinant *Salmonella enterica* serovar Typhimurium strongly affects colonization capabilities and specific CD4(+)-T-cell responses. Infect Immun. 2001;69:7493–500.
25. Bumann D, Hueck C, Aebischer T, Meyer TF. Recombinant live *Salmonella* spp. for human vaccination against heterologous pathogens. FEMS Immunol Med Microbiol. 2000;27:357–64.
26. Medina E, Paglia P, Rohde M, Colombo MP, Guzman CA. Modulation of host immune responses stimulated by *Salmonella* vaccine carrier strains by using different promoters to drive the expression of the recombinant antigen. Eur J Immunol. 2000;30:768–77.
27. Paglia P, Medina E, Arioli I, Guzman CA, Colombo MP. Gene transfer in dendritic cells, induced by oral DNA vaccination with *Salmonella typhimurium*, results in protective immunity against a murine fibrosarcoma. Blood. 1998;92:3172–6.
28. Paglia P, Terrazzini N, Schulze K, Guzman CA, Colombo MP. *In vivo* correction of genetic defects of monocyte/macrophages using attenuated *Salmonella* as oral vectors for targeted gene delivery. Gene Ther. 2000;7:1725–30.
29. Caramalho I, Lopes-Carvalho T, Ostler D, Zelenay S, Haury M, Demengeot J. Regulatory T cells selectively express toll-like receptors and are activated by lipopolysaccharide. J Exp Med. 2003;197:403–11.
30. Powrie F, Maloy KJ. Immunology. Regulating the regulators. Science. 2003;299:1030–1.
31. Steidler L, Hans W, Schotte L et al. Treatment of murine colitis by *Lactococcus lactis* secreting interleukin-10. Science. 2000;289:1352–5.
32. Cong Y, Weaver CT, Lazenby A, Elson CO. Bacterial-reactive T regulatory cells inhibit pathogenic immune responses to the enteric flora. J Immunol. 2002;169:6112–19.

Section III
Consequences of luminal antigen uptake: Induction of T cell populations

10
Role of IL-13 and NKT cells in human ulcerative colitis and oxazalone colitis in mice

F. HELLER

INTRODUCTION

The incidence of chronic inflammatory bowel diseases (IBD) is growing in industrialized countries[1]. While the pathogenesis of Crohn's disease (CD) and ulcerative colitis (UC) still remains unclear, the factors involved in starting and perpetuating the inflammatory process in CD are much better studied than in UC. In CD interleukin-12 (IL-12) plays a central role in inducing a Th1 response of the mucosal lymphocytes, and neutralization of IL-12 abrogates disease in animal models of CD[2]. Th1 lymphocytes produce tumour necrosis factor α (TNF-α) and interferon-γ (IFN-γ) when stimulated, and these cytokines can induce apoptosis of epithelial, mesenchymal and haematopoietic cells. They also activate macrophages and granulocytes, which in turn release oxygen radicals and NO. It is easily conceivable how an overwhelming Th1 inflammation in CD can lead to a transmural granulomatous and destructive inflammation, the typical histopathological picture that characterizes CD. On the contrary the disease process is much less clear in UC. Lymphocytes isolated from inflamed colon have been shown to produce Th2 cytokines (IL-4, IL-5, IL-10) and the production of Th1 cytokines is decreased[3,4]. However, the action of none of these cytokines can easily explain the pathological picture found in UC. Th2-type cytokines have been considered immunosuppressive, because they down-modulate macrophages and dendritic cells[5,6]. In contrast to CD, in UC the intestinal barrier function of the mucosa is severely impaired early on. Ulcers disrupt the mucosa, ranging in size from micro-erosions to large defects, and abscesses can be found in the base of the crypts.

OXAZALONE COLITIS

We have established an animal model for UC in mice. The animals are presensitized 5 days before induction of colitis by shaving a part of the abdominal skin and application of the hapten oxazalone on the skin. Five days later the mice are anaesthetized and receive an intrarectal enema of oxazalone dissolved in 50% ethanol. The ethanol induces toxic destruction of the colonic mucosa, which enables the oxazalone to enter into the lamina propria and induce an immune reaction. Mice that receive only ethanol without oxazalone, or that have not been presensitized to oxazalone, overcome the initial toxic reaction within 48 h and are clinically or histopathologically recovered. Sensitized mice, that receive an oxazalone enema, develop a chronic progressive colitis that leads to a significant weight loss and, in approximately 50%, to the death of the animal. The immune response in oxazalone colitis is characterized by a Th2 response. Lymphocytes isolated at different time-points produce increasing amounts of IL-13, but decreasing amounts of IL-4. IFN-γ is barely detectable[7,8]; thereby the cytokine profile – especially in later phases of disease – resembles the findings in human patients with UC.

INTERLEUKIN-13

Since IL-4 production decreased over the course of oxazalone colitis, but the production of IL-13 increased, we neutralized IL-13 in one group of mice. These mice were protected from the induction of disease. IL-13 and IL-4 both share a common receptor, a heterodimer of the IL-4Rα and the IL-13Rα1 chain; but both receptors can also form dimers with other proteins, which then form specific receptors for IL-4 (IL-4Rα + cγ-chain) or IL-13 (IL-13Rα1 + 2). Thereby both cytokines induce in part identical second messengers, but it has been shown that IL-13 has other second messengers besides JAK1 and JAK3, that are induced by the IL-4 receptor; in addition, IL-13 has a widespread expression on tissue cells. In other disease models IL-13 has been shown to play a central role. In allergic asthma the typical pathology of increased mucus production and airway hyperresponsiveness is dependent on IL-13, and IL-13 alone is sufficient to induce these changes in the lung[9,10]. In intestinal helminth infection IL-13 is essential to induce a protective immune response, which clears the infection of the gut[11].

NKT CELLS IN OXAZALONE COLITIS

When we analysed the lymphocytes that produce IL-13 during the course of the inflammation, we found that these cells are CD16-positive cells. Since CD16 is widely expressed on NK and NKT cells we depleted mice of these cells with CD161 antibodies. Depleted mice were protected from oxazalone colitis, while mice treated with control antibodies developed typical disease. These experiments indicated that either NK or NKT cells are essential for disease induction. To selectively inhibit NKT cells we blocked their activation with CD1 blocking antibodies. Treated animals did not develop any disease. We confirmed these experiments with NKT knockout mice (Jα281KO) and with CD1 knockout mice; both strains were resistant to the induction of oxazalone colitis. However, both strains are capable of inducing Th2-immune responses.

Next we stimulated lymphocytes isolated from mice with oxazalone colitis with α-galactosyl-ceramide (αGalCer) and L cells transfected with CD1. Such culture conditions provide a strong and specific stimulus to NKT cells, which are the only cell type that can respond to CD1 and glycolipids. This stimulation induced a very high IL-13 response from lymphocytes from the lamina propria and spleen. When we stimulated selected CD4$^+$ cells with αGalCer the cells produced large amounts of IL-13, even though the majority of CD4 cells was negative for CD161 by FACS staining. These experiments proved that NKT cells are essential for the induction of oxazalone colitis, and that this inflammation is mediated by IL-13 produced by NK cells.

IL-13 AND HUMAN ULCERATIVE COLITIS

Lymphocytes from human patients with UC produce large quantities of IL-13. As shown earlier, IL-4 production is virtually absent, indicating that the disease is mediated by IL-13 alone. Most likely IL-4 is only produced early in the disease process as in the animal model, and then decreases and is replaced by IL-13.

To study the influence IL-13 has on epithelial cells we utilized monolayers of HT29/B6 cells, which form *in vitro* a barrier similar to that of colonic epithelial cells *in vivo*. The integrity of this barrier can be assessed by measuring the transepithelial resistance. After the addition of 10 ng/ml IL-13 to these cultures transepithelial resistance dropped to 40% of control cultures. This effect was dose-dependent and could be enhanced by the addition of TNF-α.

Three effects mediate the influence which IL-13 has on the epithelial barrier function:

1. IL-13 induces apoptosis of epithelial cells. This single cell apotosis leaves micro-erosions in the line of epithelial cells, which dramatically impairs the barrier function, leading to the influx of luminal contents into the lamina propria.
2. Under the influence of IL-13 epithelial cells express significantly more claudin-2, while other tight junction proteins are unaffected. Claudin-2 is a pore-forming tight junction protein, which leads to a facilitated diffusion of large molecules from the luminal to the basolateral side.
3. IL-13 impairs the ability of epithelial cells to grow and close gaps between epithelial cells. Compared to control cultures, cells in IL-13-treated cultures had a 30% reduced velocity in closing 200 μm wide gaps between cells.

SUMMARY

Oxazalone colitis, an animal model of human ulcerative colitis, is mediated by IL-13. Similar to human UC lymphocytes do not produce IFN-γ, and small amounts of IL-4. The production of IL-13 increases over the course of the inflammation and is essential for the induction of the disease. IL-13 is also produced in samples from human patients with UC. In the animal model IL-13 is produced by NKT cells, which are essential for disease induction.

IL-13 has a profound effect on the intestinal barrier of human epithelial cells. IL-13 induces apoptosis of epithelial cells. Under the influence of IL-13 cells show an altered tight junction protein expression and have an impaired wound-healing velocity.

These findings suggest that neutralization of IL-13 as a treatment for severe UC might be effective.

References

1. Lashner BA. Epidemiology of inflammatory bowel disease. Gastroenterol Clin N Am. 1995;24:467–74.
2. Neurath, MF et al. Antibodies to interleukin 12 abrogate established experimental colitis in mice. J Exp Med. 1995;182:1281–90.
3. Fuss IJ et al. Disparate CD4+ lamina propria (LP) lymphokine secretion profiles in inflammatory bowel disease. Crohn's disease LP cells manifest increased secretion of IFN-gamma, whereas ulcerative colitis LP cells manifest increased secretion of IL-5. J Immunol. 1996; 157:1261–70.
4. West G et al. Interleukin-4 in inflammatory bowel disease and mucosal immune reactivity. Gastroenterology. 1996;110:1683–95.
5. Manna SK, Aggarwal BB. IL-13 suppresses TNF-induced activation of nuclear factor-kB, activation protein-1, and apoptosis. J Immunol. 1998;161:2863–72.
6. Muchamel T et al. IL-13 protects mice from lipopolysaccharide-induced lethal endotoxemia. J Immunol. 1997;158:2898–903.
7. Boirivant M et al. Oxazalone colitis: a murine model of T helper cell type 2 colitis treatable with antibodies to interleukin 4. J Exp Med. 1998;188:1929–39.
8. Heller F et al. Oxazolone colitis, a Th2 colitis model resembling ulcerative colitis, is mediated by IL-13-producing NK-T cells. Immunity. 2002;17:629–38.
9. Wills-Karp M et al. Interleukin-13: central mediator of allergic asthma. Science. 1998;282: 2258–61.
10. Gruening G et al. Requirement for IL-13 independently of IL-4 in experimental asthma. Science. 1998;282:2261–3.
11. Urban JF Jr, Noben-Trauth N, Donaldson DD, Madden KB, Morris SC, Collins AF. IL-13, IL-4 Ralpha, and Stat6 are required for the expulsion of the gastrointestinal nematode parasite *Nippostrongylus brasiliensis*. Immunity. 1998;8:255.

11
Different subsets of CD4$^+$ regulatory T cells and their role in immunoregulation

K. SIEGMUND, A. HAMANN and J. HUEHN

TOLERANCE MEDIATED BY REGULATORY T CELLS

Our immune system is well equipped to protect us against a myriad of different pathogens. The necessity to react efficiently against these foreign antigens harbours the risk that the immune system reacts destructively against self-components and that autoimmunity occurs. During T-cell development in the thymus the vast majority of autoreactive cells are eliminated in a process called negative selection. However, there is strong evidence that this central tolerance mechanism is not complete. Several studies have described the existence of self-reactive T cells as part of the normal T-cell repertoire in healthy individuals[1,2]. Nevertheless, the expression of T-cell receptors (TCR) specific for an autoantigen is not sufficient for the development of autoimmune diseases, which are estimated to affect up to 5% of the population (reviewed in ref. 3). In most individuals autoreactive T cells remain harmless and autoimmunity does not occur, since several peripheral tolerance mechanisms counter-regulate autoreactive cells recirculating through the periphery, including induction of T-cell anergy, T-cell deletion and immunological ignorance[4,5]. In addition to these 'passive' mechanisms of controlling self-reactive T cells there is strong evidence for an 'active' tolerance mechanism mediated by so-called regulatory T cells. The existence of T cells suppressing immune responses was postulated in the early 1970s[6,7], and since then has been discussed controversially because the cellular and molecular mechanisms responsible for the suppressive phenomenon remained largely unknown. In the mid-1990s Sakaguchi and co-workers demonstrated regulatory activity within a small sub-population (5–10%) of peripheral CD4$^+$ T cells constitutively expressing CD25, the α chain of the IL-2 receptor complex[8]. Transfer of CD25-depleted CD4$^+$ T cells induced multiple autoimmune diseases in immunodeficient recipients, whereas co-transfer of $CD25^+CD4^+$ T cells prevented inflammation and self-destruction in several models of autoimmunity[8]. Neonatal thymectomy (on day 3) led to the development of spontaneous multi-organ autoimmunity, which was correlated with a decrease in the number of $CD25^+CD4^+$ regulatory T cells in peripheral lymphoid tissues[9]. Studies using TCR-transgenic mice have demonstrated that the generation of $CD25^+CD4^+$ regulatory T cells depends on the expression of the model antigen in the thymus and that these cells are induced only if high-avidity ligands were presented by thymic epithelial cells (reviewed in refs 10 and 11). Furthermore, $CD25^+CD4^+CD8^-$ thymocytes displayed suppressive capacity *in vitro* and *in vivo*[9,12]. These findings led to the suggestion that $CD25^+CD4^+$ regulatory T cells are thymus-derived. However, peripheral induction of suppressive $CD4^+$ T cells upon antigen exposure under tolerogenic conditions has also been reported. For example, oral administration of antigen supported the development of regulatory T cells and the establishment of systemic tolerance (reviewed in ref. 13).

$CD25^+CD4^+$ regulatory T cells showed a partially anergic phenotype with poor proliferation upon TCR triggering *in vitro* and growth dependence on exogenous IL-2[12,14]. Furthermore, these cells produced small amounts of proinflammatory cytokines (IL-2, IL-4, IFN-γ and TNF-α) compared to other antigen-experienced $CD4^+$ T cells[14–16]. The mechanism of suppression is still discussed controversially: in some *in-vivo* models immunosuppressive cytokines, such as IL-10 and transforming growth factor β_1 (TGF-β_1), were required for the control of autoimmunity[17–19]. However, suppression *in vitro* was solely mediated by a cell–cell contact-dependent, cytokine-independent mechanism[14,20]. Several surface molecules, including CTLA-4 (cytotoxic T lymphocyte antigen-4), GITR (glucocorticoid-induced TNF receptor family-associated) and ICOS (inducible co-stimulator) were found to be associated with regulatory activity in some settings[21–23]. The usage of these and other molecules, e.g. CD45RB and CD62L, to identify regulatory T cell subsets is problematic, because their expression is strongly dependent on the activation status of the cell. CD25 expression, for example, is transiently up-regulated on activated cells and therefore cannot be used to discriminate between recently activated and regulatory T cells. The best marker currently known for $CD4^+$ regulatory T cells seems to be the recently identified transcription factor Foxp3, which has been shown to be specifically expressed in $CD25^+CD4^+$ T cells and which seemed to be required for both development and function of regulatory T cells[24–26].

THE INTEGRIN $\alpha_E\beta_7$ – A MARKER FOR UNIQUE SUBSETS OF $CD25^+$ AND $CD25^-$ REGULATORY T CELLS

Recently the integrin α_E (CD103) has been identified as a marker for regulatory $CD4^+$ T cells isolated from secondary lymphoid organs of mice[27–29]. $\alpha_E\beta_7$ was previously known as a marker for intraepithelial lymphocytes (IEL) residing in the gut wall and other epithelial compartments such as skin or lung[30,31]. The expression of $\alpha_E\beta_7$ is transcriptionally regulated by TGF-β, a cytokine produced by intestinal epithelial cells and in tissues, where chronic inflammation takes place[31], but does not change after T-cell activation.

Table 1 Characteristics of the integrin $\alpha_E\beta_7$ in the murine system

Expression on	IEL (CD8$^+$)	≈90%	Lefrancois et al.[49]
	IEL (CD4$^+$)	≈70%	Cerf-Bensussan et al.[30]
	Peripheral CD4$^+$ T cells	≈5–6%	Kilshaw and Murant[31]
	(induced by TGF-β upon activation)		Lehmann et al.[27]
Ligand	E-cadherin	(epithelial expression)	Cepek et al.[34]
Phenotype of	Reduced number of LPL and IEL		Schon et al.[35]
knockout mice	Inflammatory skin disorder		Schon et al.[36]

The precise role of $\alpha_E\beta_7$ is not fully understood (Table 1). In contrast to the related integrin $\alpha_4\beta$, which acts as a homing receptor for mucosa-seeking lymphocytes by recognizing mucosal addressin cell adhesion molecule-1 (MAdCAM-1)[32] $\alpha_E\beta_7$ seems to play no role in the migration of lymphocytes into mucosal or epithelial sites[33]. However, the interaction between $\alpha_E\beta_7$ and its ligand E-cadherin, which is expressed on epithelial cells but not on endothelium[34], might be involved in the retention of lymphocytes within epithelial compartments. This is supported by the phenotype of α_E-deficient mice, which showed a reduction in the number of mucosal T lymphocytes[35]. Furthermore, these mice develop mild cutaneous inflammatory disorders[36], which led to the suggestion that the integrin might be important for the control of autoimmunity in the skin (Table 1).

In addition to intraepithelial lymphocytes the integrin α_E is expressed on a small subpopulation of about 5–6% CD4$^+$ T cells from secondary lymphoid organs. Initial characterization of this subset in our laboratory revealed that the vast majority of this subpopulation co-expresses CD25 and is localized within the CD45RB^{low} compartment (Figure 1A and ref. 27). Since both markers were known to identify regulatory T cells we analysed whether the α_E-expressing subsets exhibit suppressive capacity. Functional studies both *in vitro* (suppression of naïve T cell proliferation) and *in vivo* (inhibition of induced SCID colitis) revealed that α_E^+ T cell subsets irrespective of their CD25 expression showed regulatory activity (Figure 1B). Throughout all settings, α_E^+CD25$^+$ cells turned out to be the most potent suppressors. *In vitro* the α_E^+CD25$^-$ subpopulation displayed only moderate suppressive activity comparable to total CD45RB^{low} CD4$^+$ cells. Almost complete inhibition of proliferation was observed at a regulator/target ratio of 1:3 for the α_E^-CD25$^+$ subset, whereas α_E^+CD25$^-$ cells showed complete suppression only if used at a 1:1 ratio. However, α_E^+CD25$^-$ cells were potent regulators *in vivo*; they were found to be as effective as α_E^-CD25$^+$ cells in inhibiting the development of SCID colitis[27]. Furthermore, Foxp3 mRNA, which has recently been reported as a unique marker for CD25$^+$ regulatory T cells, was present in all three regulatory T cell subsets. This finding underlines the regulatory function of α_E^-CD25$^+$, α_E^+CD25$^+$ as well as α_E^+CD25$^-$ T cells.

Since expression of $\alpha_E\beta_7$ is a hallmark for intraepithelial lymphocytes and since $\alpha_E\beta_7$ expression is induced by TGF-β, which is known to be a key factor for the development of regulatory T cells, the presence of α_E on highly effective regulatory T cells from secondary lymphoid organs might indicate their previous

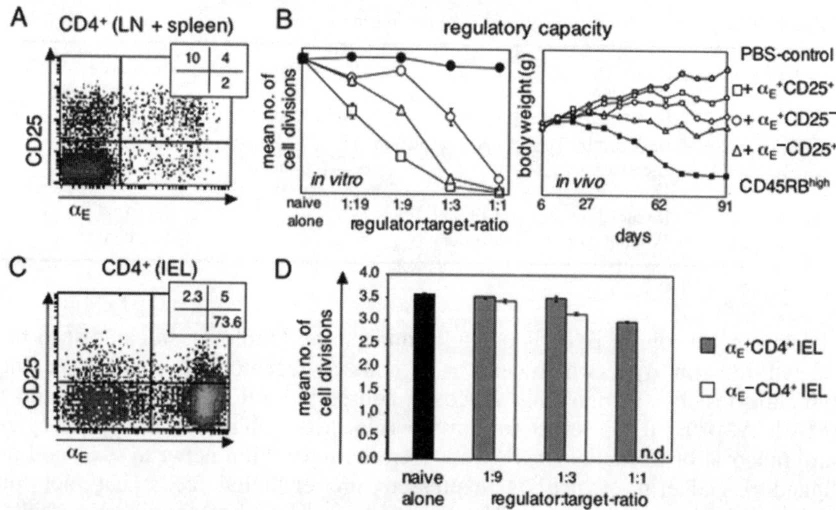

Figure 1 The integrin $\alpha_E\beta_7$ is a marker for regulatory CD4$^+$ T cells. **A**: Expression of α_E and CD25 on mixed CD4$^+$ lymphocytes form lymph nodes (LN) and spleen analysed by flow cytometry. **B**: CD4$^+$ T-cell subsets characterized by the expression of α_E and CD25 displayed regulatory activity: the regulatory T cells were able to suppress proliferation of naive CD4$^+$ T cells (*in vitro*) and were protective in a model of SCID colitis (*in vivo*). **C**: The majority of CD4$^+$ intraepithelial lymphocytes (IEL) expressed the integrin $\alpha_E\beta_7$, whereas only a few CD25-positive cells were found in this subset. **D**: $\alpha_E{}^+$CD4$^+$ IEL showed no suppressive activity on the proliferation of naive T cells *in vitro*. (A–C reprinted with permission from Lehmann et al., Proc Natl Acad Sci. 2002; 99:13031. Copyright 2000, National Academy of Sciences, USA)

maturation in a TGF-β-rich milieu. To test the hypothesis that $\alpha_E{}^+$ regulatory T cells shuttle as 'heralds of tolerance' between epithelial and lymphoid sites transferring tolerogenic potential, we analysed α_E-expressing CD4$^+$ IELs by flow cytometry and functional studies and observed almost no CD25 co-expression and only negligible suppressive capacity *in vitro* (Figure 1C, D). However, we cannot yet exclude the existence of subsets of $\alpha_E{}^+$CD4$^+$ IEL that exhibit regulatory activity.

To unravel the molecular basis for the observed difference in the regulatory capacity between $\alpha_E{}^-$CD25$^+$, $\alpha_E{}^+$CD25$^+$ and $\alpha_E{}^+$CD25$^-$ subsets from secondary lymphoid organs, we further characterized these regulatory subsets by analysing their cytokine expression (Table 2). Whereas $\alpha_E{}^-$CD25$^+$ and especially $\alpha_E{}^+$CD25$^+$ cells fulfilled the hallmark of regulatory T cells by expressing only low frequencies of both proinflammatory (TNF-α, IFN-γ and IL-2) and Th2-type cytokines (IL-4, IL-5, IL-10 and IL-13) upon restimulation, the $\alpha_E{}^+$CD25$^-$ subset showed a rather peculiar cytokine expression pattern. These cells expressed IL-2 and IFN-γ at frequencies comparable to those of classical CD4$^+$CD45RB^{low} memory cells. Strikingly, the frequencies for IL-4, IL-5 and especially IL-13 were even enhanced. Thus, $\alpha_E{}^+$CD25$^-$ cells represent a unique subset, in which production of IL-2 and other cytokines is not conflicting with

Table 2 Expression of cytokines and immunomodulatory molecules on CD4$^+$ regulatory T cells. The table shows the percentage of positive cells determined by intracellular (cytokines and CTLA-4) and surface (ICOS) staining followed by flow cytrometric analysis

	$\alpha_E^- CD25^+$	$\alpha_E^+ CD25^+$	$\alpha_E^+ CD25^-$
IL-2	12.8 ($\pm$4.4)	5.4 ($\pm$3.4)	34.9 ($\pm$11.1)
TNF-α	14.4 ($\pm$3.2)	4.0 ($\pm$2.6)	22.9 ($\pm$14.1)
IFN-γ	4.6 ($\pm$1.4)	2.4 ($\pm$2.4)	19.7 ($\pm$9.7)
IL-4	2.3 ($\pm$1.2)	1.6 ($\pm$2.7)	4.1 ($\pm$1.4)
IL-5	1.9 ($\pm$1.7)	1.6 ($\pm$2.6)	5.6 ($\pm$1.4)
IL-13	2.1 ($\pm$1.6)	1.6 ($\pm$2.7)	11.0 ($\pm$2.8)
IL-10	2.6 ($\pm$1.5)	3.6 ($\pm$2.0)	2.3 ($\pm$0.9)
CTLA-4	6.8 ($\pm$3.2)	18.8 ($\pm$5.7)	17.6 ($\pm$5.7)
ICOS	1.3 ($\pm$0.5)	10.7 ($\pm$3.3)	13.7 ($\pm$3.8)

suppressive function either *in vitro* or *in vivo*. Next we analysed the expression of the immunomodulatory molecules CTLA-4 and ICOS that have both been shown to be involved in the function of regulatory T cells in certain models[21,23]. We observed that both molecules showed the highest expression in the α_E-expressing subsets (Table 2). These findings led to the conclusion that CTLA-4 and ICOS are predominantly correlated with α_E and not with CD25 in the regulatory compartment.

The considerable heterogeneity in the regulatory T-cell pool with respect to the suppressive capacity, cytokine profile and surface expression of immuno-modulatory molecules suggests that these distinct subsets mediate suppression via different mechanisms.

GENE EXPRESSION PROFILING DISPLAYS A HIGH DEGREE OF HETEROGENEITY BETWEEN THE REGULATORY T CELL SUBSETS

cDNA microarray technology is a powerful tool to unravel differences in the mRNA expression level between cell subsets and to obtain a comprehensive picture of the phenotype of the population of interest. We performed gene expression profiling (affymetrix microarray) to identify molecular differences between $\alpha_E^- CD25^+$, $\alpha_E^+ CD25^+$ and $\alpha_E^+ CD25^-$ regulatory CD4$^+$ T cells. Strikingly, many molecules associated with effector/memory differentiation and migration behaviour turned out to be differentially expressed. Confirmation of the gene profiling data by quantitative RT-PCR and flow cytometry revealed that the phenotype of $\alpha_E^- CD25^+$ cells resembles that of naive T cells, whereas both α_E-expressing subsets displayed an effector/memory phenotype (Table 3). In general the largest differences were found between $\alpha_E^- CD25^+$ and $\alpha_E^+ CD25^-$, whereas $\alpha_E^+ CD25^+$ often displayed an intermediate phenotype. Both α_E-expressing subsets showed significantly lower CD45RB levels than $\alpha_E^- CD25^+$ cells. However, differences in developmental stage were much more obvious when L-selectin (CD62L) and CD44 were used as markers for the naive versus effector/memory

Table 3 α_E-expressing regulatory T cells display an effector/memory phenotype, whereas CD25 single positive cells resemble naive T cells. The table summarizes results obtained from DNA microarray, quantitative RT-PCR, flow cytometry and chemotaxis assays

α_E positive > CD25 single positive	CD25 single positive > α_E positive
CD44	L-selectin, CD45RB
P-/E-selectin binding ligands	CCR7
ICAM-1, LFA-1, β_1 integrin	
CXCR3, CCR4, CCR6	

status of CD4$^+$ T cells. The α_E^-CD25$^+$ cells expressed almost exclusively high levels of CD62L, which enables entry into lymph nodes via high endothelial venules and is crucial for the recirculation of naive T cells. In contrast, within both α_E-expressing subsets a substantial fraction has down-regulated L-selectin expression and additionally these subsets showed increased expression levels of CD44. Furthermore, α_E-positive cells expressed high levels of E- and P-selectin-binding ligands as well as other adhesion molecules such as ICAM-1, LFA-1 and β_1-integrin, which are required to extravasate into inflamed sites.

CHEMOTACTIC RESPONSIVENESS AND MIGRATORY BEHAVIOUR OF REGULATORY T-CELL SUBSETS

So far, the question of where regulatory T cells exert their suppressive function *in vivo* has not been answered satisfactorily. Are they required in secondary lymphoid organs in order to inhibit the initiation of immune responses or is their presence in the affected tissue critical to suppress inflammation during the effector phase? The capacity of regulatory T cells to suppress activation and proliferation of naive T cells[37] and the capability of the CD62L^{high} subset of CD25$^+$CD4$^+$ regulatory T cells to inhibit the initiation of autoimmune diseases in certain models[38,39] led to the suggestion that regulatory T cells can operate in a lymphoid environment. Nevertheless, other studies have reported that regulatory T cells can respond to inflammatory chemokines[40,41], can be isolated from effector sites, i.e. from the synovial fluid of patients with rheumatoid arthritis[42], and can ameliorate ongoing inflammation in a murine model of colitis[43]. These findings suggested that regulatory T cells are indeed able to enter inflamed tissue and act directly at effector sites. Both scenarios seem to apply, depending on the subtype of regulatory T cells.

To prove whether the observed differences in adhesion molecule and chemokine receptor expression were of any significance for the localization of regulatory T-cell subsets we performed chemotaxis assays as well as *in-vivo* homing experiments under homeostatic and inflammatory conditions (Figure 2). We observed that α_E^-CD25$^+$ cells showed a significantly higher migratory response than α_E-expressing cells towards CCL19, a ligand for CCR7, which is involved in the migration of immune cells into lymph nodes. A contrasting pattern was found for chemotaxis towards the inflammatory chemokines CXCL9, CCL17 and CCL20, which bind to the receptors CXCR3, CCR4 and CCR6,

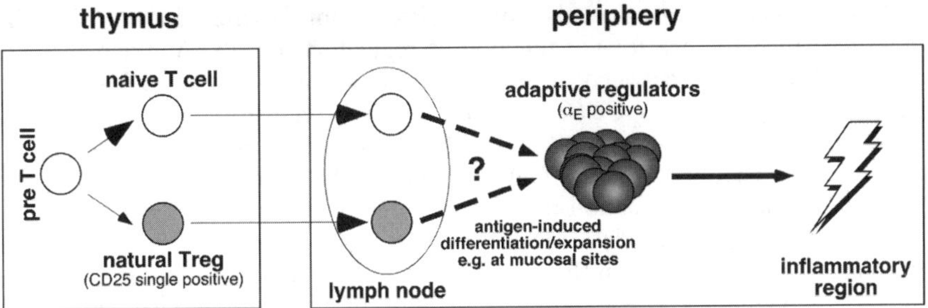

Figure 2 Model of an existing dichotomy among CD4$^+$ regulatory T cells in regard to development, antigen specificity and site where regulation takes place (see text for description)

respectively. These chemokines preferentially attracted α_E-expressing cells. Finally, *in-vivo* homing experiments, in which radioactively labelled T-cell subsets were injected into naive mice, revealed that $\alpha_E^-CD25^+$ cells predominantly migrate into peripheral and mesenteric lymph nodes, whereas both α_E-expressing subsets showed only minor migration into lymph nodes, but preferentially accumulated in the liver, an organ where activated and effector/memory T cells are known to be trapped[44]. Striking differences between the analysed subsets were observed with respect to their ability to immigrate into inflamed sites. Homing experiments in a model of acute skin inflammation demonstrated that only $\alpha_E^+CD25^-$ cells efficiently migrated into the inflamed skin. Chemokine responsiveness, as well as migration properties under homeostatic and inflammatory conditions, demonstrated the high degree of heterogeneity within the pool of regulatory T cells with respect to the site of suppression, and this supports the idea of functionally diverse subsets of regulators. These results revealed that α_E-expressing subsets are prototypes of inflammation-seeking regulatory T cells, whereas $\alpha_E^+CD25^+$ cells represented a recirculating population with a poor capacity to enter inflamed tissue.

REGULATORY ACTIVITY IS CORRELATED WITH THE ABILITY TO MIGRATE INTO EFFECTOR SITES

The importance of regulatory CD4$^+$ T cells for the maintenance of self-tolerance has been shown during the past few years in several autoimmune models. However, most of the experiments were performed in immunodeficient mice (i.e. nu/nu or SCID) that were reconstituted with subpopulations of regulatory T cells (reviewed in ref. 45). To date these experiments have been discussed controversially, since the lymphopenic situation of the recipients does not allow a precise analysis of the suppressive capacity of the regulatory T-cell subsets. It has been suggested that lymphopenia, although not sufficient to induce autoimmunity, may represent a major contributing factor[10]. Furthermore, recently published data suggested that T-cell regulation might be only a side-effect of homeostasis and competition[46].

Results obtained *in vivo* also often differ from *in-vitro* findings, i.e. the relevance of cytokines for the function of regulatory T cells. Another example for the discrepancy between *in-vitro* and *in-vivo* data was the analysis of the suppressive potential of $CD62L^{high}$ $CD25^+CD4^+$ regulatory T cells. Whereas *in-vitro* studies did not reveal a higher suppressive capacity of $CD62L^{high}$ compared to $CD62L^{low}$ $CD25^+CD4^+$ T cells[28], the $CD62L^{high}$ subset was the only regulatory subpopulation that was capable of suppressing development of diabetes in the NOD model[39]. These findings indicated that the localization of regulatory T cells *in vivo* influences their inhibitory function. We analysed the impact of regulatory T-cell subset localization on their suppressive capacity in murine antigen-induced arthritis, a non-lymphopenic model of acute and chronic inflammation[47], and we observed a strong correlation of the suppressive capacity with the preferential migration of the regulatory T-cell subsets into the sites of inflammation. Only those regulatory T-cell subsets that expressed the integrin $\alpha_E\beta_7$, and that were equipped with a whole set of adhesion molecules and chemokine receptors to enter inflamed regions, showed significantly enhanced migration into the affected knee joint and were able to inhibit signs of inflammation (reduction of knee joint swelling in the acute phase and suppression of mononuclear cell infiltrates and tissue destruction in the chronic phase). In contrast, $\alpha_E^-CD25^+$ cells showed no preferential migration into the inflamed sites and therefore had no curative effect in this model.

CONCLUSION

Several mechanisms contribute to the maintenance of self-tolerance. Beyond negative selection in the thymus, mechanisms of peripheral tolerance, including the active suppression by regulatory T cells, control autoreactive cells. Although much effort has been put into the characterization of regulatory T cells, there are still many open questions concerning their *in-vivo* action: Where do they develop? What signals maintain a functional regulatory T cell pool? What antigens do they recognize? Where do they act?

Recently, Bluestone and Abbas proposed a dichotomy among the regulatory T-cell pool with the existence of two different types of regulatory $CD4^+$ T cells named natural and adaptive regulators. These cells were thought to differ with regard to development, effector mechanism and antigen specificity (Figure 2)[48]. This model might explain the different findings regarding regulatory T cells in recent years. According to their proposals, natural regulators are generated during the normal process of T-cell maturation in the thymus in response to self-antigen locally presented on medullary epithelial cells. This subset is thought to be most effective under non-inflammatory settings, suppressing autoreactive cells and maintaining self-tolerance. In contrast, adaptive regulatory T cells develop under conditions of antigenic stimulation either from naive T cells or from the naturally occurring regulatory T cells. These adaptive regulatory T cells, which are variable in the level of CD25 expression, are thought to exert their inhibitory function *in vivo* via immunosuppressive cytokines. The role of adaptive regulators in immunoregulation can be envisioned in the control of inflammatory autoimmune diseases that are more similar to infectious settings (e.g. IBD) as well as in the inhibition of inflammatory reactions against foreign antigens.

Our extensive phenotyping and the functional analyses of regulatory T-cell subsets led to the suggestion that α_E^-CD25$^+$ and α_E-expressing cells can be regarded as prototypes of natural and adaptive regulatory T cells, respectively. In line with the concept of Bluestone and Abbas, the regulatory T-cell pool can be subdivided in naive-like, recirculating and effector/memory-like inflammation-seeking regulators. One can predict, based on the findings mentioned above, that α_E-expressing subsets, by combining high suppressive capacity with the ability to migrate into inflamed sites, might have a strong therapeutic potential in the treatment of established autoimmune diseases.

References

1. Wekerle H, Bradl M, Linington C, Kaab G, Kojima K. The shaping of the brain-specific T lymphocyte repertoire in the thymus. Immunol Rev. 1996;149:231–43.
2. Goldrath AW, Bevan MJ. Selecting and maintaining a diverse T-cell repertoire. Nature. 1999;402:255–62.
3. Sakaguchi S. Regulatory T cells: key controllers of immunologic self-tolerance. Cell. 2000;101:455–8.
4. Arnold B, Schonrich G, Hammerling GJ. Multiple levels of peripheral tolerance. Immunol Today. 1993;14:12–14.
5. van Parijs L, Perez VL, Abbas AK. Mechanisms of peripheral T cell tolerance. Novartis Found Symp. 1998;215:5–14; discussion 14–20, 33–40.
6. Gershon RK, Kondo K. Cell interactions in the induction of tolerance: the role of thymic lymphocytes. Immunology. 1970;18:723–37.
7. Ha TY, Waksman BH. Role of the thymus in tolerance. X. 'Suppressor' activity of antigen-stimulated rat thymocytes transferred to normal recipients. J Immunol. 1973;110:1290–9.
8. Sakaguchi S, Sakaguchi N, Asano M, Itoh M, Toda M. Immunologic self-tolerance maintained by activated T cells expressing IL-2 receptor alpha-chains (CD25). Breakdown of a single mechanism of self-tolerance causes various autoimmune diseases. J Immunol. 1995;155: 1151–64.
9. Itoh M, Takahashi T, Sakaguchi N et al. Thymus and autoimmunity: production of CD25+CD4+ naturally anergic and suppressive T cells as a key function of the thymus in maintaining immunologic self-tolerance. J Immunol. 1999;162:5317–26.
10. Maloy KJ, Powrie F. Regulatory T cells in the control of immune pathology. Nat Immunol. 2001;2:816–22.
11 Annacker O, Pimenta-Araujo R, Burlen-Defranoux O, Bandeira A. On the ontogeny and physiology of regulatory T cells. Immunol Rev. 2001;182:5–17.
12. Papiernik M, de Moraes ML, Pontoux C, Vasseur F, Penit C. Regulatory CD4 T cells: expression of IL-2R alpha chain, resistance to clonal deletion and IL-2 dependency. Int Immunol. 1998;10:371–8.
13. von Herrath MG, Harrison LC. Antigen-induced regulatory T cells in autoimmunity. Nat Rev Immunol. 2003;3:223–32.
14. Thornton AM, Shevach EM. CD4$^+$CD25$^+$ immunoregulatory T cells suppress polyclonal T cell activation *in vitro* by inhibiting interleukin 2 production. J Exp Med. 1998;188:287–96.
15. Asano M, Toda M, Sakaguchi N, Sakaguchi S. Autoimmune disease as a consequence of developmental abnormality of a T cell subpopulation. J Exp Med. 1996;184:387–96.
16. Papiernik M, Banz A. Natural regulatory CD4 T cells expressing CD25. Microbes Infect. 2001;3:937–45.
17. Powrie F, Carlino J, Leach MW, Mauze S, Coffman RL. A critical role for transforming growth factor-beta but not interleukin 4 in the suppression of T helper type 1-mediated colitis by CD45RB(low) CD4$^+$ T cells. J Exp Med. 1996;183:2669–74.
18. Groux H, O'Garra A, Bigler M et al. A CD4$^+$ T-cell subset inhibits antigen-specific T-cell responses and prevents colitis. Nature. 1997;389:737–42.

19. Asseman C, Powrie F. Interleukin 10 is a growth factor for a population of regulatory T cells. Gut. 1998;42:157–8.
20. Takahashi T, Kuniyasu Y, Toda M et al. Immunologic self-tolerance maintained by CD25+CD4+ naturally anergic and suppressive T cells: induction of autoimmune disease by breaking their anergic/suppressive state. Int Immunol. 1998;10:1969–80.
21. Read S, Malmstrom V, Powrie F. Cytotoxic T lymphocyte-associated antigen 4 plays an essential role in the function of CD25(+)CD4(+) regulatory cells that control intestinal inflammation. J Exp Med. 2000;192:295–302.
22. Shimizu J, Yamazaki S, Takahashi T, Ishida Y, Sakaguchi S. Stimulation of CD25(+)CD4(+) regulatory T cells through GITR breaks immunological self-tolerance. Nat Immunol. 2002;3:135–42.
23. Akbari O, Freeman GJ, Meyer EH et al. Antigen-specific regulatory T cells develop via the ICOS–ICOS-ligand pathway and inhibit allergen-induced airway hyperreactivity. Nat Med. 2002;8:1024–32.
24. Khattri R, Cox T, Yasayko SA, Ramsdell F. An essential role for Scurfin in CD4$^+$CD25$^+$ T regulatory cells. Nat Immunol. 2003;4:337–42.
25. Fontenot JD, Gavin MA, Rudensky AY. Foxp3 programs the development and function of CD4+CD25+ regulatory T cells. Nat Immunol. 2003;4:330–6.
26. Hori S, Nomura T, Sakaguchi S. Control of regulatory T cell development by the transcription factor Foxp3. Science. 2003;299:1057–61.
27. Lehmann J, Huehn J, Rosa MDL et al. Expression of the integrin alphaEbeta7 identifies unique subsets of CD25+ as well as CD25- regulatory T cells. Proc Natl Acad Sci USA. 2002;99:13031–6.
28. McHugh R, Whitters MJ, Piccorillo CA et al. CD4$^+$CD25$^+$ immunoregulatory T cells: gene expression analysis reveals a functional role for the glucocorticoid-induced TNF receptor. Immunity. 2002;16:311–23.
29. Banz A, Peixoto A, Pontoux C, Cordier C, Rocha B, Papiernik M. A unique subpopulation of CD4+ regulatory T cells controls wasting disease, IL-10 secretion and T cell homeostasis. Eur J Immunol. 2003;33:2419–28.
30. Cerf-Bensussan N, Jarry A, Brousse N, Lisowska-Grospierre B, Guy-Grand D, Griscelli C. A monoclonal antibody (HML-1) defining a novel membrane molecule present on human intestinal lymphocytes. Eur J Immunol. 1987;17:1279–85.
31. Kilshaw PJ, Murant SJ. Expression and regulation of beta 7(beta p) integrins on mouse lymphocytes: relevance to the mucosal immune system. Eur J Immunol. 1991;21:2591–7.
32. Hamann A, Andrew DP, Jablonski-Westrich D, Holzmann B, Butcher EC. Role of a4-integrins in lymphocyte homing to mucosal tissues *in vivo*. J. Immunol. 1994;152:3282–93.
33. Austrup F, Rebstock S, Kilshaw PJ, Hamann A. TGF beta1-induced expression of the mucosa-related integrin alpha E on lymphocytes is not associated with mucosa-specific homing. Eur J Immunol. 1995;25:1487–91.
34. Cepek KL, Shaw SK, Parker CM et al. Adhesion between epithelial cells and T lymphocytes mediated by E-cadherin and the alpha E beta 7 integrin. Nature. 1994;372:190–3.
35. Schon MP, Arya A, Murphy EA et al. Mucosal T lymphocyte numbers are selectively reduced in integrin alpha E (CD103)-deficient mice. J Immunol. 1999;162:6641–9.
36. Schon MP, Schon M, Warren HB, Donohue JP, Parker CM. Cutaneous inflammatory disorder in integrin alphaE (CD103)-deficient mice. J Immunol. 2000;165:6583–9.
37. Annacker O, Pimenta-Araujo R, Burlen-Defranoux O, Barbosa TC, Cumano A, Bandeira A. CD25$^+$CD4$^+$ T cells regulate the expansion of peripheral CD4 T cells through the production of IL-10. J Immunol. 2001;166:3008–18.
38. Herbelin A, Gombert JM, Lepault F, Bach JF, Chatenoud L. Mature mainstream TCR alpha beta$^+$CD4$^+$ thymocytes expressing L-selectin mediate 'active tolerance' in the nonobese diabetic mouse. J Immunol. 1998;161:2620–8.
39. Szanya V, Ermann J, Taylor C, Holness C, Fathman CG. The subpopulation of CD4$^+$CD25$^+$ splenocytes that delays adoptive transfer of diabetes expresses L-selectin and high levels of CCR7. J Immunol. 2002;169:2461–5.
40. Goulvestre C, Batteux F, Charreire J. Chemokines modulate experimental autoimmune thyroiditis through attraction of autoreactive or regulatory T cells. Eur J Immunol. 2002;32:3435–42.

41. Iellem A, Colantonio L, D'Ambrosio D. Skin-versus gut-skewed homing receptor expression and intrinsic CCR4 expression on human peripheral blood CD4[+]CD25[+] suppressor T cells. Eur J Immunol. 2003;33:1488–96.

42. Cao D, Malmstrom V, Baecher-Allan C, Hafler D, Klareskog L, Trollmo C. Isolation and functional characterization of regulatory CD25brightCD4[+] T cells from the target organ of patients with rheumatoid arthritis. Eur J Immunol. 2003;33:215–23.

43. Mottet C, Uhlig HH, Powrie F. Cutting edge: Cure of colitis by CD4(+)CD25(+) regulatory T cells. J Immunol. 2003;170:3939–43.

44. Klugewitz K, Topp S, Dahmen U et al. Differentiation-dependent and subset-specific recruitment of T-helper cells into the liver. Hepatology. 2002;35:568–78.

45. McHugh RS, Shevach EM, Thornton AM. Control of organ-specific autoimmunity by immunoregulatory CD4(+)CD25(+) T cells. Microbes Infect. 2001;3:919–27.

46. Barthlott T, Kassiotis G, Stockinger B. T cell regulation as a side effect of homeostasis and competition. J Exp Med. 2003;197:451–60.

47. Brackertz D, Mitchell GF, Mackay IR. Antigen-induced arthritis in mice. Arthritis Rheum. 1977;20:841.

48. Bluestone JA, Abbas AK. Natural versus adaptive regulatory T cells. Nat Rev Immunol. 2003;3:253–7.

49. Lefrancois L, Parker CM, Olson S, Muller W, Wagner N, Puddington L. The role of beta7 integrins in CD8 T cell trafficking during an antiviral immune response. J Exp Med. 1999;189:1631–8.

12
Regulatory T cells in animal models: therapeutic potential

C. O. ELSON, Y. CONG, A. KONRAD, N. IQBAL
and C. T. WEAVER

INTRODUCTION

The intestine is the major interface between the host and the external environment. In addition to food antigens the mucosal immune system must deal with a huge number of antigens and adjuvant molecules produced by the enteric microbiota. Despite this enormous antigenic challenge the immune response in the intestine, although substantial, remains relatively limited, indicating that the immune response there is tightly regulated. Until recent years the cellular and molecular mechanisms maintaining such immune homeostasis in the intestine have been obscure. In the past decade there has been a leap forward in our understanding of the key pathways involved in immune homeostasis, particularly from experiments involving gene-targeted mice. Hundreds of different genes encoding immune molecules have either been selectively deleted or transgenically overexpressed in mice. A small number of such 'induced mutant' mice have gone on to develop inflammatory bowel disease. A common feature in these induced mutant mice that develop colitis has been that CD4$^+$ T cells are the effector cell in most of them, and secondly that the bacterial microbiota is the stimulus driving the inflammatory disease (reviewed in ref. 1).

It has become clear from such experiments that the immune response to the bacterial microbiota is tightly regulated, and that this regulation occurs at multiple levels, including both innate and acquired immune mechanisms. Many different cell types contribute to intestinal immune regulation, including CD4$^+$ and CD8$^+$ T cells, NK-T cells, B cells, and $\gamma\delta$T cells. These have all been demonstrated to have some beneficial effect in different models of intestinal inflammation. However, most prominent among these regulatory cells are the CD4$^+$ T cell lineage which itself includes multiple subsets, including T-regulatory-1[2], T-helper-3[3], and the CD25$^+$CD4$^+$ (reviewed in refs 4 and 5) T cell subsets. The identification of these subsets has led to reinterpretation of the current paradigm in which T-helper-1 (Th1) cells are thought to regulate T-helper-2 (Th2) cells and vice-versa. An emerging concept is that Th1 and Th2 cells are both effector subsets able to cause disease. That is certainly true in the intestine, where both Th1 and Th2 cells have been shown to be able to cause colitis[6]. CD4$^+$ T-regulatory cell subsets appear able to control both Th1 and Th2 responses[7,8]. Based on this new paradigm many of the experimental models of IBD can be classified as representing either impaired regulatory cell activity or as representing excessive T cell effector function which overcomes a normal level of immune regulation (Table 1).

Among the models classified as representing impaired T cell regulation, some molecular pathways to IBD can be identified. For example, mice with induced mutations of the IL-10 gene[9], the IL-10 receptor gene (CRF2–4)[10], or the gene encoding the transcription factor STAT-3 in macrophages and neutrophils[11], all result in a similar phenotype of colitis, thus defining an IL-10 pathway. In a similar fashion mice deficient in either TGF-β_1 gene[12], the TGF-β receptor II gene[13], or in the transcription factor SMAD3[11] display diffuse inflammation including colitis. Thus the IL-10 pathway and the TGF-β pathway both seem to be crucial for maintenance of intestinal immune homeostasis and for the prevention of excessive responses to the antigens of the intestinal microbiota. Interestingly, these pathways appear to reflect the activity of two subsets of CD4$^+$ T-regulatory subsets, namely the Tr1 subset that produces large amounts of IL-10 and the Th3 subset that produces large amounts of TGF-β_1. These two subsets have been implicated as mediating oral tolerance, and both have been shown able to inhibit induction of colitis in adoptive hosts. It remains unclear whether these are two separate subsets or the same subset that produces large amounts of TGF-β_1 under some circumstances and large amounts of IL-10 under others. It is clear that these two cytokines are interrelated, and that each is able to induce the production of the other.

Table 1 Mechanistic clustering of mouse models of IBD

Impaired T cell regulation	*Excessive T cell effector function*
CD45RB transfer model	Stat 4 transgenic
IL-2, IL-2Rα-deficient	IL-7 transgenic
BM$\rightarrow$ Tgϵ26 transfer model	TNF-α 'knock-in'
	? TCR-α-deficient
IL-10-deficient	CD40L transgenic*
CRF 2–4-deficient (IL-10Rβ)	
Mϕ-PMN Stat 3-deficient	
TGF-β-deficient	
TGFβRII-deficient	
SMAD3-deficient	

Selected experimental models can be assigned to either a category of 'impaired T cell regulation' or to a category of 'excessive T cell effector function', as shown. The net effect of either is the same; i.e. chronic intestinal inflammation. Within the impaired regulation group several models can be clustered further into an IL-10 pathway, and others into a TGF-β pathway, in which deficiency of the cytokine, its receptor, or its key intracellular signalling molecule can all result in disease. * Diffuse inflammation not limited to the intestine.

WHERE ARE T-REGULATORY CELLS GENERATED, PARTICULARLY THOSE THAT REGULATE IMMUNE RESPONSES TO THE ENTERIC MICROBIOTA?

This remains an open question. The $CD4^+CD25^+$ lineage is known to be generated in the thymus early in life. This subset comprises some 5–10% of both thymic and peripheral $CD4^+$ T cells in adults. This subset clearly plays an important role in maintenance of tolerance to autoantigens, such as those in the stomach, thyroid and adrenals; indeed, depletion of this subset in mice, for example by thymectomy on day 3 of life, results in autoimmunity in these organs later in life[14]. However, such thymectomy has not been reported to induce colitis; thus it is unclear whether this subset, generated in a sterile thymus, induces cells that are able to regulate responses to exogenous antigens such as those of the enteric bacteria. Indeed, T-regulatory cells can be generated in the periphery, in addition to in the thymus. Using transgenic technology aberrant expression of antigen on thymic stromal cells generated $CD4^+CD25^+$ T-regulatory cells. However, aberrant expression of the same antigen by non-activated haematopoietic cells peripherally produced $CD4^+CD25^-$ T-regulatory cells[15]. Indeed, a recent paper has described a dendritic cell subset that is able to induce Tr1 cell differentiation *in vivo*. This dendritic cell subset is normally less than 1% of the total dendritic cell population and is marked by expression of $CD11c^{lo}CD45RB^{hi}$ surface markers[16]. These cells have a plasmacytoid morphology and would be considered an immature phenotype of dendritic cells. They secrete IL-10 upon activation and are able to induce the generation of antigen-specific T-regulatory-1 cells and tolerance *in vivo*[16]. Whether such dendritic cells are preferentially located in the intestine or draining lymph nodes is as yet unknown; however, intestinal $CD4^+$ T cells with Tr1-like activity, and that are reactive to enteric bacterial antigens, have been identified in both humans and mouse[17,18].

CAN T-REGULATORY CELLS PREVENT COLITIS?

The answer to this question is unequivocally yes for $CD4^+$ T-regulatory cells; each of the subsets mentioned above, including $CD4^+CD25^+$, $CD4^+$ Th3 cells and $CD4^+$ Tr1 cells, have been shown to prevent colitis in different model systems. One of the earliest demonstrations of this was in the $CD45RB^{hi}$ adoptive transfer model. In this model $CD4^+CD45RB^{hi}$ naive T cells are adoptively transferred into RAG-1-deficient mice or SCID mice. As these expand and develop in the new host they develop an unrestrained reactivity against antigens of the enteric microbiota and induce colitis. In the experiment in question, Tr1 cells reactive to ovalbumin were co-transferred with the potentially pathogenic $CD4^+CD45RB^{hi}$ T cells. The OVA-specific Tr1 cells were able to prevent the induction of colitis if the mice were fed low amounts of OVA antigen in order to trigger the Tr1 cells[7]. There was no effect if the animals were not fed the ovalbumin. This experiment demonstrates that T-regulatory cells are specific in regard to their activation but non-specific in their inhibitory phase once activated. In this instance, OVA-specific regulatory cells were suppressing the reactivity to antigens of the enteric bacteria unrelated to OVA, a phenomenon which has been called bystander suppression. A Tr1 subset reactive to the enteric bacteria has also been shown to be able to inhibit colitis induced by a memory effector T cell subset that was reactive to the enteric bacteria also in the C3H/HeJBir model[18]. Thus, Tr1 cells were able to inhibit both naive and memory T cell responses to the enteric bacteria.

CAN T-REGULATORY CELLS TREAT AN ESTABLISHED COLITIS?

This is an important question in relation to the potential translation of regulatory T cell therapy for humans with IBD, because patients generally present at the clinic with established active disease. There is not much data on this point, but recent studies in the CD45RB[hi] transfer model have demonstrated the ability of T-regulatory cells to actively treat an ongoing colitis[19]. Much less is known about such T-regulatory subsets in humans; thus it is unclear whether human T-regulatory subsets would be able to treat active disease, or even whether they would be able to prevent relapse of inactive disease.

WHAT IS THE MECHANISM OF T-REGULATORY CELL ACTION?

This remains somewhat controversial and variable, depending on how the regulation is being measured; however, three mechanisms have been identified to date: the production of large amounts of IL-10 which is particularly evident in Tr1 cells, the production of large amounts of TGF-β_1 which is a hallmark of the Th3 subset, and a cytokine-independent cell contact mechanism. In *in-vitro* systems, particularly with CD4$^+$CD25$^+$ T cells, the cell contact mechanism appears sufficient on its own, and neither IL-10 nor TGF-β is required[14]. The presence of TGF-β_1 on the surface of CD4$^+$CD25$^+$ cells has been reported as a mechanism of such cognate inhibition[20]; however this observation has not yet been reproduced. The situation *in vivo* is obviously more complex with the effector and regulatory cells dispersed and not in close apposition. Not surprisingly, T-regulatory cell inhibition *in vivo* appears to require inhibitory cytokines such as IL-10 and/or TGF-β_1 (reviewed in ref. 21). The cellular target of T-regulatory activity is also a bit dependent on experimental conditions. Some T-regulatory subsets appear able to directly inhibit effector cells such as Th1 cells *in vitro*; however, the Tr1 subset, particularly the one identified in C3H/HeJBir mice that is reactive to enteric bacteria, inhibit antigen-presenting cells such as dendritic cells rather than having a direct effect on Th1 cells[22]. It seems likely that all three mechanisms, namely IL-10, TGF-β_1 and cell contact, operate simultaneously, and the relative predominance of any one of the mechanisms depends on the conditions and microenvironment involved.

CAN T-REGULATORY CELLS BE USED FOR THE TREATMENT OF HUMAN IBD?

The answer to this question is unknown, and will clearly lie in future research; however, on a theoretical basis stimulation of antigen-specific T-regulatory cells would represent a potentially ideal therapy; one that could suppress the pathogenic response while leaving the rest of the immune system intact (Figure 1). A key question yet to be answered is whether bystander inhibition by T-regulatory cells is a robust phenomenon and can be demonstrated in other experimental systems and in humans. To date, bystander inhibition of experimental colitis has been shown only in a system using cells from a T cell receptor transgenic mouse[7]. It will be particularly important to determine whether bystander inhibition can be triggered by defined enteric bacterial antigens that would be present locally in the gut. This will be crucial, particularly in humans, because in most patients we will not be able to identify exactly what antigens are driving the pathogenic response.

A potential therapeutic paradigm is as follows: a T-regulatory cell reactive to a common environmental antigen of the enteric bacteria will encounter its antigen on dendritic cells that have phagocytosed and processed it. This dendritic cell is likely to be in the intestine or draining nodes, and almost certainly would have phagocytosed and processed other bacterial antigens as well, including those that are driving the pathogenic process. Once the Tr1 cell is activated by exposure to its specific antigen it will begin producing IL-10 and/or TGF-β, and activate the cell contact inhibitory mechanism. In so doing, the T-regulatory cell will inhibit not only the response to its own antigen, but will also inhibit T cell responses to

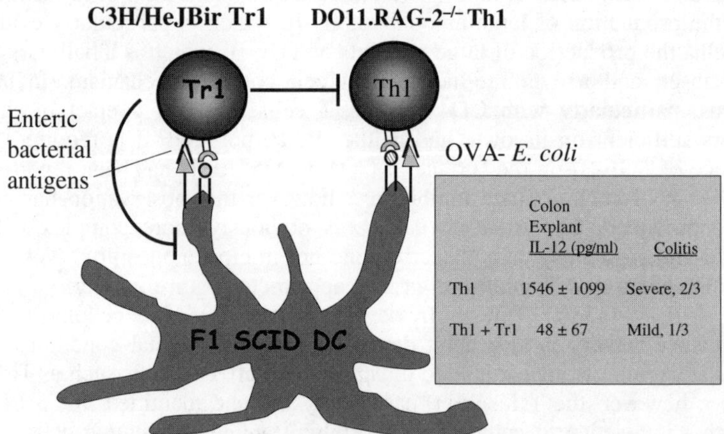

	Colon Explant IL-12 (pg/ml)	Colitis
Th1	1546 ± 1099	Severe, 2/3
Th1 + Tr1	48 ± 67	Mild, 1/3

Figure 1 Bystander inhibition as a potential therapeutic approach to IBD. The T regulatory cell interacts with a dendritic cell (DC) via TCR:MHC interactions. This results in inhibition of the DC such that it is unable to present antigen or provide cytokine costimulation to a pathogenic Th1 cell. The latter either fails to expand or more likely undergoes apoptosis in the absence of DC stimulation. Some preliminary data are presented in the box insert, using a variation of a previously described antigen-specific model of colitis[6]. In this experiment C3H/HeJBir Tr1 cells specific for enteric bacterial antigens were co-transferred with DO11.RAG-2⁻/⁻ Th1 effector cells, specific for OVA, into a (C3H × BALB)F1 scid/scid recipient mouse. The box insert shows the results at sacrifice 8 weeks later. IL-12 production by colon explant cultures and histological colitis were both substantially reduced in the group receiving both Tr1 and Th1 cells compared to recipients of only the pathogenic Th1 cells. If these preliminary data can be reproduced they will provide proof of principle that bystander inhibition/regulation can be a therapeutic modality in IBD

other antigens that had been taken up by that dendritic cell. Th1 effector cells encountering that T-regulatory cell-inhibited dendritic cells will either not be activated or may even undergo apoptosis, in that they would have been deprived of an important growth factor such as IL-12 in the case of Th1 cells[23].

How might this work in practice? One can envisage a variety of approaches to this therapeutic approach. One would be the *ex-vivo* induction and expansion of autologous cells for reinfusion. This might take the form of expansion of immature dendritic cells that are loaded with the commensal bacterial antigen and reinfused; or perhaps expansion of the T-regulatory cells themselves *in vitro* with subsequent reinfusion. Other possibilities would be therapeutic interventions to enhance T-regulatory numbers or function; the means to do this are as yet unknown. A third possibility is gene therapy with a transcription factor that drives T-regulatory cell development, for example Foxp3 which has recently been shown to be crucial for the development of the $CD4^+CD25^+$ subset[24,25]. Lastly, it may be possible to deviate the pathogenic immune response into one that is beneficial by some form of oral immunization of high-risk individuals using immunodominant enteric bacterial antigens, that is an 'IBD vaccine'. One of the major problems limiting the translation of these approaches to humans with IBD is the lack of clinical markers that identify T-regulatory cells in patients or suitable assays to measure their activity in order to guide development of these novel therapies.

References

1. Elson CO, Weaver CT. Experimental mouse models of inflammatory bowel disease: new insights into pathogenic mechanisms. In: Targan SR, Shanahan F, Karp LC, editors. Inflammatory Bowel Disease: From Bench to Bedside, 2nd edn. Dordrecht: Kluwer, 2003:67–99.
2. Levings MK, Roncarolo MG. T-regulatory 1 cells: a novel subset of CD4 T cells with immunoregulatory properties. J Allergy Clin Immunol. 2000;106:S109–12.
3. Fukaura H, Kent SC, Pietrusewicz MJ, Khoury SJ, Weiner HL, Hafler DA. Induction of circulating myelin basic protein and proteolipid protein-specific transforming growth factor-beta1-secreting Th3 T cells by oral administration of myelin in multiple sclerosis patients. J Clin Invest. 1996;98:70–7.
4. Asano M, Toda M, Sakaguchi N, Sakaguchi S. Autoimmune disease as a consequence of developmental abnormality of a T cell subpopulation. J Exp Med. 1996;184:387–96.
5. Takahashi T, Tagami T, Yamazaki S et al. Immunologic self-tolerance maintained by CD25(+)CD4(+) regulatory T cells constitutively expressing cytotoxic T lymphocyte-associated antigen 4. J Exp Med. 2000;192:303–10.
6. Iqbal N, Oliver JR, Wagner FH, Lazenby AS, Elson CO, Weaver CT. T helper 1 and T helper 2 cells are pathogenic in an antigen-specific model of colitis. J Exp Med. 2002;195:71–84.
7. Groux H, O'Garra A, Bigler M et al. A $CD4^+$ T cell subset inhibits antigen-specific T-cell responses and prevents colitis. Nature. 1997;389:737–42.
8. Cottrez F, Hurst SD, Coffman RL, Groux H. T-regulatory cells 1 inhibit a Th2-specific response *in vivo*. J Immunol. 2000;165:4848–53.
9. Kuhn R, Lohler J, Rennick D, Rajewsky K, Muller W. Interleukin-10-deficient mice develop chronic enterocolitis. Cell. 1993;75:263–74.
10. Spencer SD, Di Marco F, Hooley J et al. The orphan receptor CRF2–4 is an essential subunit of the interleukin 10 receptor. J Exp Med. 1998;187:571–8.
11. Yang X, Letterio JJ, Lechleider RJ et al. Targeted disruption of SMAD3 results in impaired mucosal immunity and diminished T cell responsiveness to TGF-beta. EMBO J. 1999; 18:1280–91.
12. Kulkarni AB, Ward JM, Yaswen L et al. Transforming growth factor-beta 1 null mice. An animal model for inflammatory disorders. Am J Pathol. 1995;146:264–75.

13. Gorelik L, Flavell RA. Abrogation of TGFβ signaling in T cells leads to spontaneous T cell differentiation and autoimmune disease. Immunity. 2000;12:171–81.
14. Shevach EM. Certified professionals: CD4(+)CD25(+) suppressor T cells. J Exp Med. 2001;193:F41–6.
15. Apostolou I, Sarukhan A, Klein L, von Boehmer H. Origin of regulatory T cells with known specificity for antigen. Nat Immunol. 2002;3:756–63.
16. Wakkach A, Fournier N, Brun V, Breittmayer JP, Cottrez F, Groux H. Characterization of dendritic cells that induce tolerance and T-regulatory 1 cell differentiation *in vivo*. Immunity. 2003;18:605–17.
17. Khoo UY, Proctor IE, Macpherson AJ. CD4+ T cell down-regulation in human intestinal mucosa: evidence for intestinal tolerance to luminal bacterial antigens. J Immunol. 1997;158:3626–34.
18. Cong Y, Weaver CT, Lazenby A, Elson CO. Bacterial-reactive T-regulatory cells inhibit pathogenic immune responses to the enteric flora. J Immunol. 2002;169:6112–19.
19. Mottet C, Uhlig HH, Powrie F. Cutting edge: cure of colitis by CD4(+)CD25(+) regulatory T cells. J Immunol. 2003;170:3939–43.
20. Nakamura K, Kitani A, Strober W. Cell contact-dependent immunosuppression by CD4(+)CD25(+) regulatory T cells is mediated by cell surface-bound transforming growth factor beta. J Exp Med. 2001;194:629–44.
21. Asseman C, Mauze S, Leach MW, Coffman RL, Powrie F. An essential role for interleukin 10 in the function of regulatory T cells that inhibit intestinal inflammation. J Exp Med. 1999;190:995–1004.
22. Cong Y, Weaver CT, Lazenby A, Elson CO. T-regulatory-1 (Tr1) cells that prevent CD4+ T cell colitis inhibit the antigen-presenting function and IL-12 production of dendritic cells. Gastroenterology. 2001;120:A38.
23. Fuss IJ, Marth T, Neurath MF, Pearlstein GR, Jain A, Strober W. Anti-interleukin 12 treatment regulates apoptosis of Th1 T cells in experimental colitis in mice. Gastroenterology. 1999;117:1078–88.
24. Fontenot JD, Gavin MA, Rudensky AY. Foxp3 programs the development and function of CD4+CD25+ regulatory T cells. Nat Immunol. 2003;4:330–6.
25. Hori S, Nomura T, Sakaguchi S. Control of regulatory T cell development by the transcription factor Foxp3. Science. 2003;299:1057–61.

13
Regulation of mucosal inflammation by TGF-β_1 plasmid

A. KITANI

LIMITATION OF NATURALLY OCCURRING SUPPRESSOR CELLS

In recent years evidence has accumulated that naturally occurring T regulatory cells (T_{reg}) producing TGF-β and/or IL-10 can prevent or even reverse Th1 cell-mediated inflammation models. Several kinds of T_{reg} have been described. One cell, which is identified by its expression of CD25 prior to activation and recently shown to express an intracellular protein called Foxp3, acts *in vitro* via cell–cell contact and *in vivo*, directly or indirectly via production of TGF β[1,2]. We have published data showing this cell (commonly referred to as the CD4$^+$CD25$^+$ T_{reg}) expresses TGF-β and produces TGF-β and IL-10 when appropriately stimulated *in vitro*[3]. This cell may thus be similar to the Th3 regulatory cell occurring during oral tolerance induction and also producing TGF-β. A second type of regulatory cell, called a Tr1 cell, appears to affect suppression via secretion of IL-10 alone, since it produces little or no TGF-β[4]. One important difference between these cells other than cytokine secretion is that CD25$^+$ cells arise in the thymus in response to self antigens, and Tr1 cells appear to be responding to exogenous antigens; thus the two types of cell may provide regulation under different conditions. However, chronic inflammation is considered as a result of impaired expansion of such naturally occurring regulatory cells *in vivo*[5]. Moreover, transfer of regulatory cell obtained from normal donors may cause an allogenic response, especially in the clinical setting[6]; therefore we have attempted to generate TGF-β and/or IL-10 producing cells by gene engineering *in vivo*.

DEVELOPMENT OF NEW GENE TRANSFER METHOD TO GENERATE SUPPRESSOR CELLS

We introduce here a simple one-gene non-viral gene transfer method which demonstrates efficient generation of TGF-β production *in vivo*. Moreover, the

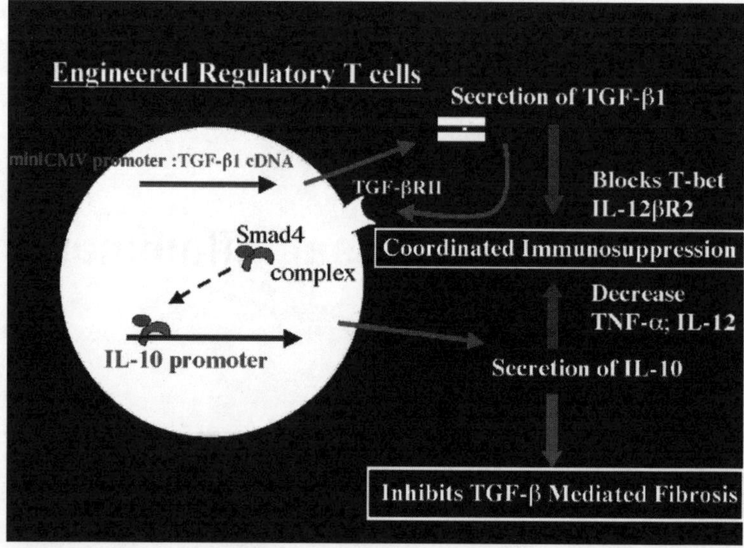

Figure 1 pTet-On-TGF-β transfected T cells secrete active TGF-β_1 under miniCMV promoter activated by the binding of Tet-On protein in the presence of doxycycline. Secreted TGF-β_1 binds to TGF-β receptor II and signal is delivered to Smad 4 complex to activate IL-10 promoter. Thus, TGF-β_1 and IL-10 are co-produced and exert coordinated suppression; TGF-β_1 blocks T bet and IL-12 β_2 receptor expression, and IL-10 decreases TNF-α and IL-12. IL-10 also facilitates inhibition of TGF-β-mediated fibrosis development

method we have developed also accomplishes a doxycycline tightly regulated safe gene therapeutic strategy[7]. The non-viral plasmid producing TGF-β (pTet-On-TGF-β) is equipped with two protein expression units: (1) Tet-On protein under a CMV promoter, and (2) active (mature) TGF-β under a miniCMV promoter which is activated by Tet-On protein binding in the presence of doxycycline[8,9].

INTRANASAL DELIVERY OF TGF-β PLASMID INDUCES IL-10 PRODUCTION *IN VIVO*

When pTet-On-TGF-β is administered with the concomitant injection of doxycycline, not only TGF-β but also IL-10 is rapidly induced *in vivo*, and this IL-10 production is continued even after the production of TGF-β is decreased by the cessation of doxycycline. This observation is consonant with previous findings showing that TGF-β_1 and IL-10 secretion tend to occur together by T_{regs}[10–13].

We examined the effect of pTet-On-TGF-β in a TNBS-induced colitis model, and found that this plasmid, when activated in the presence of doxycydine, quite effectively prevented disease, evaluated by body weight curves, pathology findings and cytokine profiles in inflamed colons. We confirmed that lamina propria mononuclear cells produce both TGF-β and IL-10, and inhibited IFN-γ and IL-12 production, suggesting the suppressive effect of Th1 inflammation. TGF-β_1 blocks T bet and IL-12 β_2 receptor expression, and consequently suppressed IFN-γ production[8,14]. It is considered that IL-10 decreases IL-12 and TNF-α production[15] (Figure 1). Facilitation of co-production of TGF-β and IL-10 could occur through IL-10 enhancement of TGF-β_1 signalling. This possibility is supported by Cottrez et al. who showed that IL-10 maintains TGF-β_1RII expression on activated cells that would otherwise down-regulate this receptor[16]. In addition, it is known that Th1 cytokines such as IFN-γ and TNF-α up-regulate Smad7, a cytosolic intermediate that inhibits TGF-β_1 signalling via other Smads[5], and it is thus possible (but not yet proven) that IL-10 inhibits such Smad7 up-regulation.

MOLECULAR MECHANISM OF IL-10 INDUCTION BY THE TGF-β PLASMID

We further examined how IL-10 induction associates with TGF-β production. We infected retrovirus Th1 developing cells[17] with encoding GFP and active TGF-β *in vitro*. Flow cytometric analysis showed that IL-10 is produced by both TGF-β positive and negative Th1 cells in the culture infected with TGF-β retrovirus. We searched the murine IL-10 promoter region for a Smad-binding element (SBE) as a TGF-β signalling molecule. We found an 'SBE variant' site GTCCAGAC at −901 that closely resembled the consensus SBE, GTCTAGAC and contains overlapping CAGA sequences (termed a CAGA box)[18]. We observed that addition of anti-Smad4 caused supershift with the SBE variant oligo in the electromobility shift assay, and that the mutation of this sequence abrogated TGF-β-mediated IL-10 promoter activity by luciferase assay.

CO-PRODUCTION OF IL-10 IS A UNIQUE CHARACTER FOR T$_{reg}$ CELLS AND PREVENTS FIBROSIS IN pTet-On-TGF-β GENE TRANSFER

We found that TGF-β_1 plasmid administration somewhat paradoxically reverses bleomycin-induced pulmonary fibrosis in wild-type mice, and such reversal is IL-10-dependent because it does not occur in IL-10-deficient mice in which the plasmid does not induce IL-10. This suggests that the association of TGF-β_1 and IL-10 secretion has advantages not only in relation to immunological suppression but also in relation to the ability of TGF-β_1 to mediate fibrosis[19]. The co-production activity is limited to T cells and macrophages among the various types of cells and cell lines, such as epithelial, squamous, and fibroblast cell lines from colon, lung and other tissues. This is important because it shows that administration of TGF-β with a delivery system that does not target these cells specifically is likely to be associated with unacceptable fibrosis. Overall, our method described here calls attention to the feasibility of inducing T$_{reg}$ cells for use in many forms of inflammation.

Acknowledgements

I thank Drs Fuss I, Nakamura K, Kumaki F, Usui T and Strober W for valuable help and advice.

References

1. Sakaguchi S, Sakaguchi N, Shimizu J et al. Immunologic tolerance maintained by CD25+CD4+ regulatory T cells: their common role in controlling autoimmunity, tumor immunity, and transplantation tolerance. Immunol Rev. 2001;182:18–32.
2. Hori S, Nomura T, Sakaguchi S. Control of regulatory T cell development by the transcription factor Foxp3. Science. 2003;299:1057–61.
3. Nakamura K, Kitani A, Strober W. Cell contact-dependent immunosuppression by CD4(+)CD25(+) regulatory T cells is mediated by cell surface-bound transforming growth factor beta. J Exp Med. 2001;194:629–44.
4. Groux H, O'Garra A, Bigler M et al. A CD4+ T-cell subset inhibits antigen-specific T-cell responses and prevents colitis. Nature. 1997;389:737–42.
5. Ulloa L, Doody J, Massague J. Inhibition of transforming growth factor-beta/SMAD signalling by the interferon-gamma/STAT pathway. Nature. 1999;397:710–13.
6. Jonuleit H, Schmitt E, Stassen M, Tuettenberg A, Knop J, Enk AH. Identification and functional characterization of human CD4(+)CD25(+) T cells with regulatory properties isolated from peripheral blood. J Exp Med. 2001;193:1285–94.
7. Gossen, M, Freundlieb S, Bender G, Muller G, Hillen W, Bujard H. Transcriptional activation by tetracyclines in mammalian cells. Science. 1995;268:1766–9.
8. Kitani A, Fuss I, Nakamura K, Schwartz OM, Usui T, Strober W. Treatment of experimental (trinitrobenzene sulfonic acid) colitis by intranasal administration of transforming growth factor (TGF)β1 plasmid: TGF-β1-mediated suppression of T helper cell type 1 response occurs by interleukin (IL)-10 induction and IL-12 receptor β2 chain downregulation. J Exp Med. 2000;192:41–52.
9. Kitani A, Fuss I, Nakamura K, Kumaki F, Usui T, Strober W. TGF-β1-producing regulatory T cells induce Smad-mediated IL-10 secretion that facilitates coordinated immunoregulatory activity and amelioration of TGF-β1-mediated fibrosis. J Exp Med. 2003;198:1179–88.
10. Fuss, IJ, Boirivant M, Lacy B, Strober W. The interrelated roles of TGF-beta and IL-10 in the regulation of experimental colitis. J Immunol. 2002;168:900–8.
11. Kitani A, Chua K, Nakamura K, Strober W. Activated self-MHC-reactive T cells have the cytokine phenotype of Th3/T regulatory cell 1 cells. J Immunol. 2000;165:691–702.
12. Maloy KJ, Salaun L, Cahill R, Dougan G, Saunders NJ, Powrie F. CD4+CD25+ T(R) cells suppress innate immune pathology through cytokine-dependent mechanisms. J Exp Med. 2003;197:111–19.
13. Asseman C, Mauze S, Leach MW, Coffman RL, Powrie F. An essential role for interleukin 10 in the function of regulatory T cells that inhibit intestinal inflammation. J Exp Med. 1999;190:995–1004.
14. Gorelik L, Constant S, Flavell RA. Mechanism of transforming growth factor beta-induced inhibition of T helper type 1 differentiation. J Exp Med. 2002;195:1499–505.
15. Segal BM, Dwyer BK, Shevach EM. An interleukin (IL)-10/IL-12 immunoregulatory circuit controls susceptibility to autoimmune disease. J Exp Med. 1998;187:537–46.
16. Cottrez F, Groux H. Regulation of TGF-beta response during T cell activation is modulated by IL-10. J Immunol. 2001;167:773–8.
17. Usui T, Nishikomori R, Kitani A, Strober W. GATA-3 suppresses Th1 development by downregulation of STAT-4, not through effects on IL-12Rβ2 chain or T bet. Immunity. 2003;18:415–28.
18. Denissova NG, Pouponnot C, Long J, He D, Liu F. Transforming growth factor β-inducible independent binding of SMAD to the Smad7 promoter. Proc Natl Acad Sci USA. 2000;97:6397–402.
19. Coker RK, Laurent GJ, Shahzeidi S et al. Transforming growth factors-beta 1, -beta 2, and -beta 3 stimulate fibroblast procollagen production *in vitro* but are differentially expressed during bleomycin-induced lung fibrosis. Am J Pathol. 1997;150:981–91.

14
Human CD25$^+$ regulatory T cells: suppression of self and intestinal antigens

S. LUNDIN, A. LUNDGREN, S. RAGHAVAN,
A.-M. SVENNERHOLM, K. WING, S. LINDGREN
and E. SURI-PAYER

INTRODUCTION

The past decade has led to a renewed interest in suppressor cells. Multiple populations of CD4 T cells have been isolated and analysed for their capacity to suppress proliferation and cytokine production of CD4 T helper (Th) and CD8 cytotoxic cells. Regulatory T cells can be divided into two groups. The 'naturally occurring' CD25$^+$ regulatory T cells (T$_{reg}$), which constitute 5–10% of the CD4 T cells in mice and rats and approximately 3% in humans[1]. CD25$^+$ cells originate in the thymus[2], but may be further activated in the periphery. Additionally, CD4$^+$CD25$^-$ T cells with T cell-suppressive function have been described in different experimental systems[3–5]. These could possibly be derived from CD25$^+$ T$_{reg}$ that lost CD25 expression. The second group of regulatory T cell populations can be induced *in vivo* or *in vitro*. Interleukin-10 (IL-10) secretion by dendritic cells in the course of infections or the stimulation of CD4 T cells *in vitro* in the presence of IL-10 induces T regulatory 1 (Tr1) cells[6]. Ovalbumin-specific Tr1 cells can prevent colitis via bystander suppression[7]. Oral application of antigen leads to generation of T helper 3 (Th3) cells, which in turn lead to the manifestation of oral tolerance[8].

The relation between the different regulatory T cell populations is not yet clear. Tr1 cells seem to be independent of CD25$^+$ T$_{reg}$ and do not develop out of CD25$^+$ cells[9]. The situation is less clear for regulatory cells that are responsible for oral tolerance. Oral feeding of antigen may activate and expand CD25$^+$ T$_{reg}$[10], or may induce regulatory cells out of CD4$^+$CD25$^-$ cells[11].

The mechanism of suppression varies between the different regulatory T cells and the experimental system used. Briefly, induced Tr1 and Th3 cells suppress via secretion of IL-10 and TGF-β, while natural $CD25^+$ T_{reg} seem to function in a cytokine-independent manner[1]. However, as they may induce such cytokines in the suppressed T cells (or other host cells *in vivo*), IL-10 and TGF-β nevertheless play a role in the prevention of some autoimmune diseases via CD25 T_{reg}[12–14].

Despite the vast interest in $CD25^+$ T_{reg} cells, many fundamental questions are still unresolved:

1. Are all $CD25^+$ cells T_{reg} or how can $CD25^+$ T_{reg} be distinguished phenotypically from $CD25^+$ effector T cells?
2. What is the functional mechanism of suppression?
3. Which antigen(s) is (are) recognized by the $CD25^+$ T_{reg} or how are T_{reg} activated *in vivo*?
4. Are T_{reg} defective in human autoimmune diseases?

Some of these issues have been discussed in excellent recent reviews[1,15]. We will concentrate on human T_{reg} and also describe the role of $CD25^+$ T_{reg} in inflammatory diseases of the gastrointestinal tract in murine models.

$CD25^+$ T_{reg} IN THE SUPPRESSION OF AUTOIMMUNITY: COMPARISON OF GASTRITIS AND COLITIS

$CD25^+$ cells were discovered by their virtue of preventing organ-specific autoimmune diseases such as autoimmune gastritis, thyroiditis and oophoritis. The injection of spleen or lymph node cells that were depleted of $CD25^+$ cells into T cell-deficient animals leads to the development of these various autoimmune diseases. The coinjection of $CD25^+$ cells blocks the activation of the self-reactive Th cells and thus prevents autoimmunity[15]. This protection is

Table 1 Functional characteristics of $CD25^+$ T_{reg} *in vitro* and *in vivo*

	In vitro	*Gastritis*	*Colitis*	*References*
Model	Proliferation	Pernicious anaemia	Colitis ulcerosa	
Induction	$CD4^+CD25^-$	$CD4^+CD25^-$ naive	$CD4^+CD45RB^{high}$ naive	2, 14
Prevention	$CD25^+$	$CD25^+$	$CD45RB^{low}/CD25^+$	2, 14
Cure		?	Yes	20
Germfree mice		+++	No	2, 14
Antigen for T_{eff}	Any	H/K ATP-ase	Enteral bacteria	19, 21
Antigen for T_{reg}	Any ?	?	Enteral bacteria	21
Mechanism:				
IL-4	–	–	–	1, 14, 16, 17
IL-10	–	–	+	1, 14, 16, 17
TGF-β	–	–	+	1, 14, 17
CTLA-4	–	+/–	+	1, 14, 15, 17

independent of the presence of B and CD8 cells, and does not involve secretion of IL-4, IL-10 and TGF-β from the CD25$^+$ T$_{reg}$[16,17]. Whether CTLA-4 signalling is needed for suppression of gastritis is in dispute[15,17] (Table 1). The main target autoantigen in murine gastritis and human pernicious anaemia is the proton pump (H/K ATP-ase α and β chain)[18–20]. It is unclear if the same antigen is recognized by CD25$^+$ T$_{reg}$.

Autoimmune colitis ensues in scid mice receiving CD45RB^{hi} cells as well as in mice deficient for IL-10, and it is used as a model for colitis ulcerosa[14]. In contrast to autoimmune gastritis, colitis is strictly dependent on the presence of bacterial flora, and effector T cells in colitis recognize bacterial or faecal antigens[21]. While no common pathogen that induces colitis has yet been identified, the severity of colitis is markedly enhanced by *Helicobacter hepaticus*[14]. We are not aware of any report demonstrating gut wall self-antigen-specific T cells in colitis; it could thus be called an 'infectious' rather than an autoimmune disease.

CD45RB^{low} cells, as well as CD25$^+$ cells that constitute a subpopulation of the CD45RB^{low} cells, protect from and even cure colitis[22]. This protection can be abrogated by the injection of anti-IL-10, anti-IL-10R or anti-TGF-β (but not anti-IL-4) monoclonal antibodies[14]. This shows a clear difference between the protection from autoimmune gastritis and bacterially induced colitis (Table 1). In RAG2$^{-/-}$ mice CD25 T$_{reg}$ were also shown to directly suppress the innate immune system[23]. Thus, IL-10 and/or TGF-β may be needed to counteract the activation of the innate immune system by bacteria.

Immune competent mice do not show an activation of the immune system in the form of an inflammatory response against the bacterial flora. The mechanisms that prevent this activation are not yet resolved. CD4 cells from the lamina propria (LP) of normal mice do not proliferate in response to bacterial (faecal) antigens; in fact they are able to suppress the antibacterial response of the LP CD4 cells from mice with colitis[21]. LP T cells, LN and splenic T cells of normal mice showed significant proliferation to enteral antigens after depletion of CD25$^+$ cells[24]. This indicates that T helper cells specific for bacterial antigens are present in the gut and the peripheral lymphoid system. Purified CD25$^+$ cells from LP as well as the LN could block the activation of CD4 cells to bacterial antigens. These experiments demonstrate that CD25$^+$ cells prevent the activation of Th cells against the enteric antigens. Interestingly, CD25$^+$ cells from germfree mice were also able to suppress responses to bacterial antigens (personal communication M. Claesson, Copenhagen) and CD45RB^{low} cells from germfree mice could protect from colitis in specific pathogen-free mice[25]. Further work should clarify how T$_{reg}$ cells are selected for these enteral antigens.

Other models in which CD25$^+$ T$_{reg}$ inhibit or ameliorate autoimmunity are diabetes and experimental autoimmune encephalomyelitis[26,27]. Further, CD25$^+$ T$_{reg}$ play a role in transplantation tolerance, and they dampen the immune response to infections[15,28]. Taken together, T$_{reg}$ are clearly beneficial for the organism through their ability to preserve the immune homeostasis by preventing an 'over-reaction' of the immune system and aberrant pathology. However, the downside of T$_{reg}$ is that they can suppress the immune reaction towards malignant cells and consequently allow cancer to develop[2].

CHARACTERIZATION AND FUNCTION OF T_{reg} *IN VITRO* (MURINE AND HUMAN)

$CD25^+$ T_{reg} are characterized by the constitutive expression of CD122 (CD25β chain), glucocorticoid-induced TNF receptor family-related gene (GITR), and they contain intracellular stores for CD152 (CTLA-4, cytotoxic T-lymphoctye antigen-4)[1]. However, these antigens are also expressed on recently activated effector T cells[1]. This makes it difficult to characterize a T_{reg} by phenotype, and requires functional tests to determine if the cell in question really has regulatory function. Therefore, the recent discovery of exclusive expression of the transcription factor scurfin, which is encoded by the Foxp3 gene, on T_{reg} and not on other CD4 T cells, was greeted with great enthusiasm. In addition, transfection of $CD4^+CD25^-$ T cells with Foxp3 converted them into T_{reg} cells, indicating that this gene plays a role in the function of T_{reg}[29].

The discovery that T_{reg} do not proliferate *in vitro* (they are anergic), but suppress the proliferation and cytokine production of naive T cells, made it possible to learn more about the mechanism of suppression. In addition, it enabled the identification of $CD25^+$ T_{reg} in human peripheral blood. Isolated $CD4^+CD25^+$ cells inhibited the proliferation of $CD4^+CD25^-$ cells in cultures stimulated with allogenic antigen-presenting cells (APC) or mitogens (ConA, PHA, soluble anti-CD3 plus APC, anti-CD3 plus anti-CD28) (reviewed in ref. 30). As to the functional mechanism of suppression *in vitro*, many groups have confirmed that $CD25^+$ cells need to be activated in order to suppress, that cell contact to $CD25^-$ cells is required and that anti-IL-10, anti-IL-10R, anti-TGF-β and anti-CTLA-4 antibodies do not block the suppression, indicating that these molecules are dispensable for suppression[1] (Table 1). Further, blocking the PD-1/PDL-1 interaction only slightly reduces suppression[31]. Suppression can be abrogated by 'turning off' T_{reg} via GITR signalling[32]. Once activated through its TCR a T_{reg} can suppress T cells of other specificities (bystander suppression) and a T_{reg} that has been fixed after TCR activation can suppress proliferation of Th cells[1,13]. The molecular mechanism of suppression is presently unknown. $CD25^+$ T_{reg} down-regulate the production of IL-2 and many other cytokines (IFN-γ, IL-4, IL-5, IL-13, TNF-α) but can induce IL-10 and or TGF-β production in the suppressed cells[13,31]. The addition of exogenous IL-2 restores the proliferation of the naive T cells and strong TCR stimulation such as high concentration of crosslinked anti-CD3 mAb or the use of PMA/ionomycin also overcome suppression[1,31,33].

The staining of murine $CD4^+$ cells with anti-CD25 (interleukin 2 receptor (IL-2R) α chain) shows two distinct cell populations, $CD25^-$ cells and $CD25^+$ cells which constitute approximately 5–10% of the CD4 cells (Figure 1A). This result is identical for lymph node cells, spleen cells and blood cells. When human peripheral cells are stained for CD25 then three populations of $CD4^+$ cells emerge. $CD25^-$ cells, cells displaying an intermediate density of CD25 antigens ($CD25^{int}$ cells) and cells displaying a high density of CD25 antigens ($CD25^{++}$ cells). Most $CD25^+$ cells belong to the $CD25^{int}$ category (about 40%), while only 1–3% of CD4 T cells stain brightly for CD25 (Figure 1B)[34]. Further phenotypic and functional analysis revealed that only the $CD25^{++}$ cells express CD122, GITR and CD152 (CTLA-4) (Figure 1C–E). $CD25^{++}$ cells are small, and display a memory phenotype ($CD45RA^-$, $CD45RO^+$, $CD69^-$, partly

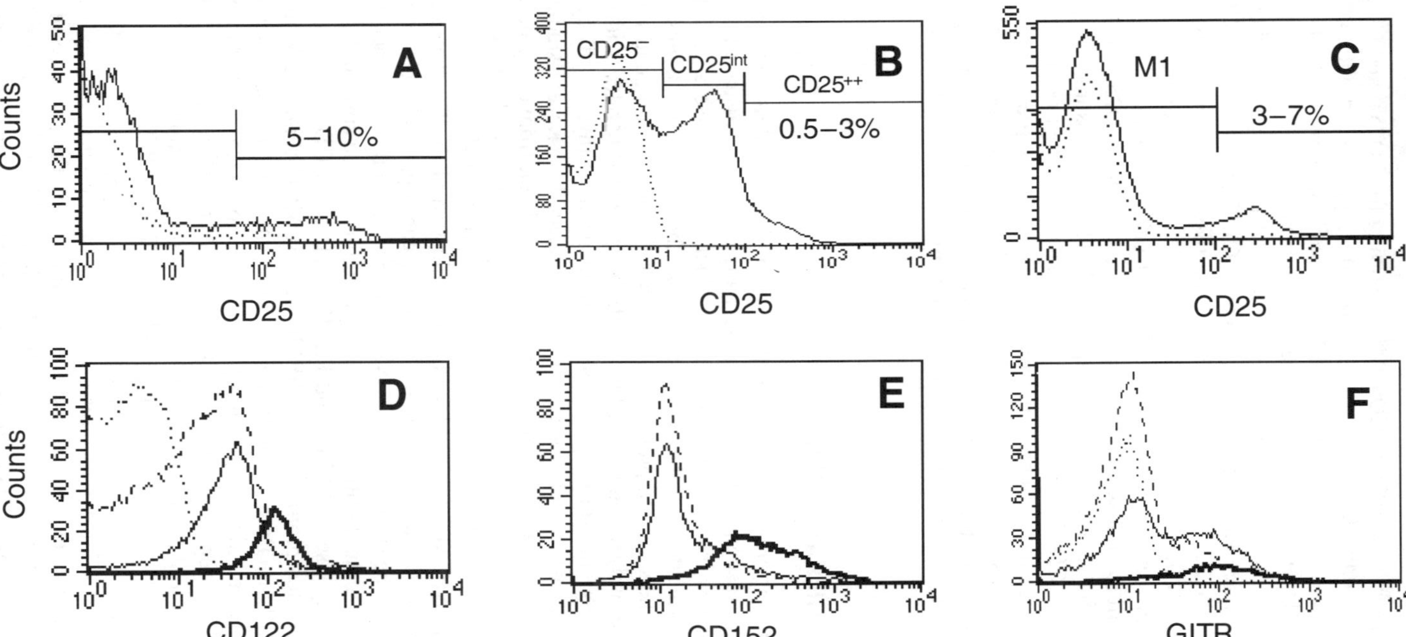

Figure 1 Phenotype of human CD25$^+$ T$_{reg}$. **A–C** show the CD25 staining of purified CD4$^+$ T cells from the lymph nodes of mice (**A**), human adult peripheral blood (**B**) and cord blood (**C**). Adult peripheral blood contains a sizeable fraction of CD25^{int} cells and only up to 3% of CD4 T cells express high levels of CD25 (CD25^{++}). Only these CD25^{++} cells (bold lines) express increased levels of CD122 (**D**), intracellular CD152 (**E**) and nearly all of these cells express GITR (**F**). CD25$^-$ and CD25^{int} cells expressed low levels of CD122 and did not contain intracellular CTLA-4 stores (dotted and thin line, respectively)

$CD62L^{low}$, $CD38^{low}$, $CD45RB^{low}$, $CD95^{high}$)[34]. Sorting for $CD25^{int}$ and $CD25^{++}$ cells revealed that only the $CD25^{++}$ cells potently suppressed proliferation of $CD25^{-}$ cells (data not shown and ref. 31). $CD25^{int}$ cells are most probably effector/memory T cells while $CD25^{-}$ cells are mainly naive T cells[34].

Cord blood does not contain a sizeable fraction of $CD25^{int}$ cells and therefore $CD25^{+}$ cells are more easily discernible (Figure 1C). These cord blood $CD25^{+}$ cells expressed CD122 and CD152 like T_{reg}[34], but they had lower expression of GITR and CD45RO than their adult counterparts[35]. In addition, though we were able to detect suppressive activity in cord blood cells when using polyclonal stimuli, they seem to be less potent when compared to adult $CD25^{++}$ cells and they did not inhibit antigen-specific responses[35]. Thus, we assume that, after leaving the thymus, $CD25^{+}$ cells need to be stimulated with their respective antigen (self-antigen) in the periphery and then acquire their suppressive function. This interpretation fits with the fact that $CD25^{+}$ cells from adult blood only suppress when they are of the CD45RO phenotype[36,37]. Nevertheless, using polyclonal stimulation, $CD25^{+}$ cells from the murine and human thymus are suppressive[38–40].

ANTIGEN SPECIFICITY OF T_{reg}

While the studies of prevention of gastritis, oophoritis, thyroiditis, etc., suggest that $CD25^{+}$ T_{reg} recognize the same tissue antigens as the disease-inducing effector T cells, this has not been proven. The fact that T_{reg} have a polyclonal TCR repertoire indicates that they could recognize the same self-antigens as Th cells. Studies on the selection process indicate that T_{reg} possess a high affinity to the selecting self-antigen. However, these data have been generated with TCR transgenic mice engineered to express foreign antigens in the thymus[5]. They give no indication as to which self-antigens naturally select T_{reg}. Recent studies on the expression of tissue antigens in the thymus revealed that from every organ at least one antigen is ectopically expressed on thymic epithelial cells. This thymic expression of, e.g., myelin oligodendrocyte glycoprotein (MOG) or glutamic acid decarboxylase (GAD)-65 could lead to the selection of the T_{reg} that eventually prevents the host from autoimmunity[41]. As T_{reg} can suppress T cells of other specificity it should be sufficient if T_{reg} can recognize one self-antigen per organ.

In order to determine if human $CD25^{+}$ T_{reg} recognize tissue specific antigens, we studied the response of PBMC and PBMC depleted of $CD25^{+}$ T_{reg} to self-antigens. We detected proliferation of PBMC against MOG (Figure 2A) and β-lactoglobulin (β-LG). Both these responses were enhanced in the absence of $CD25^{+}$ cells. The addition of purified $CD25^{+}$ cells to $CD25^{-}$ cells that were activated by CD3 depleted irradiated PBMC and MOG leads to a dose-dependent reduction of the proliferation and IFN-γ production by the $CD25^{-}$ T cells (Figure 2B). In the absence of T_{reg} both $CD45RA^{+}CD62L^{+}$ naive T cells and to a higher extent memory T cells proliferated in response to MOG. This indicates that effector T cells recognize the self-antigen even in healthy volunteers, but they are prevented from inducing pathology by the presence of T_{reg}. Because we could not detect MOG-specific T_{reg} in cord blood, we assume that T_{reg} need to be primed by MOG in the periphery in order to obtain their suppressive

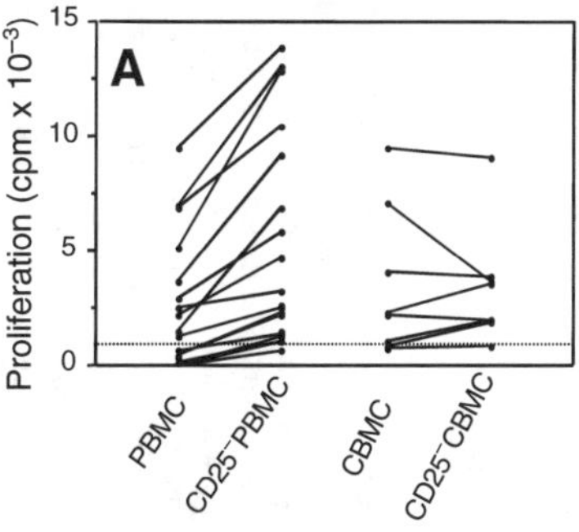
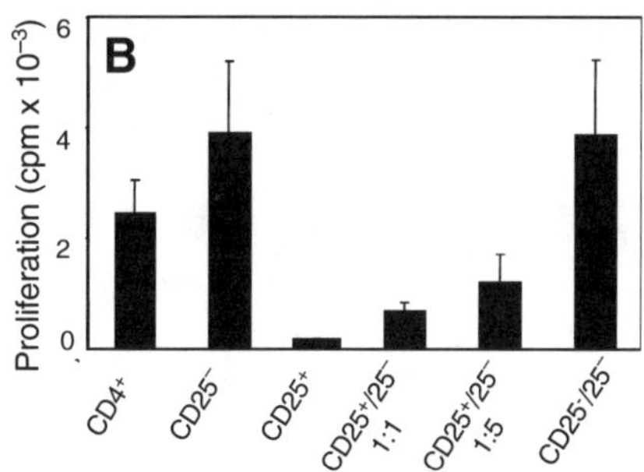

Figure 2 Human CD25$^+$ cells suppress the MOG-specific proliferation of CD4$^+$CD25$^-$ cells. **A:** Total PBMC (2×10^5) or PBMC depleted of CD25$^+$ cells via magnetic beads (CD25$^-$ PBMC) were cultured in the presence of 10 µg/ml human MOG^{IgD} for 7 days. The depletion of CD25$^+$ cells led to an increase in proliferation in all 18 subjects tested (left side). In contrast, depletion of CD25$^+$ cells in cord blood mononuclear cells (CBMC) did not increase the proliferation (right side). **B:** Purified CD4$^+$ cells from adult volunteers (10^5), CD4$^+$CD25$^-$ cells and a mixture of CD25$^+$ and CD25$^-$ cells at 1:1 and 1:5 ratio were stimulated with MOG and irradiated CD3-depleted PBMC for 7 days. While the depletion of CD25$^+$ cells increased proliferation the addition of CD25$^+$ cells led to a dose-dependent decrease in the proliferation of CD25$^-$ cells. CD25$^+$ cells themselves did not proliferate in response to MOG and APC. IFN-γ production was also measured and was similarly suppressed as was proliferation

function. This idea is supported by the finding that rats lacking thyroids lose thyroid-specific regulatory cells while they retain cells protecting from insulitis[42].

A screen of multiple proteins by Taams et al. showed that human CD25$^+$ T$_{reg}$ do not only recognize self-antigens (heat-shock protein), but also reduce responses to bacterial antigens (tetanus toxoid, purified protein derivate) and food antigens (ovalbumin and milk protein)[36]. T$_{reg}$ specific for infectious agents were also detected in mice, e.g. against *Leishmania* antigens[43]. Depletion of CD25$^+$ cells leads to an overwhelming, sometimes lethal, inflammatory reaction after infection with *Pneumocystis carinii*, *Candida albicans* or *Leishmania major* (reviewed in ref. 28).

REGULATION OF *HELICOBACTER* INFECTION BY T$_{reg}$

We have studied the role of T$_{reg}$ in *Helicobacter pylori* infections in mice and humans. *H. pylori* is a spiral Gram-negative bacterium that colonizes the gastric and duodenal mucosa and causes chronic gastritis[44]. About 15% of infected individuals develop peptic ulcer, mucosa-associated lymphoid tissue lymphoma or gastric adenocarcinoma. Colonization of the mucosa leads to local inflammation with infiltration of neutrophils, macrophages and T and B cells specific for *H. pylori* antigens.

The reconstitution of nude mice with LN cells containing T$_{reg}$ reduced the bacterial load two-fold, while in the absence of CD25$^+$ T$_{reg}$ the load was further reduced 9-fold (Figure 3A–C). This indicated an increased activation of

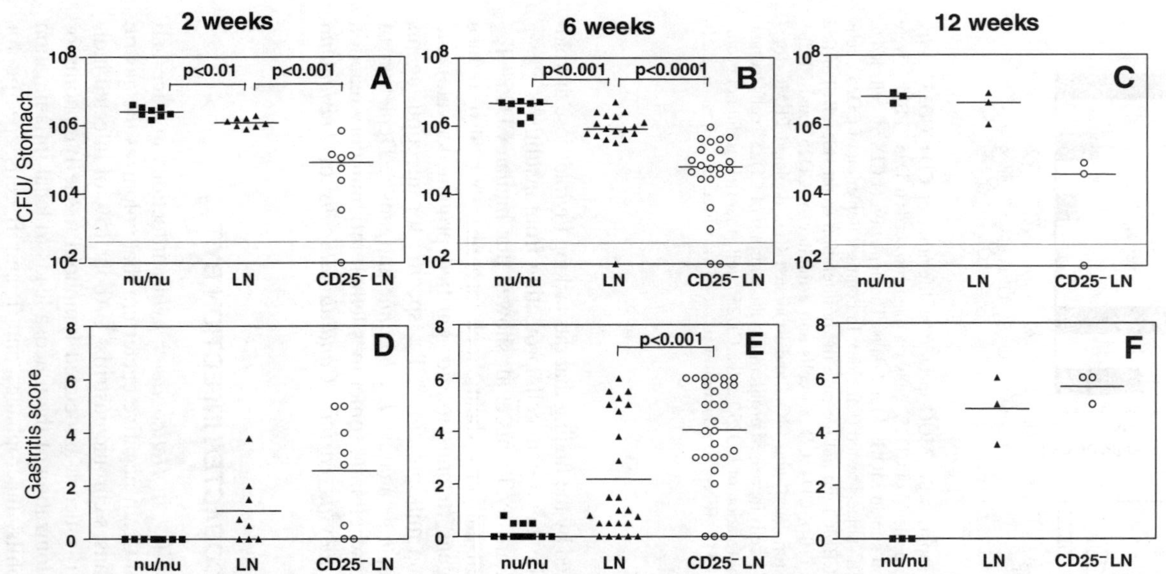

Figure 3 CD25$^+$ cells suppress the immune response against *H. pylori* in mice as evidenced by reduced bacterial clearance and reduced gastritis. C57BL/6 *nu/nu* mice were reconstituted with LN or CD25$^-$ LN cells (containing 2×10^6 CD4 T cells) purified from C57BL/6 mice. After 3 weeks mice were infected with 3×10^8 CFU *H. pylori* SS1 strain and mice were sacrificed 2, 6 and 12 weeks after infection. The stomach was divided longitudinally and half of the stomach was used to determine the bacterial colonization (**A–C**) and half was cut into longitudinal stripes, sectioned and stained with H&E (**D–F**). Athymic mice contained a high bacterial load with no histological changes in the gastric mucosa for the entire observation period of 12 weeks. The reconstitution with T cells led to a 2–3-fold reduction of bacterial counts; bacterial growth was further depressed 9-fold in the absence of CD25 cells. First signs of gastritis were detected as early as 2 weeks after infection; this was mild, consisting mainly of lymphocytic infiltration in the group receiving LN cells (grade 2–3), but much more severe in mice receiving CD25-depleted LN cells where destruction of chief and parietal cells was evident (grade 3–5). At 6 weeks only a few mice receiving LN cells proceeded to severe gastritis, and more than half had not yet developed gastritis. In contrast, the incidence and severity of gastritis in mice that received CD25-depleted LN cells was very high. Most mice had a completely destroyed mucosal architecture with no parietal cells or chief cells left, and replacement of the mucosa by mucus-producing neck cells and concomitant hyperplasia (grade 6). In keeping with the literature stating that C57BL/6 mice are resistant to the development of autoimmune gastritis, C57BL/6 *nu/nu* mice that received CD25$^-$ LN cells in the absence of bacterial infection did not develop gastritis[45]

H. pylori-reactive T cells. Indeed, DTH responses to *H. pylori* antigen, as well as the proliferation and IFN-γ production of purified T cells in response to bacterial antigens and the degree of CD4 T cell infiltration into the gastric mucosa, were all significantly higher in mice lacking T$_{reg}$[45]. In addition, preliminary co-culture experiments revealed an increased proliferation of CD4$^+$CD25$^-$ T cells in response to *H. pylori* antigens in comparison to CD4 T cells, and suppression of these responses when CD25$^+$ cells from the mesenteric lymph nodes (MLN) of the same infected mice were added to the culture. This indicates that CD25$^+$ T cells from the MLN recognize *H. pylori* antigen. We speculate that CD25$^+$ T$_{reg}$ are activated during the course of infection and down-regulate the response of antigen-specific effector T cells. Indeed, the absence of T$_{reg}$ *in vivo* had severe consequences in the infected mucosa. While mice that received LN cells had a slow onset of mild gastritis, absence of T$_{reg}$ was coupled with a fast development of severe gastritis (Figure 3D,E). Therefore it seems that T$_{reg}$ dampen the immune response in order to avoid overwhelming pathology and thus symptoms[28].

This theory was further strengthened in our study of *H. pylori*-infected asymptomatic persons. CD4 T cells were isolated from PBMC and then sorted into naive (CD45RA$^+$CD62L$^+$) and memory T cells (CD45RA$^-$ and CD45RA$^+$ CD62L$^-$) and stimulated by dendritic cells pulsed with *H. pylori* membrane preparations. We found that memory T cells from asymptomatic individuals proliferated poorly compared to naive T cells from the same individual (Figure 4A). The dampened responses of memory T cells was due to suppression by T$_{reg}$ as the addition of IL-2 or the depletion of CD25$^+$ cells led to a significant increase in proliferation (Figure 4B). Most importantly, the addition of sorted CD25^{++} cells to CD25$^-$ cells markedly decreased the proliferation in response to *H. pylori* membrane antigens (Figure 4C). Because the suppressive function of T$_{reg}$ is evident only after stimulation through their TCR these data imply that T$_{reg}$ were activated in these cultures by *H. pylori* antigen. Since control cultures using TT as antigen showed normal responses in the asymptomatic carriers, and were not significantly affected by the depletion of T$_{reg}$, we conclude that T$_{reg}$ specific for *H. pylori* are activated or expanded in the *H. pylori*-infected asymptomatic carriers. T$_{reg}$ activated by the infectious agent may then inhibit any local tissue-destructive response by controlling the effector function of tissue antigen-specific effector T cells in the same local site, and at the same time contribute to the chronicity of the infection by dampening a protective T-cell response to the bacteria.

CD25$^+$ T$_{reg}$ IN HUMAN DISEASES

Since organ-specific autoimmune, as well as inflammatory bowel diseases, are controlled by CD25$^+$ T$_{reg}$ in animal studies, there is great interest in determining if patients suffering from autoimmune diseases have a defect in T$_{reg}$. At present there are only scant data, and these do not allow for definitive conclusions. Patients with a recent onset of type I diabetes, as well as those with long-standing diabetes, show decreased numbers of CD25$^+$ cells in the circulation[46]. Since gating for 'real' T$_{reg}$ on the basis of CD25 expression is difficult (if not impossible) in the human system, it is crucial to confirm those findings with

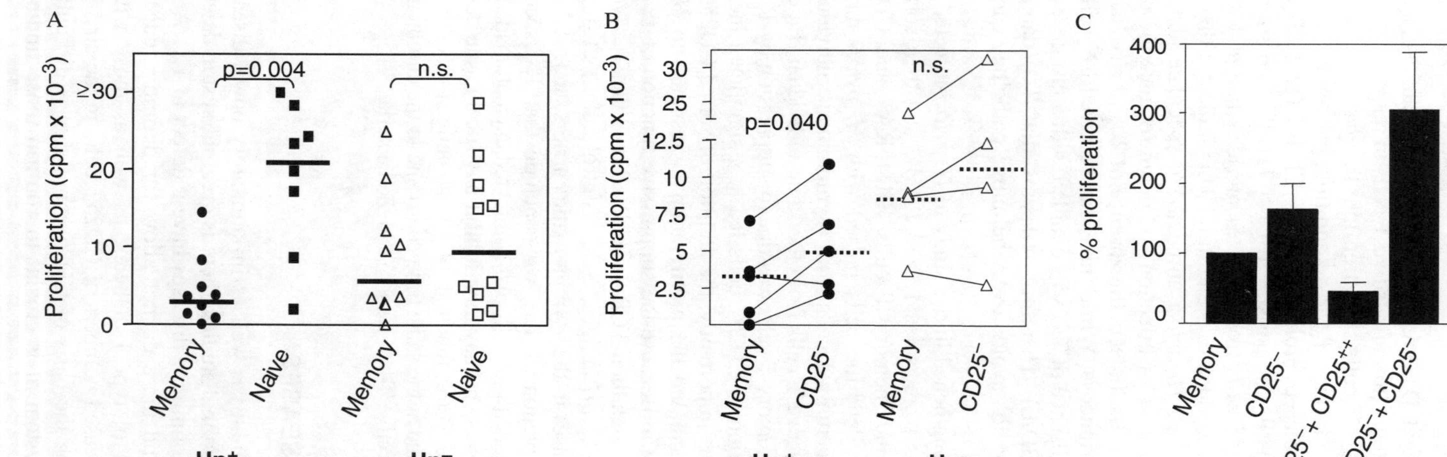

Figure 4 CD25$^+$ cells control the response of human *H. pylori*-specific memory T cells. PBMC from asymptomatic carriers of *H. pylori* (Hp+) and from *H. pylori*-negative control individuals (Hp−) were sorted into CD4$^+$ CD45RA$^+$CD62L$^+$ naive T cells, CD4$^+$ CD45RA$^-$ memory and CD4$^+$ CD45RA$^-$ CD25$^-$ memory T cells. A total of 10^5 cells were stimulated with monocyte-derived mature DC that had been pulsed with a membrane preparation of *H. pylori* strain Hel 305. Cell proliferation and IFN-γ production were measured after 5 days. **A**: While naive T cells from *H. pylori*-infected individuals displayed a significant antigen-specific proliferation towards *H. pylori* antigens, the memory T cells did not proliferate; nor did they secrete IFN-γ. **B**: Upon removal of CD25$^+$ cells there was a significant increase in the proliferation of memory T cells in the infected patients and a small non-significant increase in uninfected controls. **C**: The addition of CD25^{++} cells to CD25$^-$ cells at a 1 : 1 ratio resulted in suppression of the *H. pylori*-specific memory T cell proliferation. IFN-γ secretion mimicked the proliferation data[55]

functional assays showing the suppressive capacity of the T cells. Such studies are being attempted in MS patients. While numbers of CD25$^+$ cells are not altered their suppressive capacity after anti-CD3 stimulation is reduced[47]. Drawbacks of this study are that blood cells have been studied yielding little insight into the situation in the central nervous system and that MS-specific or self-antigens have not been included.

The opposite finding has been reported in rheumatoid arthritis. CD25$^+$ T$_{reg}$ are expanded in the synovium and suppress the helper T cell responses[48]. Activation and expansion of T$_{reg}$ has also been reported in cancer patients[49,50]. The timing of this activation, the antigen specificity of T$_{reg}$ in malignant diseases and their role in immune suppression in cancer await further studies. In mice depletion of T$_{reg}$, or a combination therapy of T$_{reg}$ depletion, activation of APC and blocking of CTLA-4 signalling, allowed for tumour eradication[15,51]. Further work is needed to determine the optimal combination of treatments that might in the long run be able to turn the immune suppression around and enable the immune system to fight cancer. However, this may lead to an activation of autoimmune diseases and overwhelming pathology in case of infections.

Patients with a defect in the Foxp3 gene show a severe activation of the immune system leading to lymphadenopathy and multiple autoimmune manifestations (immune dysregulation, polyendocrinopathy, enteropathy, X-linked syndrome, IPEX)[29]. The Foxp3 gene product scurfin has been shown to be essential for T$_{reg}$ function[29]. Since mice lacking scurfin due to a mutation in the Foxp3 gene lack CD25$^+$ T$_{reg}$ and develop a similar syndrome as do IPEX patients[52], it is very likely that these individuals lack functional T$_{reg}$. Signalling via the IL-2R is needed for the survival and/or function of CD25$^+$ T$_{reg}$ in the periphery and therefore IL2$^{-/-}$, CD25$^{-/-}$ and CD122$^{-/-}$ mice all lack functional T$_{reg}$ and develop a similar multiorgan inflammation and colitis[53]. Patients with IL-2Rα deficiency similarly develop infiltration in many organs[54]; thus, is it also conceivable that humans lacking CD25 develop their inflammatory diseases due to the absence of functional T$_{reg}$?

SYNOPSIS

The multitude of open questions regarding CD25$^+$ T$_{reg}$ has led many laboratories to work with CD25$^+$ cells. The questions span from the characterization of the suppressive 'subpopulation' and its molecular characterization, via the mechanism of suppression *in vitro* and *in vivo*, to studies of disease prevention and treatment in many different models of autoimmune diseases, transplantation tolerance, infectious immunity and cancer research. The possibility to transfer purified cells between mice, and to use various genetically manipulated animals, greatly facilitates these studies. In contrast, it is very difficult to study T$_{reg}$ in human disease. Only very few CD25$^+$ T$_{reg}$ can be isolated from human blood, and to isolate them from tissue biopsies is almost impossible. For the reliable analysis of the function of human T$_{reg}$ and their alteration in various human diseases new and easier techniques to test for T$_{reg}$ function are needed. To this end a T$_{reg}$ specific marker and an 'easy' functional test are required. With these tools we will hopefully understand the alterations in T_{reg} in human diseases. Further, the elucidation of the suppressive mechanism will hopefully provide fresh ideas for the development of new therapies for patients with autoimmune diseases that can actually cure these patients.

Acknowledgements

This work was supported by the Swedish Medical Research Council (MFR) Grant Nr. 71X-13487, the Swedish Cancer Society, FRF Stiftelse, SEB Banken, Konung Gustav V:s 80 Arsfond, and the Göteborg University Vaccine Research Institute (GUVAX).

References

1. Shevach EM. CD4[+] CD25[+] suppressor T cells: more questions than answers. Nat Rev Immunol. 2002;2:389–400.
2. Sakaguchi S, Takahashi T, Yamazaki S et al. Immunologic self tolerance maintained by T-cell-mediated control of self-reactive T cells: implications for autoimmunity and tumor immunity. Microbes Infect. 2001;3:911–18.
3. Lehmann J, Huehn J, de la Rosa M et al. Expression of the integrin alpha Ebeta 7 identifies unique subsets of CD25[+] as well as CD25[−] regulatory T cells. Proc Natl Acad Sci USA. 2002;99:13031–6.
4. Furtado GC, Olivares-Villagomez D, Curotto de Lafaille MA, Wensky AK, Latkowski JA, Lafaille JJ. Regulatory T cells in spontaneous autoimmune encephalomyelitis. Immunol Rev. 2001;182:122–34.
5. Apostolou I, Sarukhan A, Klein L, von Boehmer H. Origin of regulatory T cells with known specificity for antigen. Nat Immunol. 2002;3:756–63.
6. Roncarolo MG, Bacchetta R, Bordignon C, Narula S, Levings MK. Type 1 T regulatory cells. Immunol Rev. 2001;182:68–79.
7. Groux H, O'Garra A, Bigler M et al. A CD4[+] T-cell subset inhibits antigen-specific T-cell responses and prevents colitis. Nature. 1997;389:737–42.
8. Weiner HL. Induction and mechanism of action of transforming growth factor-beta-secreting Th3 regulatory cells. Immunol Rev. 2001;182:207–14.
9. Levings MK, Sangregorio R, Sartirana C et al. Human CD25[+]CD4[+] T suppressor cell clones produce transforming growth factor beta, but not interleukin 10, and are distinct from type 1 T regulatory cells. J Exp Med. 2002;196:1335–46.
10. Zhang X, Izikson L, Liu L, Weiner HL. Activation of CD25[+]CD4[+] regulatory T cells by oral antigen administration. J Immunol. 2001;167:4245–53.
11. Thorstenson KM, Khoruts A. Generation of anergic and potentially immunoregulatory CD25[+]CD4 T cells *in vivo* after induction of peripheral tolerance with intravenous or oral antigen. J Immunol. 2001;167:188–95.
12. Dieckmann D, Bruett CH, Ploettner H, Lutz MB, Schuler G. Human CD4[+]CD25[+] regulatory, contact-dependent T cells induce interleukin 10-producing, contact-independent type 1-like regulatory T cells [corrected]. J Exp Med. 2002;196:247–53.
13. Jonuleit H, Schmitt E, Kakirman H, Stassen M, Knop J, Enk AH. Infectious tolerance: human CD25[+] regulatory T cells convey suppressor activity to conventional CD4[+] T helper cells. J Exp Med. 2002;196:255–60.
14. Singh B, Read S, Asseman C et al. Control of intestinal inflammation by regulatory T cells. Immunol Rev. 2001;182:190–200.
15. Sakaguchi S, Sakaguchi N, Shimizu J et al. Immunologic tolerance maintained by CD25[+] CD4[+] regulatory T cells: their common role in controlling autoimmunity, tumor immunity, and transplantation tolerance. Immunol Rev. 2001;182:18–32.
16. Suri-Payer E, Cantor H. Differential cytokine requirements for regulation of autoimmune gastritis and colitis by CD4[+]CD25[+] T cells. J Autoimmun. 2001;16:115–23.
17. McHugh RS, Shevach EM, Thornton AM. Control of organ-specific autoimmunity by immunoregulatory CD4[+]CD25[+] T cells. Microbes Infect. 2001;3:919–27.

18. Suri-Payer E, Kehn PJ, Cheever AW, Shevach EM. Pathogenesis of post-thymectomy autoimmune gastritis. Identification of anti-H/K adenosine triphosphatase-reactive T cells. J Immunol. 1996;157:1799–805.

19. Suri-Payer E, Amar AZ, McHugh R, Natarajan K, Margulies DH, Shevach EM. Post-thymectomy autoimmune gastritis: fine specificity and pathogenicity of anti-H/K ATPase-reactive T cells. Eur J Immunol. 1999;29:669–77.

20. Gleeson PA, Toh BH. Molecular targets in pernicious anaemia. Immunol Today. 1991;12:233–8.

21. Gad M, Brimnes J, Claesson MH. CD4$^+$ T regulatory cells from the colonic lamina propria of normal mice inhibit proliferation of enterobacteria-reactive, disease-inducing Th1-cells from scid mice with colitis. Clin Exp Immunol. 2003;131:34–40.

22. Mottet C, Uhlig HH, Powrie F. Cutting edge: Cure of colitis by CD4$^+$CD25$^+$ regulatory T cells. J Immunol. 2003;170:3939–43.

23. Maloy KJ, Salaun L, Cahill R, Dougan G, Saunders NJ, Powrie F. CD4$^+$CD25$^+$ T(R) cells suppress innate immune pathology through cytokine-dependent mechanisms. J Exp Med. 2003;197:111–19.

24. Gad M, Brimnes J, Claesson MH. CD4$^+$ T cells react with enterobacterial antigens in the absence of CD4$^+$CD25$^+$ T cells and are regulated by naive progenitor CD4$^+$CD25$^+$ T regulatory cells. Keystone Symposium, University of Copenhagen, April 2003 (abstract).

25. Annacker O, Burlen-Defranoux O, Pimenta-Araujo R, Cumano A, Bandeira A. Regulatory CD4 T cells control the size of the peripheral activated/memory CD4 T cell compartment. J Immunol. 2000;164:3573–80.

26. Salomon B, Lenschow DJ, Rhee L et al. B7/CD28 costimulation is essential for the homeostasis of the CD4$^+$CD25$^+$ immunoregulatory T cells that control autoimmune diabetes. Immunity. 2000;12:431–40.

27. Kohm AP, Carpentier PA, Anger HA, Miller SD. Cutting edge: CD4$^+$CD25$^+$ regulatory T cells suppress antigen-specific autoreactive immune responses and central nervous system inflammation during active experimental autoimmune encephalomyelitis. J Immunol. 2002;169:4712–16.

28. Sakaguchi S. Regulatory T cells: mediating compromises between host and parasite. Nat Immunol. 2003;4:10–11.

29. Hori S, Nomura T, Sakaguchi S. Control of regulatory T cell development by the transcription factor Foxp3. Science. 2003;299:1057–61.

30. Shevach EM. Certified professionals: CD4$^+$CD25$^+$ suppressor T cells. J Exp Med. 2001;193:F41–6.

31. Baecher-Allan C, Brown JA, Freeman GJ, Hafler DA. CD4$^+$CD25^{high} regulatory cells in human peripheral blood. J Immunol. 2001;167:1245–53.

32. McHugh RS, Whitters MJ, Piccirillo CA et al. CD4$^+$CD25$^+$ immunoregulatory T cells: gene expression analysis reveals a functional role for the glucocorticoid-induced TNF receptor. Immunity. 2002;16:311–23.

33. Thornton AM, Shevach EM. CD4$^+$CD25$^+$ immunoregulatory T cells suppress polyclonal T cell activation in vitro by inhibiting interleukin 2 production. J Exp Med. 1998;188:287–96.

34. Wing K, Ekmark A, Karlsson H, Rudin A, Suri-Payer E. Characterization of human CD25$^+$CD4$^+$ T cells in thymus, cord and adult blood. Immunology. 2002;106:190–9.

35. Wing K, Lindgren S, Kollberg G et al. CD4 T cell activation by myelin oligodendrocyte glycoprotein is suppressed by adult but not cord blood CD25$^+$ T cells. Eur J Immunol. 2003;33:579–87.

36. Taams LS, Vukmanovic-Stejic M, Smith J et al. Antigen-specific T cell suppression by human CD4$^+$CD25$^+$ regulatory T cells. Eur J Immunol. 2002;32:1621–30.

37. Jonuleit H, Schmitt E, Stassen M, Tuettenberg A, Knop J, Enk AH. Identification and functional characterization of human CD4$^+$CD25$^+$ T cells with regulatory properties isolated from peripheral blood. J Exp Med. 2001;193:1285–94.

38. Stephens LA, Mottet C, Mason D, Powrie F. Human CD4$^+$CD25$^+$ thymocytes and peripheral T cells have immune suppressive activity *in vitro*. Eur J Immunol. 2001;31:1247–54.

39. Annunziato F, Cosmi L, Liotta F et al. Phenotype, localization, and mechanism of suppression of CD4$^+$CD25$^+$ human thymocytes. J Exp Med. 2002;196:379–87.

40. Itoh M, Takahashi T, Sakaguchi N et al. Thymus and autoimmunity: production of CD25$^+$CD4$^+$ naturally anergic and suppressive T cells as a key function of the thymus in maintaining immunologic self-tolerance. J Immunol. 1999;162:5317–26.

41. Kyewski B, Derbinski J, Gotter J, Klein L. Promiscuous gene expression and central T-cell tolerance: more than meets the eye. Trends Immunol. 2002;23:364–71.

42. Seddon B, Mason D. Peripheral autoantigen induces regulatory T cells that prevent autoimmunity. J Exp Med. 1999;189:877–82.
43. Belkaid Y, Piccirillo CA, Mendez S, Shevach EM, Sacks DL. CD4$^+$CD25$^+$ regulatory T cells control *Leishmania major* persistence and immunity. Nature. 2002;420:502–7.
44. Ernst PB, Gold BD. The disease spectrum of *Helicobacter pylori*: the immunopathogenesis of gastroduodenal ulcer and gastric cancer. Annu Rev Microbiol. 2000;54:615–40.
45. Raghavan S, Fredriksson M, Svennerholm A-M, Holmgren J, Suri-Payer E. Absence of CD4$^+$CD25$^+$ regulatory T cells is associated with a loss of regulation leading to increased pathology in *Helicobacter pylori*-infected mice. Clin Exp Immunol. 2003;132:393–400.
46. Kukreja A, Cost G, Marker J et al. Multiple immuno-regulatory defects in type-1 diabetes. J Clin Invest. 2002;109:131–40.
47. Viglietta V, Baecher-Allan C, Hafler D. CD4$^+$CD25$^+$ regulatory T cells have reduced function in patients with multiple sclerosis. Clin Immunol. 2003 (Suppl. 1):S175.
48. Cao D, Malmstrom V, Baecher-Allan C, Hafler D, Klareskog L, Trollmo C. Isolation and functional characterization of regulatory CD25^{bright}CD4$^+$ T cells from the target organ of patients with rheumatoid arthritis. Eur J Immunol. 2003;33:215–23.
49. Woo EY, Yeh H, Chu CS et al. Cutting edge: regulatory T cells from lung cancer patients directly inhibit autologous T cell proliferation. J Immunol. 2002;168:4272–6.
50. Wolf AM, Wolf D, Steurer M, Gastl G, Gunsilius E, Grubeck-Loebenstein B. Increase of regulatory T cells in the peripheral blood of cancer patients. Clin Cancer Res. 2003;9:606–12.
51. Sutmuller RP, van Duivenvoorde LM, van Elsas A et al. Synergism of cytotoxic T lymphocyte-associated antigen 4 blockade and depletion of CD25$^+$ regulatory T cells in antitumor therapy reveals alternative pathways for suppression of autoreactive cytotoxic T lymphocyte responses. J Exp Med. 2001;194:823–32.
52. Fontenot JD, Gavin MA, Rudensky AY. Foxp3 programs the development and function of CD4$^+$CD25$^+$ regulatory T cells. Nat Immunol. 2003;4:330–6.
53. Almeida AR, Legrand N, Papiernik M, Freitas AA. Homeostasis of peripheral CD4$^+$ T cells: IL-2R alpha and IL-2 shape a population of regulatory cells that controls CD4$^+$ T cell numbers. J Immunol. 2002;169:4850–60.
54. Roifman CM. Human IL-2 receptor alpha chain deficiency. Pediatr Res. 2000;48:6–11.
55. Lundgren A, Suri-Payer E, Enarsson K, Svennerholm AM, Lundin BS. *Helicobacter pylori*-specific CD4$^+$ CD25^{high} regulatory T cells suppress memory T-cell responses to *H. pylori* in infected individuals. Infect Immun. 2003;71:1755–62.

15
Human CD25$^+$ regulatory T cells in inflammatory bowel disease

J. MAUL, M. ZEITZ and R. DUCHMANN

INTRODUCTION

CD4$^+$CD25$^+$ T cells have been initially described in rodents as a population of immunoregulatory T cells (T$_{reg}$) that prevent the development of several autoimmune diseases by actively suppressing the activation and expansion of self-reactive lymphocytes.

In mice the injection of spleen or lymph node cells that were depleted of CD25$^+$ cells into T-cell-deficient animals leads to the development of various autoimmune diseases as autoimmune gastritis, thyroiditis and oophoritis. The coinjection of CD25$^+$ cells blocks the activation of self-reactive T cells and thus prevents autoimmunity[1].

CD4$^+$CD25$^+$ T$_{reg}$ also have potent anti-inflammatory capacity in animal models of intestinal inflammation. They not only prevent experimentally induced colitis but also reverse established pathology[2]. CD4$^+$CD25$^+$ T$_{reg}$ also control aberrant inflammatory immune responses towards microbial antigens. Thus, mice depleted of T$_{reg}$ could no longer control their T-cell response to normal intestinal flora and consequently developed chronic intestinal inflammation. Therefore, CD4$^+$CD25$^+$ T cells are likely candidates to search for inadequate counterregulation in human IBD.

CHARACTERISTICS OF CD4$^+$CD25$^+$ T$_{reg}$

In rodents nearly all CD25$^+$ T cells show regulatory properties[3]. In addition, T$_{reg}$ in rodent models have been shown to be present within the CD45RB^{low} [4] or the integrin $\alpha_E\beta_7$ positive T cell populations[5]. Human T$_{reg}$, in contrast, represent a subpopulation within the CD25$^+$ T-cell pool. They form a tail to the right on CD25$^+$ flow cytometry and can thus be identified by their high density of the IL-2 receptor

α chain[6,7]. They co-express the IL-2 receptor β chain CD122. CD25 and CD122 form the high-affinity IL-2 receptor, although it is not shown that these two molecules are really functionally associated on the cell surface of T_{reg}. Interleukin-2 seems to be required for the generation of CD25$^+$ regulatory cells since these cells are absent in IL-2-deficient animals[8]. Interestingly, addition of IL-2 *in vitro* not only breaks[5] proliferative arrest of CD4$^+$CD25$^+$ T_{reg} but also breaks their suppressive capacity[9,10].

CD25$^+$ is up-regulated on activated cells and it is neither an exclusive nor a specific marker for T_{reg}. Recent reports, however, show that the transcription factor Foxp3 might be a specific marker for CD4$^+$CD25$^+$ regulatory cells[11]. In contrast to most phenotypic markers, which are quite likely surrogate markers related to the differentiation of T_{reg}, the expression of Foxp3 seems to be crucial for their functional characteristics. This was shown by introducing the Foxp3 gene into naive CD4$^+$CD25$^-$ T cells which subsequently displayed anergic/suppressive function.

Like in their rodent counterparts, human CD4$^+$CD25$^+$ T_{reg} are characterized by their intracellular expression of CTLA-4[10,12]. However, CTLA-4-mediated suppression does not seem to be as important for CD4$^+$CD25$^+$ T_{reg} function as it is in mice. Human T_{reg} apparently mediate cell-contact-dependent suppression, which may involve PD-1[6], whereas soluble factors such as IL-10, IL-4 or TGF-β, which characterize rodent regulatory cells, do not seem to play a role[10,13,14]. However, although cytokines do not seem to be directly involved in the suppressive activity of CD4$^+$CD25$^+$ T_{reg}, two recent studies[21,22] demonstrate that cytokines may be indirectly involved in CD4$^+$CD25$^+$ T_{reg}-mediated suppression, as these cells also convey cell-contact-dependent 'catalytic/infectious' suppressor activity to conventional CD4$^+$ T cells. These 'infected' cells are subsequently able to suppress CD4$^+$ T cells in a soluble manner involving TGF-β or IL-10. Thus, few CD4$^+$CD25^{high} cells, when present in the intestine, could amplify their suppressive effects through CD4$^+$CD25$^-$ T cells. This could be an additional explanation for the unresponsiveness of normal lamina propria T cells[23] and their high production of IL-10[24].

CD4$^+$CD25$^+$ T$_{reg}$ IN HUMAN DISEASE

There is still little information on the frequency and function of T_{reg} in human diseases. First studies indicate an important role in cancer, diabetes mellitus type I and rheumatoid arthritis. In patients with epithelial malignancies, increased numbers of suppressor CD4$^+$CD25$^+$ T cells were found in the circulation[15] and in cancer tissue[16] where they might inhibit anti-tumour responses. In contrast, evidence was provided for a decrease of T_{reg} in the peripheral blood of patients with immune-mediated diabetes mellitus[17], suggesting that impairment of regulatory cells favours the development of autoimmunity. In another autoimmune disease, rheumatoid arthritis, however, CD25$^+$ T cells were normally expressed in peripheral blood but strongly enriched in synovial fluid[7].

CD4$^+$CD25$^+$ T$_{reg}$ IN IBD

IBD may be described as a dysbalance of the immune system caused by an excess of inflammatory stimuli and mediators and an inadequate function or number of cellular components that down-regulate the mucosal immune response[18]. With regard to the latter, preliminary studies from our group indicate that CD4$^+$CD25^{high} T cells maintain their highly suppressive activity in patients with IBD and effectively inhibit proliferation of CD4$^+$CD25$^-$ cells. In contrast to their preserved functionality, however, the frequency of CD4$^+$CD25$^+$ T$_{reg}$ varied with disease activity in both Crohn's disease and ulcerative colitis patients with an increase in inactive and a decrease in active disease.

The cause for this change in frequency of peripheral CD25^{high} T cells is still unclear. In addition, there are at present no data available on the frequency and function of T$_{reg}$ within normal or diseased human intestine. In principle, expansion of T$_{reg}$ might be driven by the inflammation that they regulate, and thus occur at the site of inflammation. Similar to the situation in an animal model of colitis, where transferred CD4$^+$CD25$^+$ T cells invaded the intestine, proliferated in the inflamed lamina propria, resolved the inflammation and consequently cured colits[2], one could therefore expect that an influx of regulatory cells into the site of intestinal inflammation also occurs in human IBD. In the inflamed tissue their proliferative arrest could be broken, e.g. through stimulation via their T-cell receptors (TCR) in the presence of high levels of IL-2, resulting in an expansion of T$_{reg}$ in the inflamed intestine. Although activation of T$_{reg}$ via anti-CD3 and IL-2 abrogates the suppressive capacity of T$_{reg}$, it has been shown that the expanded population regains its suppressive function. This expanded regulatory population could then contribute to resolve intestinal inflammation by restoring the balance between inflammatory and regulatory components (Figure 1).

Alternatively, T$_{reg}$ might expand in the non-inflamed intestine following stimulation through endogenous antigens, e.g. from the intestinal flora[19]. CD25$^+$ T$_{reg}$ express TCR for interaction with peptide antigen and Toll-like receptors (TLR) for interaction with conserved microbial patterns[20], and are thus amenable to differential regulation when stimulated by bacterial products (Figure 2).

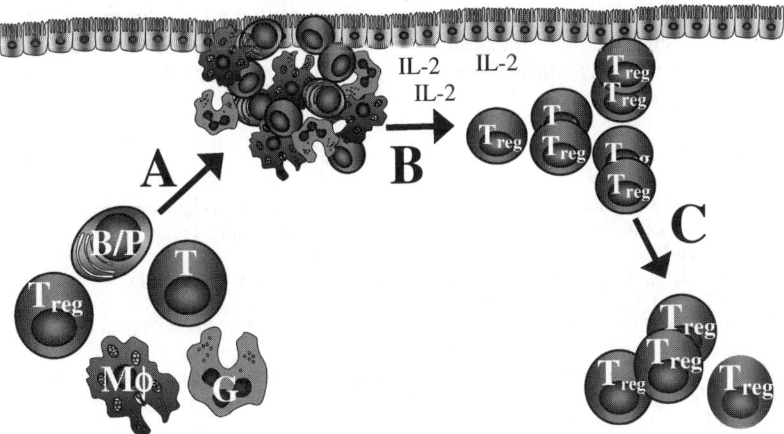

Figure 1 Expansion of regulatory T cells during inflammation. **A:** Recruitment of inflammatory cells (T$_{reg}$, regulatory T cell; T, T cell; B/P, B-/plasma cell; Mϕ, monocyte/macrophage; G, granulocyte) to the site of intestinal inflammation. **B:** Proliferation of T$_{reg}$ through high levels of IL-2 in inflammatory milieu. **C:** Resolution of inflammation and recirculation of expanded T$_{reg}$

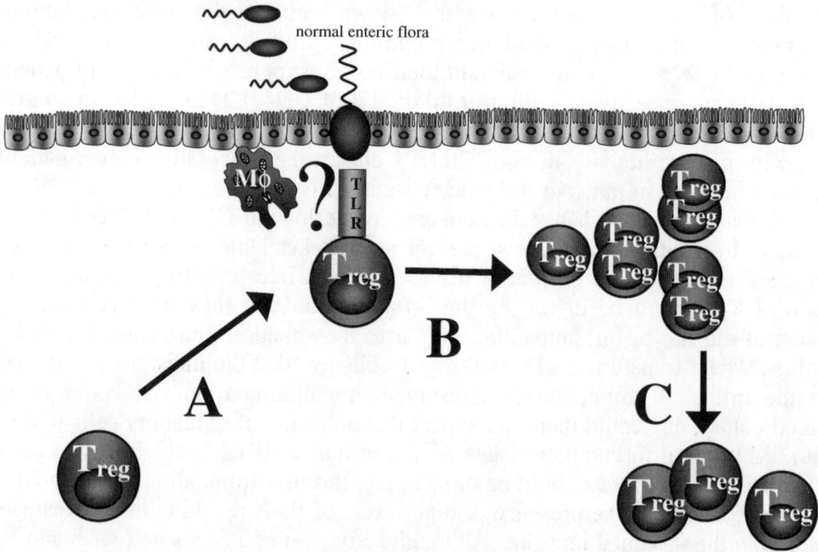

Figure 2 Expansion of regulatory T cells by interaction with normal enteric flora. **A:** Regulatory T cells (T_{reg}) circulate in the gut. T_{reg} express Toll-like-receptors (TLR) for interaction with bacterial components. In this interaction gut epithelial cells or macrophages (Mɸ) may be involved. **B:** Proliferation of T_{reg}. **C:** Recirculation of expanded T_{reg}

Intuitively, one might expect that expansion of T_{reg} at inflammatory sites represents a physiological response to shut off inflammation in infectious diseases, e.g. diverticulitis, whereas inflammation in IBD is more likely associated with a defect in the generation of T_{reg}. In that scenario the expansion of the intestinal $CD25^+$ T_{reg} pool during remission, and its contraction during relapse, would be inverse to the expansion and contraction of inflammatory, e.g. Th1 or Th2 cell, populations during these phases, and be reflected in the circulating $CD25^+$ T_{reg} pool.

References

1. Sakaguchi S, Sakaguchi N, Shimizu J et al. Immunologic tolerance maintained by $CD25^+$ $CD4^+$ regulatory T cells: their common role in controlling autoimmunity, tumor immunity, and transplantation tolerance. Immunol Rev. 2001;182:18–32.
2. Mottet C, Uhlig HH, Powrie F. Cutting edge: cure of colitis by CD4(+)CD25(+) regulatory T cells. J Immunol. 2003;170:3939–43.
3. Thornton AM, Shevach EM. Suppressor effector function of $CD4^+CD25^+$ imunoregulatory cells is antigen nonspecific. J Immunol. 2000;164:183–90.
4. Read S, Malmstrom V, Powrie F. Cytotoxic T lymphocyte-associated antigen 4 plays an essential role in the function of CD25(+)CD4(+) regulatory cells that control intestinal inflammation. J Exp Med. 2000;192:295–302.
5. Lehmann J, Huehn J, de la Rosa M et al. Expression of the integrin alpha Ebeta 7 identifies unique subsets of $CD25^+$ as well as $CD25^-$ regulatory T cells. Proc Natl Acad Sci USA. 2002;99:13031–6.
6. Baecher-Allan C, Brown JA, Freeman GJ, Hafler DA. $CD4^+$CD25high regulatory cells in human peripheral blood. J Immunol. 2001;167:1245–53.

7. Cao D, Malmstrom V, Baecher-Allan C, Hafler D, Klareskog L, Trollmo C. Isolation and functional characterization of regulatory CD25brightCD4+ T cells from the target organ of patients with rheumatoid arthritis. Eur J Immunol. 2003;33:215–23.

8. Papiernik M, de Maoraes ML, Pontoux C, Vasseur F, Penit C. Regulatory CD4 T cells: expression of IL-2R alpha chain, resistance to clonal deletion and IL-2 dependency. Int Immunol. 1998;10:371–8.

9. Ng WF, Duggan PJ, Ponchel F et al. Human CD4+CD25+ cells: a naturally occurring population of regulatory T cells. Blood. 2001;98:2736–44.

10. Jonuleit H, Schmitt E, Stassen M, Tuettenberg A, Knop J, Enk AH. Identification and functional characterization of human CD4+CD25+ T cells with regulatory properties isolated from peripheral blood. J Exp Med. 2001;193:1285–94.

11. Hori S, Nomura T, Sakaguchi S. Control of regulatory T cell development by the transcription factor FOXP3. Science. 2003;299:1057–61.

12. Wing K, Ekmark A, Karlsson H, Rudin A, Suri-Payer E. Characterization of human CD25+CD4+ T cells in thymus, cord and adult blood. Immunology. 2002;106:190–9.

13. Taams LS, Smith J, Rustin MH, Salmon M, Poulter LW, Akbar A. Human anergic/suppressive CD4+CD25+ T cells: a highly differentiated and apoptosis-prone population. J Immunol. 2001;31:1122–31.

14. Levings MK, Sangregorio R, Roncarolo M-G. Human CD25+CD4+ T regulatory cells suppress naive and memory T cell proliferation and can be expanded in vitro without loss of function. J Exp Med. 2001;193:1295–301.

15. Wolf AM, Wolf D, Steurer M, Gastl G, Gunsilius E, Grubeck-Loebenstein B. Increase of regulatory T cells in the peripheral blood of cancer patients. Clin Cancer Res. 2003;9:606.

16. Woo EY, Yeh H, Chu CS et al. Cutting edge: regulatory T cells from lung cancer patients directly inhibit autologous T cell proliferation. J Immunol. 2002;168:4272–6.

17. Kukreja A, Cost G, Marker J et al. Multiple immuno-regulatory defects in type-1 diabetes. J Clin Invest. 2002;109:131–40.

18. Strober W, Fuss IJ, Blumberg RS. The immunology of mucosal models of inflammation. Annu Rev Immunol. 2002;20:495–549.

19. Duchmann R, Kaiser I, Hermann E, Mayet W, Ewe K, Meyer zum Buschenfelde KH. Tolerance exists towards resident intestinal flora but is broken in active inflammatory bowel disease (IBD). Clin Exp Immunol. 1995;102:448–55.

20. Sakaguchi S. Control of immune responses by naturally arising CD4+ regulatory T cells that express Toll-like receptors. J Exp Med. 2003;197:397–401.

21. Dieckmann D, Bruett CH, Ploettner H, Lutz MB, Schuler G. Human CD4(+)CD25(+) regulatory, contact-dependent T cells induce interleukin 10-producing, contact-independent type 1-like regulatory T cells [corrected]. J Exp Med. 2002;196:247–53.

22. Jonuleit H, Schmitt E, Kakirman H, Stassen M, Knop J, Enk AH. Infectious tolerance: human CD25(+) regulatory T cells convey suppressor activity to conventional CD4(+) T helper cells. J Exp Med. 2002;196:255–60.

23. Zeitz M, Quinn T, Graeff A, James S. Mucosal T cells provide helper function but do not proliferate when stimulated by specific antigen in lymphogranuloma venereum proctitis in nonhuman primates. Gastroenterology. 1988;94:353–66.

24. Braunstein J, Qiao L, Autschbach F, Schurmann G, Meuer S. T cells of the human intestinal lamina propria are high producers of interleukin-10. Gut. 1997;41:215–20.

Section IV
Modulation of mucosal immune responses by targeting cytokines and accessory molecules

16
The Smad signalling pathway in Crohn's disease and ulcerative colitis

T. T. MACDONALD and G. MONTELEONE

INTRODUCTION

Mice lacking TGF-β_1 develop widespread inflammation including the gut[1], and it is generally considered that TGF-β is a master negative regulator of intestinal inflammation. TGF-β is made by many cell types, but particular attention has been paid to its production by T cells, so-called regulatory cells. There is now evidence in a number of systems that TGF-β_1-secreting T cells or membrane-bound TGF-β_1 on regulatory cells can prevent inflammation, including experimental colitis[2–5].

This work, however, presents a problem when translated into clinical inflammatory bowel disease since, in inflamed gut, TGF-β is made by many different cell types and is present in abundance in inflamed tissue. In this situation it is very difficult to imagine how T-cell-specific TGF-β_1 could down-regulate inflammation in the mucosa. There is the possibility that Th3 cells mediate their activity in gut-associated lymphoid tissues at the inductive phase of colitogenic T cells, but this is not amenable for study in humans. We have therefore been interested in the control of TGF-β_1 signalling in normal and inflamed human intestinal mucosa.

Smad SIGNALLING

TGF-β_1 initiates signalling through the ligand-dependent activation of a complex of heterodimeric transmembrane serine/threonine kinases, consisting of type I (TGF-β_1RI) and type II (TGF-β_1RII) receptors (Figure 1). Upon TGF-β_1 binding the receptors rotate relatively within the complex, resulting in phosphorylation and activation of TGF-β_1RI by the constitutively active and auto-phosphorylated

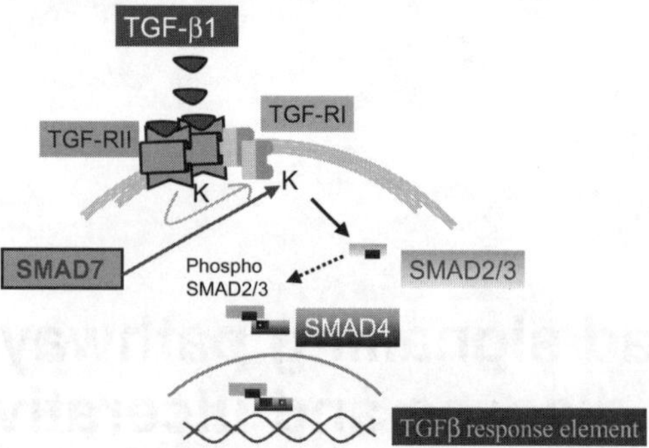

Figure 1 Diagrammatic illustration of the TGF-β signalling pathway and its inhibition by Smad7. For details, see text

TGF-β_1RII[6]. TGF-β_1 signals from the receptor to the nucleus using a set of proteins, termed Smads, based on their high homology to the *Drosophila* Mad and the *Caenorhabditis elegans* Sma proteins. To date, nine different Smad genes which fall into three distinct functional sets have been identified: signal-transducing receptor-activated Smads, which include Smad1, 2, 3, 5, 8 and 9; a single common mediator, Smad4, and inhibitory Smad6 and 7[7,8]. Activated TGF-β_1RI directly phosphorylates Smad2 and Smad3 at serine residues in the carboxy-terminal SSXS sequence[8,9]. Once activated, Smad2 and Smad3 associate with Smad4 and translocate to the nucleus where Smad protein complexes participate in transcriptional control of target genes[8–10]. Importantly, targeted disruption of the Smad3 gene is associated with diminished cell responsiveness[11] to TGF-β_1. Mutant mice exhibit a massive infiltration of T cells and pyogenic abscess formation in the stomach and intestine, supporting the view that Smad3 is an essential mediator of the TGF-β_1-induced anti-inflammatory and suppressive activities[11]. The inhibitory Smad7 acts by occupying ligand-activated TGF-β_1RI and interfering with the phosphorylation of Smad2/Smad3 (Figure 1). Up-regulation of Smad7 has been associated with an inhibition of TGF-β_1-induced signalling[12,13]. Although the mechanisms that regulate Smad7 production are not fully known, recent studies have shown that activators of either NFκB (e.g. TNF-α and IL-1β) or STAT-1 (e.g. IFN-γ) pathway can enhance Smad7 expression[14,15].

Smad SIGNALLING IN IBD

We have provided evidence for defective Smad signalling in chronic gut inflammation in the colon in IBD[16] and the stomach in *Helicobacter pylori* gastritis[17]. The inhibitory Smad-Smad7- is over-expressed in IBD mucosa and purified mucosal T cells, and in both whole tissue and isolated cells there is defective TGF-β_1 signalling as measured by reduced phospho-Smad3 immunoreactivity. Specific anti-sense oligonucleotides for Smad7 reduce Smad7 protein in cells isolated from IBD patients, and the cells then become responsive to exogenous TGF-β_1. TGF-β_1 cannot inhibit proinflammatory cytokine production in isolated lamina

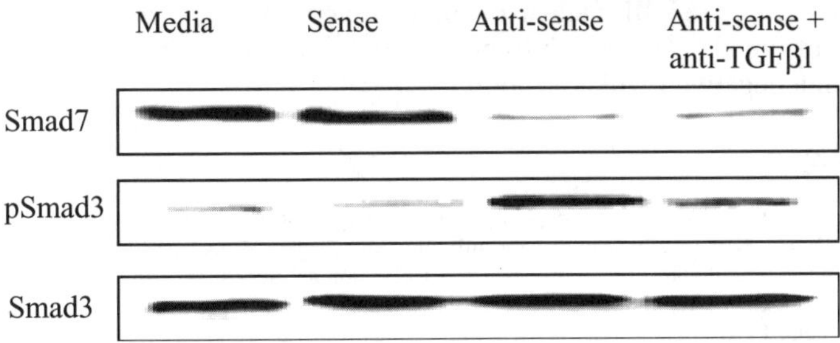

Figure 2 Western blot analysis of lamina propria mononuclear cells from a patient with Crohn's disease treated overnight in medium alone, with a sense oligonucleotide to Smad7, an anti-sense to Smad7 and an anti-sense to Smad7, along with neutralizing goat anti-TGF-β_1 antibody. The anti-sense reduces Smad7 protein. At the same time, phosphorylated Smad3 is increased in the same cells. The increase in pSmad3 is inhibited by anti-TGF-β_1, showing that it is endogenous TGF-β_1 in the culture which is inducing pSmad3

propria mononuclear cells (LPMC) from Crohn's disease (CD) patients, but inhibition of Smad7 with anti-sense oligonucleotides restores TGF-β_1 signalling and allows TGF-β_1 to inhibit cytokine production. In inflamed mucosal tissue explants from CD patients, inhibition of Smad7 also restores p-Smad3 (Figure 2) and decreases proinflammatory cytokine production, an effect which is partially blocked by anti-TGF-β_1. We have extended these studies to examine the interactions between Smad signalling and NFκB activation in inflamed gut[18]. While TGF-β_1 is a potent inhibitor of TNF-α-induced NFκB activation in normal gut, it has no activity in inflamed gut. This can be attributed to over expression of Smad7, since treatment of cells from inflamed gut with anti-sense to Smad7 allows TGF-β_1 to rapidly down-regulate NFκB activation.

Our recent studies on *H. pylori* gastritis[17] have further emphasized the role of Smad7 in promoting gut inflammation; however, in this model we are able to show that blocking IFN-γ lowers Smad7 in gastric biopsies from *H. pylori*-infected patients. Furthermore, IFN-γ on its own induces Smad7 in normal gastric biopsies.

REGULATION OF Smad7 IN INFLAMED GUT

The implication of these results is, therefore, that if it becomes possible to specifically inhibit Smad7, then endogenous TGF-β_1 in the inflamed gut can negatively regulate proinflammatory cytokine production and NFκB activation, the major components of the immune overactivity which drives tissue injury in IBD. At the same time, however, it is important to discover the factors which control Smad7 expression in inflamed gut. Furthermore, cell-specific expression of Smad7 will be important because TGF-β_1 has different effects on different cell types. Thus while blocking Smad7 will allow TGF-β_1 to reduce proinflammatory cytokine production by T cells and macrophages, in myofibroblasts it may allow TGF-β_1 to increase collagen production, resulting in fibrosis. However, at the moment we are still unclear of the relative importance in the gut of known inducers of Smad7 such as IFN-γ or TNF-α[14,15], or even if TGF-β_1 itself induces Smad7 in a negative regulatory loop[19].

References

1. Shull MM, Ormsby I, Kier AB et al. Targeted disruption of the mouse transforming growth factor-beta 1 gene results in multifocal inflammatory disease. Nature. 1992;359:693–9.
2. Nakamura K, Kitani A, Strober W. Cell contact-dependent immunosuppression by CD4(+)CD25(+) regulatory T cells is mediated by cell surface-bound transforming growth factor beta. J Exp Med. 2001;194:629–44.
3. Fuss IJ, Boirivant M, Lacy B, Strober W. The interrelated roles of TGF-beta and IL-10 in the regulation of experimental colitis. J Immunol. 2002;168:900–8.
4. Oida T, Zhang X, Goto M et al. CD4$^+$CD25$^-$ T cells that express latency-associated peptide on the surface suppress CD4$^+$CD45 RB^{high}-induced colitis by a TGF-β-dependent mechanism. J Immunol. 2003;170:2516–22.
5. Powrie F, Carlino J, Leach MW, Mauze S, Coffman RL. A critical role for transforming growth factor-beta but not interleukin 4 in the suppression of T helper type 1-mediated colitis by CD45RB(low) CD4$^+$ T cells. J Exp Med. 1996;183:2669–74.
6. Piek E, Heldin CH, Ten Dijke P. Specificity, diversity, and regulation in TGF-beta superfamily signaling. FASEB J. 1999;13:2105–24.
7. Heldin CH, Miyazono K, Ten Dijke P. TGF-beta signalling from cell membrane to nucleus through SMAD proteins. Nature. 1997;390:465–71.
8. Derynck R, Zhang Y, Feng XH. Smads: transcriptional activators of TGF-beta responses. Cell. 1998;95:737–40.
9. Abdollah S, Macias-Silva M, Tsukazaki T, Hayashi H, Attisano L, Wrana JL. TbetaRI phosphorylation of Smad2 on Ser465 and Ser467 is required for Smad2-Smad4 complex formation and signaling. J Biol Chem. 1997;272:27678–85.
10. Dennler S, Itoh S, Vivien D, Ten Dijke P, Huet S, Gauthier JM. Direct binding of Smad3 and Smad4 to critical TGF beta-inducible elements in the promoter of human plasminogen activator inhibitor-type 1 gene. EMBO J. 1998;17:3091–100.
11. Yang X, Letterio JJ, Lechleider RJ et al. Targeted disruption of SMAD3 results in impaired mucosal immunity and diminished T cell responsiveness to TGF-beta. EMBO J. 1999;18:1280–91.
12. Hayashi H, Abdollah S, Qiu Y et al. The MAD-related protein Smad7 associates with the TGFbeta receptor and functions as an antagonist of TGFbeta signaling. Cell. 1997;89:1165–73.
13. Nakao A, Afrakhte M, Moren A et al. Identification of Smad7, a TGFbeta-inducible antagonist of TGF-beta signalling. Nature. 1997;389:631–5.
14. Bitzer M, von Gersdorff G, Liang D et al. A mechanism of suppression of TGF-beta/SMAD signaling by NF-kappa B/RelA. Genes Dev. 2000;14:187–97.
15. Ulloa L, Doody J, Massague J. Inhibition of transforming growth factor-beta/SMAD signalling by the interferon-gamma/STAT pathway. Nature. 1999;397:710–13.
16. Monteleone G, Kumberova A, Croft NM, McKenzie C, Steer HW, MacDonald TT. Blocking Smad7 restores TGF-beta1 signaling in chronic inflammatory bowel disease. J Clin Invest. 2001;108:601–9.
17. Monteleone G, Mann J, Monteleone I et al. A failure of TGFβ1 negative regulation maintains sustained NK-KB activation in gut inflammation. J Biol Chem. (in press).
18. Monteleone G, Del Vecchio Blanco G et al. Defective TGFb1 signaling associates with high Smad7 in the gastric mucosa of patients with *H. pylori* infection. Gastroenterology (in press).
19. von Gersdorff G, Susztak K, Rezvani F, Bitzer M, Liang D, Bottinger EP. Smad3 and Smad4 mediate transcriptional activation of the human Smad7 promoter by transforming growth factor beta. J Biol Chem. 2000;275:11320–6.

17
Regulation of Th1 polarization in mucosal CD4$^+$ T-cell responses

J. REIMANN

INTRODUCTION

More than 90% of the challenges of the immune system with antigens (or pathogenic microorganisms) take place at mucous membranes. A first line of defence in the mucosa are cells of the innate immune system and specific, T-cell receptor (TCR) αβ-expressing T cells. The mucosal T cells display specific recognition, mediate a large spectrum of effector functions and are assumed to play the key role in the regulation of mucosal, innate and specific immune responses. Individual T-cell responses primed and restimulated *in vivo* tend to be polarized and only rarely express a balanced cytokine expression profile. Polarization is evident by the exclusive or preferential expression of signature (or hallmark) cytokines by CD4$^+$ T cells, i.e. IFN-γ and TNF (IL-2, LTα/β) by Th1 T cells, and IL-4 and IL-13 (IL-5, IL-9) by Th2 T cells (Figure 1). A balance of polarizations of the T-cell responses continuously going on in the mucosa of the lungs and the gut is essential for the integrity of these fragile tissues. Clinical experience suggests that, in the lung, deregulated T-cell responses tend to default towards a Th2 pattern (giving rise to asthma) while, in the gut, deregulated T-cell responses tend to default towards a Th1 pattern (giving rise to different syndromes of inflammatory bowel disease, IBD). It has been proposed that the declining incidence of either virus infections of the airways[1], or helminth infestations of the intestine[2,3] may play a role in the increasingly observed, deregulated polarization of mucosal T-cell responses leading to important and widespread immunopathologies.

Many preclinical models are available in mice and rats for the study of IBD. An observation emerging from most (but not all) studies on the immunopathogenesis of colitis in these models is a key role of CD4$^+$ T cells responding to antigens from the gut flora[4]. The study of the dysregulation of this interaction that leads to overwhelming Th1-biased mucosal T-cell responses is at the centre of many

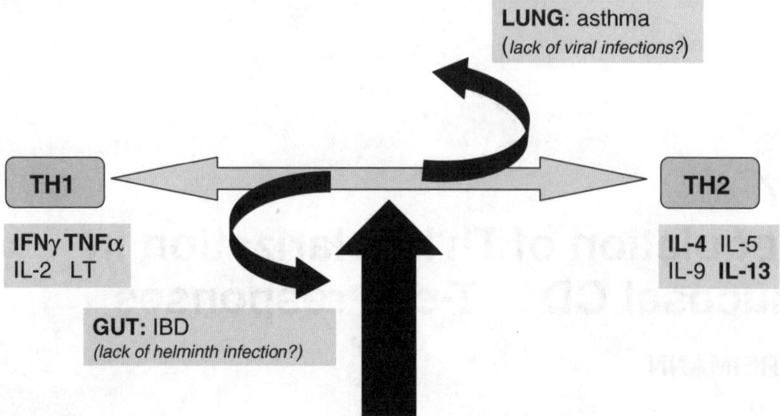

Figure 1   Mucosa-associated T-cell immunity. Multispecific T-cell responses in mucous membranes are supposed to show a balanced pattern of Th1 and Th2 cytokines. Pathologies arise from the deviation from a balanced cytokine release pattern. In the lung, T-cell responses tend to deviate more frequently towards a Th2 pattern (leading to asthma). In the gut, T-cell responses often deviate towards a Th1 pattern (leading to IBD). The signature cytokines for Th1 are interferon-γ (IFN-γ), tumour necrosis factor-α (TNF-α), interleukin (IL)-2 and lymphotoxin (LT); signature cytokines for Th2 are IL-4, IL-5, IL-9 and IL-13

research strategies. No consensus exists on the nature of the four key players in this response, i.e. (a) the triggering bacterial antigen recognized by T cells; (b) the responding CD4$^+$ T-cell subset that develops pathogenic effector functions; (c) the presenting cell that stimulates or modulates the response; and (d) the regulatory cells that determine the phenotype of the presenting and/or responding cells.

The processes involved in early triggering of pathogenic, mucosal T-cell responses are largely unresolved. Unless a structural lesion of the epithelial barrier initiates the disease process, antigen has to pass intestinal epithelial cells (IEC) to access the mucosal T-cell system (step 1 in Figure 2). Antigen can be delivered to antigen-presenting cells (APC) in the lamina propria (LP) or in organized, inductive sites (e.g. Peyer's patches, PP, or intestinal lymph follicles, ILF) either directly, or by a cross-priming event. Evidence for the latter has been reported[5,6]. Homing of T cells to subepithelial clusters of dendritic cells (DC) at the interface of the LP and the mucosa has been described in transfer colitis models[7,8]. Priming or restimulation of CD4$^+$ T cells by DC (step 2 in Figure 2) may take place *in situ* (in PP, ILF or the LP), or in regional mesenteric lymph nodes (MLN). The extensive heterogeneity of phenotypes of DC, effector T cells and regulatory T cells in the LP and MLN makes it exceedingly difficult to identify the early interactions that initiate the pathogenic T-cell reactivity.

This chapter will discuss current concepts addressing three issues related to priming and regulating pathogenic CD4$^+$ T cell responses in the mucosa. These are:

1. What regulates and maintains Th1 polarization of CD4$^+$ T cell responses?
2. What are the effector CD4$^+$ T cells in IBD-inducing cellular immune responses?
3. What are putative regulator CD4$^+$ T cells, the failure (or absence) of which allow the manifestation of the IBD-inducing potential of pathogenic CD4$^+$ T cells?

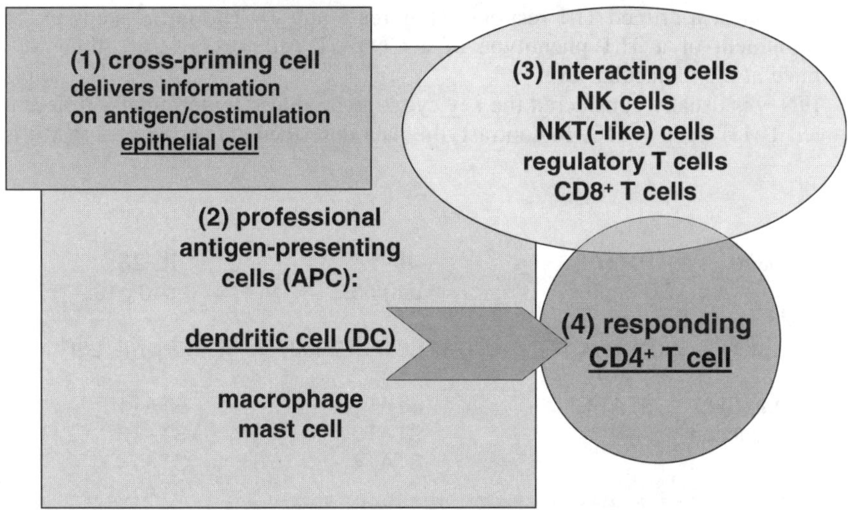

Figure 2 Mucosal T cell priming. (1) Antigen usually accesses the mucosa through the epithelial barrier; hence T-cell activation operates through cross-priming. (2) The professional antigen-presenting cell (APC) involved is probably a specialized dendritic cell (DC). (3) Regulatory cells operate at the level of the APC and/or at the level of the responding T cell; a variety of immune cell subsets have been shown to be able to exert regulatory effects on mucosal T-cell responses. (4) The responding T cells receive input from the cross-priming antigen and APC, as well as T_R cells that control its further development

Th1 POLARIZATION OF CD4$^+$ T CELL RESPONSES

Initiation of Th1 development of CD4$^+$ T cells operates in a comparatively simple way: IFN-γ binding to the IFNGR (together with TCR/CD3 and WSX-1/TCCR) generates a signal that STAT1 transduces; and that switches on the master regulator of Th1 polarization, T-bet (the only T box gene specifically expressed in lymphoid cells)[9,10]. There is ample evidence that supports this notion. T-bet$^{-/-}$ knockout mice do not develop Th1 CD4$^+$ T cell immunity. T-bet expression redirects differentiation of polarized Th2 CD4$^+$ T cells into IFN-γ-producing Th1 cells (thereby explaining the dominance of Th1- over Th2-driving stimuli). T-bet expression down-regulates development of regulatory (suppressive) T_R cells (as LP T_R cells from T-bet$^{-/-}$ knockout mice produce more TGF-β that can down-regulate pathogenic Th1 T cell responses). T-bet expression is induced by signals originating from the TCR/CD3 and the IFN-γ/IFNGR receptor complexes. These signals activate STAT1 (but not IL-12/IL-12R/STAT4) signals. T-bet induces IL-12Rβ2 expression (thereby allowing IL-12/STAT4 signalling). In addition to Th1 polarization of CD4$^+$ T cells, T-bet is required for optimal production of IFN-γ and antigen-specific T-cell activation by DC[11]. A member of the IL-12 family participates in priming naive T cells in synergy with IFN-γ, i.e. IL-27 (EBI3/p28) that induces proliferation of naive but not memory CD4$^+$ T cells[12–14]. IL-27 signals through the WSX-1/TCCR receptor (a homologue of the IL-12Rβ2 and IL-23R receptor chains). IL-27 is a co-stimulator in early CD4$^+$ T-cell priming but not required for further clonal expansion of a primed Th1 response (Figures 3 and 4). The initial steps in the development of a Th1 phenotype of a $CD4^+$ T cell response are thus well defined at the molecular level.

IFN-γ is usually considered the key cytokine produced by terminally differentiated Th1 T cells or DC. In contrast, the data described above indicate that it is

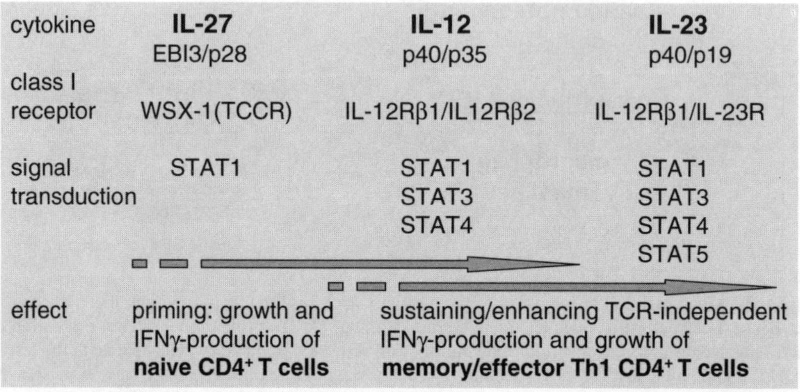

Figure 3 IL-12 family members. The three members of the IL-12 family are IL-12, IL-23 and IL-27. The heterodimeric cytokines, their receptors and signal transduction, and their effect on T-cell priming are schematically shown

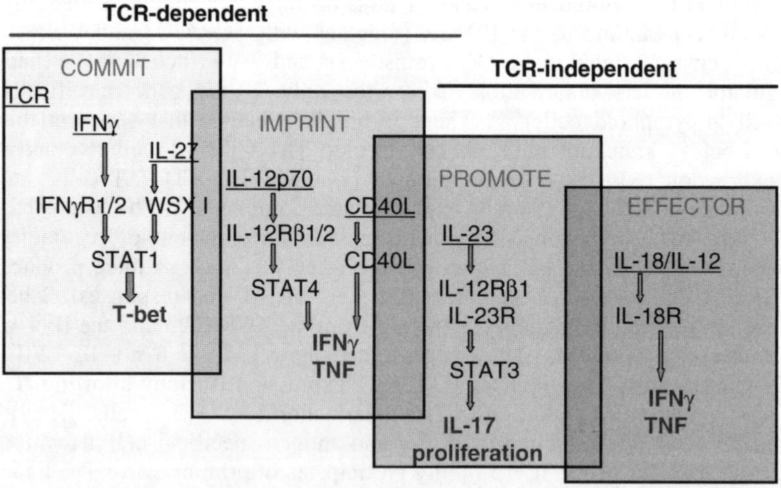

Figure 4 Hypothetical model of Th1 T-cell priming. The initial TCR-dependent and subsequent TCR-independent steps of $CD4^+$ T-cell priming are divided into four steps: (1) initial commitment to engage in specific activation; (2) imprinting of the Th1 polarization; (3) clonal expansion and beginning effector cell differentiation; and (4) terminal effector cell differentiation

also the key 'early' trigger that initiates Th1 differentiation. This raises the question regarding the cellular source of 'early' IFN-γ. Recent studies have identified many sources of 'early' lymphoid or myeloid cell-derived IFN-γ. Lymphoid cell-derived IFN-γ is released by $CD8^+$ T cells, γδ T cells or NK cells (that produce IFN-γ in a T-bet-independent way). Myeloid cell-derived IFN-γ is generated by DC or macrophages in an autoregulatory (self-amplifying) loop triggered by TLR-stimulated IL-12, IL-18, IL-1 and/or IFN-αβ. 'Early' IFN-γ is thus available from many different cells of the innate or adaptive immune system, although its origin in priming colitogenic $CD4^+$ T cell responses is not defined.

Once primed, how is the Th1 development of T cells stabilized? The course of specifically primed T-cell differentiation depends largely on the nature of the APC and the cytokine milieu that prevails at the site of APC/T cell interaction. Members of the IL-12 and IL-1/IL-18 families are involved in driving and tightly regulating multiple checkpoints in Th1 development. Recent data have revealed a considerable complexity in the sequential interactions of three different members of the IL-12 family in this process (Figures 3 and 4), i.e. IL-27, IL-12 and IL-23. These heterodimers use partially overlapping receptor subunits but different STAT molecules to convey their signals[13].

IL-12 p70 (p40/p35) produced by DC in response to TLR or CD40L signals induces IFN-γ. IL-12 signals through a high-affinity, heterodimeric IL-12 receptor (IL-12R) that exhibits low affinity for each ligand (i.e. p40 binds the IL-12Rβ1 subunit; p35 binds the IL-12Rβ2 subunit). IL-12 plays a key role in inducing and/or sustaining intestinal inflammation in different murine colitis models[15–17]. Recently, DC-derived IL-23, composed of IL-12 p40 and (p35-homologous) p19, has been identified[18]. This cytokine binds to a receptor containing the IL-12Rβ1 subunit associated with the (IL-12Rβ2-homologous) IL-23R subunit 19. IL-23-triggered signal transduction depends on STAT4[18]. Different clearance of bacterial infections in $p35^{-/-}$ versus $p40^{-/-}$, and $IL-12R\beta1^{-/-}$ versus $IL-12R\beta2^{-/-}$ knockout mice indicate that IL-23 plays a non-redundant role in Th1 T cell responses *in vivo* that differs from the role of IL-12 p70[20 23]. IL-23 and IL-12 have overlapping, but distinct, effects on murine T cells and DC[24,25]. In contrast to IL-12, IL-23 provides proliferative signals to memory T cells but is a poor IFN-γ inducer; it further induces proinflammatory IL-17 production by mouse memory T cells[18]. As T cells in the intestinal LP are predominantly of the memory phenotype, and colitis-associated $CD4^+$ T cells in the LP in clinical disease or preclinical models have exclusively a memory phenotype, an abundance of potential targets for IL-23 is available *in situ*. We have shown that expression of this cytokine is preferentially up-regulated in LP DC from mice with colitis[26]. Further studies are necessary to elucidate the relative importance of IL-12 versus IL-23 in the pathogenesis of IBD. This question is of practical importance because many therapeutic protocols focus on neutralizing IL-12.

The available data have generated a tentative model to describe initiation, expansion and differentiation of Th1 $CD4^+$ T-cell responses. In simplified terms the process involves the following four steps (Figure 4): (a) specific priming (mediated by TCR, IFN-γ and IL-27 signals); (b) driving Th1 polarization (mediated by CD40 ligation and IL-12); (c) clonally expanding the response (mediated by IL-23); and (d) differentiating Th1 effector functions (mediated by IL-18,

IL-12 and other factors). It should be stressed that this model is hypothetical, and mucosal CD4$^+$ T-cell responses may well be submitted to other or additional constraints. The advantage of these models is that they may reveal many new potential targets for therapeutic interventions that can be tested in preclinical animal models.

EFFECTOR CD4$^+$ T CELLS IN IBD

Epitope recognition by CD4$^+$ $\alpha\beta$ T cells is usually MHC-II-restricted. The small subset of CD4$^+$ $\alpha\beta$ T cells found in MHC-II-deficient (A$\alpha^{-/-}$ or A$\beta^{-/-}$ knockout) mice indicates that development of a minor subset of CD4$^+$ $\alpha\beta$ T cells is MHC-II-independent. MHC-II-independent CD4$^+$ $\alpha\beta$ T cells are thymically derived, appear early in ontogeny, localize preferentially to B-cell rather than T-cell areas in peripheral lymphoid organs, exhibit a phenotype of (resting or activated) memory T cells, have a diverse TCR$\alpha\beta$ repertoire and are functional[27,28]. These CD4$^+$ T-cell populations are apparently heterogeneous with respect to phenotype, specificity for peptides and/or glycolipids, and restriction elements used for specific recognition[29–32]. The only well-defined subset within the MHC-II-independent CD4$^+$ T-cell population are CD1d-restricted NKT cells[33,34] that express an invariant Vα14-Jα281 Vβ8.2 TCR, recognize the glycolipid α-GalCer in the context of CD1d, and rapidly release IFN-γ and IL-4 after stimulation. We have transferred splenic CD4$^+$ $\alpha\beta$ T cells from either normal, or MHC-II-deficient (A$\alpha^{-/-}$ or A$\beta^{-/-}$ knockout), or MHC-I-deficient (β2m$^{-/-}$ or CD1d$^{-/-}$) B6 donor mice into congenic, severely immunodeficient RAG1$^{-/-}$ B6 hosts to test their IBD-inducing potential. Unexpectedly, the adoptively transferred MHC-II-independent CD4$^+$ T-cell population was most efficient at inducing a colitis[35,36]. This observation indicates that MHC-II-independent CD4$^+$ T cells can efficiently trigger inflammatory Th1-type reactions in the mucosa. We reported in addition the inefficient induction of IBD by CD4$^+$ $\alpha\beta$ T cells from MHC-I-deficient (β2m$^{-/-}$) mice. It seems that conventional MHC-II-restricted CD4$^+$ T cells expand polyclonally but do not induce IBD in the adoptive host as they default to a Th2-biased reactivity. Co-transfer of genetically labelled, MHC-I-dependent and MHC-II-independent CD4$^+$ T cells demonstrated that conventional CD4$^+$ T cells need MHC-II-independent CD4$^+$ T cells to induce IBD. It is not known how MHC-II-independent CD4$^+$ T cells promote IBD development induced by CD4$^+$ T cells from normal donors. Clarification of this question is impeded by the lack of reliable markers for MHC-II-independent CD4$^+$ T-cell subsets.

Clarification of this issue is relevant because factors regulating Th1 differentiation in different immune cell subsets differ. The factors described above that drive Th1 differentiation in conventional (MHC class II-restricted) CD4$^+$ T cells are not necessarily involved in directing Th1 polarization of unconventional ($\gamma\delta$ T cells, MHC-II-independent CD4$^+$ T cells, NKT cells) T cells, conventional CD8$^+$ T cells or NK cells. Identification of the major colitogenic effector T-cell subset is therefore of interest to understand the biology of the disease, but also to define targets for a rational therapeutic strategy.

REGULATOR CD4$^+$ T CELLS ATTENUATING THE COLITOGENIC POTENTIAL OF EFFECTOR CD4$^+$ T CELLS

A key factor in IBD development seems to be a defect in the regulatory control of mucosal T-cell responses. Different candidate regulatory T (T_R) cells have been described that down-modulate or suppress T-cell responses. The best-known T_R cell subset are CD25$^+$CD4$^+$ T_R cells, a unique marker of which is the expression of the transcription factor Foxp3[37,38] (Table 1). CD25$^+$CD4$^+$ T_R cells are selected in the thymus by MHC class II-restricted epitopes[39]. These T_R cells regulate mucosal immunity as they prevent development of murine gastritis after neonatal thymectomy[40,41], are specifically induced in Peyer's patches[42], control induction of transfer colitis[43–45], and cure established colitis[46]. CD25$^+$CD4$^+$ T_R are particularly suited for a sentinel role at body surfaces because they express two kinds of receptor, i.e. clonally diverse TCR for specific antigen recognition, and Toll-like receptors (TLR) that sense conserved molecular patterns of microbes (or 'danger signals' elicited by their invasion)[47]. Other (CD25$^+$ or CD25$^-$) CD4$^+$ T_R cell subsets have been shown to control transfer colitis (Table 1). CD103 (integrin α_E)$^+$ (CD25$^+$ or CD25$^-$) $\alpha\beta$ T_R cells that express CTLA-4, protect mice from colitis, pointing to CD103 as a marker for a T_R cell subset apparently specialized for crosstalk with epithelial environments[48]. Activated, membrane TGF-β-expressing (CD25$^+$ or CD25$^-$) T_R cells suppress the manifestation of transfer colitis[49]. IL-10-producing CD4$^+$ T_{R1} suppress proliferation of CD4$^+$ T cells in response to antigen and prevent colitis induced in immunodeficient mice by transfer of CD4$^+$CD45RB^{high} T cells[50]. Hence, different CD4$^+$ T_R cell subsets have been shown to control development of murine colitis.

The mechanism of action of T_R cells in priming, expansion and differentiation of T-cell responses is unresolved. T_R may operate at the DC or the effector T cell level. Major interest has focused on 'suppressive' T_R cell subsets although amplifying T_R cell subsets may well exist, as suggested by the enhancing effect of MHC-II-independent CD4$^+$ T cells described above. An interesting, recently described model proposes that T_R suppressor cells are suppressed at the level of

Table 1 Regulatory T (T_R) cells controlling mucosal T-cell immunity

Surface phenotype	TCR	Effector	Reference
Epithelial compartment			
CD4$^+$ CD8$\alpha\alpha^+$	$\alpha\beta$	IL-10	53
CD4$^-$ CD8$^+$ CD103$^+$ CD101$^+$	$\alpha\beta$	?	54
CD4$^-$ CD8$^{+/-}$	$\gamma\delta$	?KGF	55
Lamina propria			
CD4$^+$ CD25$^+$ CD8$^-$	$\alpha\beta$	?	37,46
CD4$^+$ CD103$^+$ CD25$^{+/-}$ CD8$^-$	$\alpha\beta$	?	48
CD4$^+$ LAV/mTGFβ^+ CD25$^{+/-}$	$\alpha\beta$	TGFβ	49
CD4$^+$ CD8$^-$ (Th3)	$\alpha\beta$	TGFβ	56,57
CD4$^+$ CD8$^-$ (Tr1)	$\alpha\beta$	IL-10	50

the DC to allow effector T-cell activation[51]. This model is attractive for the study of mucosal $CD4^+$ T-cell responses as it assigns a prominent role to pathogen-associated molecular proteins (PAMP) that activate TLR. PAMP stimulating DC and T_R cells modulate specific activation of effector T cells through three independent signalling pathways: (a) they enhance restricted epitope presentation by DC in the context of costimulation; (b) they suppress T_R cell-mediated suppression (through an independent signalling pathway in DC); and (c) they directly modulate T_R cell activity (Figure 5). Microbial products activating different TLR pathways thus block suppressive effects of $CD4^+CD25^+$ T_R cells allowing activation of pathogen-specific adaptive immune responses. This block of suppressor activity is dependent in part on IL-6 which is induced by TLR upon recognition of microbial products[51]. A T-cell response to a specific (non-self) epitope is thus enabled by (non-self) PAMP that mature antigen presentation and costimulation by APC and down-modulate their ability to activate T_R cells; furthermore, they directly down-modulate T_R cell suppression. As the TLR expression pattern of effector $CD4^+$ T cells, $CD25^+CD4^+$ T_R cells and DC differs[47,52], different TLR ligands can influence the three cell interactions at distinct checkpoints. Although the model has not been critically tested for its relevance for IBD, some data suggest its interest as a hypothesis for formulating new concepts for mucosal $CD4^+$ T-cell priming. In experimental IBD induction, anti-IL-6R mAb protect against IBD induction, IBD is difficult to induce in $IL\text{-}6^{-/-}$ knockout mice hosts, and Th2 (but not Th1) $CD4^+$ T-cell responses are readily induced in $gp130^{-/-}$ knockout mice.

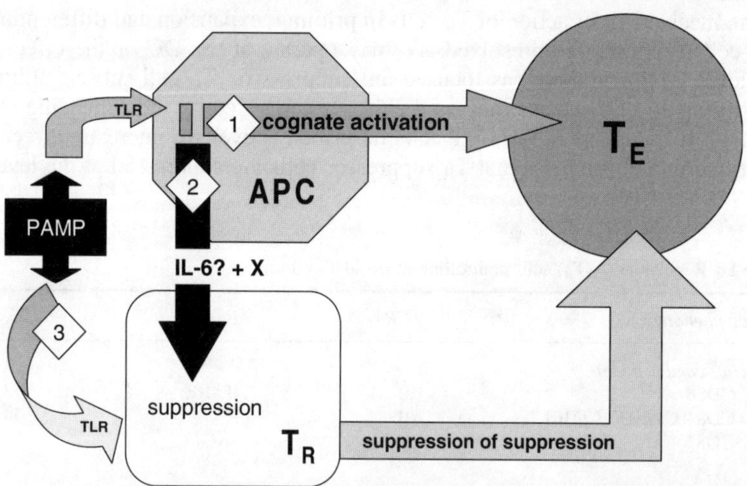

Figure 5 Hypothesis: priming is relief from T_R cell suppression as well as specific activation of T cells. (Non-self) pathogen-associated molecular patterns or proteins (PAMP) operate through Toll-like receptors (TLR) at three distinct levels to support priming of a specific response of T effector (T_E) cells. (1) They facilitate restricted epitope presentation by antigen-presenting cells (APC) in the context of costimulation. (2) They activate in APC a separate pathway that 'neutralizes' suppression by T_R cells. (3) They directly down-modulate the suppressive activity of T_R cells. Activation thus involves specific stimulation as well as suppression of suppression

CONCLUDING REMARKS

An impressive amount of data has been accumulated over the past decade on the immunopathogenesis of IBD, largely due to the emergence of fascinating new preclinical models of colitis. Detailed knowledge is available on molecular defects that trigger IBD, the mechanism of action of new therapies, and revised models of polarized T-cell priming. Despite this plethora of new data, our understanding of mucosal T-cell priming, the relevant APC, the factors driving its expansion and differentiation, and the *in-situ* control by T_R cell subsets are insufficient to generate a convincing, conceptual framework. In this situation innovative working hypotheses that select interesting facets of the T-cell response, and can be validated in preclinical experiments, are needed.

Acknowledgements

This work was supported by grants from the IZKF/A5 (University of Ulm) and the Deutsche Forschungsgemeinschaft (Re 549/9-2) to J.R.

References

1. Herrick CA, Bottomly K. To respond or not to respond: T cells in allergic asthma. Nat Rev Immunol. 2003;3:405–12.
2. Blumberg RS, Strober W. Prospects for research in inflammatory bowel disease. J Am Med Assoc. 2001;285:643–7.
3. Strober W, Fuss IJ, Blumberg RS. The immunology of mucosal models of inflammation. Annu Rev Immunol. 2002;20:495–549.
4. Iqbal N, Oliver JR, Wagner FH, Lazenby AS, Elson CO, Weaver CT. T helper 1 and T helper 2 cells are pathogenic in an antigen-specific model of colitis. J Exp Med. 2002;195:71–84.
5. Blanas E, Davey GM, Carbone FR, Heath WR. A bone marrow-derived APC in the gut-associated lymphoid tissue captures oral antigens and presents them to both $CD4^+$ and $CD8^+$ T cells. J Immunol. 2000;164:2890–6.
6. Huang FP, Platt N, Wykes M et al. A discrete subpopulation of dendritic cells transports apoptotic intestinal epithelial cells to T cell areas of mesenteric lymph nodes. J Exp Med. 2000;191:435–44.
7. Leithäuser F, Trobonjaca Z, Möller P, Reimann J. Clustering of colonic lamina propria $CD4^+$ T cells to subepithelial dendritic cell aggregates precedes the development of colitis in a murine adoptive transfer model. Lab Invest. 2001;81:1339–49.
8. Leithäuser F, Trobonjaca Z, Reimann J, Möller P. *In situ* characterization of genetically targeted (green fluorescent) single cells and their microenvironment in an adoptive host. Am J Pathol. 2001;158:1975–83.
9. Szabo SJ, Sullivan BM, Peng SL, Glimcher LH. Molecular mechanisms regulating Th1 immune responses. Annu Rev Immunol. 2003;21:713–58.
10. Neurath MF, Finotto S, Glimcher LH. The role of Th1/Th2 polarization in mucosal immunity. Nat Med. 2002;8:567–73.
11. Lugo-Villarino G, Maldonado-Lopez R, Possemato R, Penaranda C, Glimcher LH. T-bet is required for optimal production of IFN-g and antigen-specific T cell activation by dendritic cells. Proc Natl Acad Sci USA. 2003;100:7749–54.
12. Omata F, Birkenbach M, Matsuzaki S, Christ AD, Blumberg RS. The expression of IL-12 p40 and its homologue, Epstein–Barr virus-induced gene 3, in inflammatory bowel disease. Inflamm Bowel Dis. 2001;7:215–20.
13. Brombacher F, Kastelein RA, Alber G. Novel IL-12 family members shed light on the orchestration of Th1 responses. Trends Immunol. 2003;24:207–12.
14. Takeda A, Hamano S, Yamanaka A et al. Role of IL-27/WSX-1 signaling for induction of T-bet through activation of STAT1 during initial Th1 commitment. J Immunol. 2003;170:4886–90.

15. Neurath MF, Fuss I, Kelsall BL, Stuber E, Strober W. Antibodies to interleukin 12 abrogate established experimental colitis in mice. J Exp Med. 1995;182:1281–90.
16. Davidson NJ, Hudak SA, Lesley RE, Menon S, Leach MW, Rennick DM. IL-12, but not IFN-g, plays a major role in sustaining the chronic phase of colitis in IL-10-deficient mice. J Immunol. 1998;161:3143–9.
17. Camoglio L, Juffermans NP, Peppelenbosch M et al. Contrasting roles of IL-12p40 and IL-12p35 in the development of hapten-induced colitis. Eur J Immunol. 2002;32:261–9.
18. Oppmann B, Lesley R, Blom B et al. Novel p19 protein engages IL-12p40 to form a cytokine, IL-23, with biological activities similar as well as distinct from IL-12. Immunity. 2000;13:715–25.
19. Parham C, Chirica M, Timans J et al. A receptor for the heterodimeric cytokine IL-23 is composed of IL-12Rβ1 and a novel cytokine receptor subunit, IL-23R. J Immunol. 2002;168:5699–708.
20. Holscher C, Atkinson RA, Arendse B et al. A protective and agonistic function of IL-12p40 in mycobacterial infection. J Immunol. 2001;167:6957–66.
21. Cooper AM, Kipnis A, Turner J, Magram J, Ferrante J, Orme IM. Mice lacking bioactive IL-12 can generate protective, antigen-specific cellular responses to mycobacterial infection only if the IL-12 p40 subunit is present. J Immunol. 2002;168:1322–7.
22. Elkins KL, Cooper A, Colombini SM, Cowley SC, Kieffer TL. *In vivo* clearance of an intracellular bacterium, *Francisella tularensis* LVS, is dependent on the p40 subunit of interleukin-12 (IL-12) but not on IL-12 p70. Infect Immun. 2002;70:1936–48.
23. Lehmann J, Bellmann S, Werner C, Schroder R, Schutze N, Alber G. IL-12p40-dependent agonistic effects on the development of protective innate and adaptive immunity against *Salmonella enteritidis*. J Immunol. 2001;167:5304–15.
24. Aggarwal S, Ghilardi N, Xie MH, De Sauvage FJ, Gurney AL. Interleukin 23 promotes a distinct CD4 T cell activation state characterized by the production of interleukin 17. J Biol Chem. 2002;278:1910–14.
25. Belladonna ML, Renauld JC, Bianchi R et al. IL-23 and IL-12 have overlapping, but distinct, effects on murine dendritic cells. J Immunol. 2002;168:5448–54.
26. Krajina T, Leithäuser F, Möller P, Trobonjaca Z, Reimann J. Colonic lamina propria dendritic cells in mice with CD4$^+$ T cell-induced colitis. Eur J Immunol. 2003;33:1073–83.
27. Kontgen F, Suss G, Stewart C, Steinmetz M, Blüthmann H. Targeted disruption of the MHC class II Aa gene in C57BL/6 mice. Int Immunol. 1993;5:957–64.
28. Cardell S, Tangri S, Chan S, Kronenberg M, Benoist C, Mathis D. CD1-restricted CD4$^+$ T cells in major histocompatibility complex class II-deficient mice. J Exp Med. 1995;182:993–1004.
29. Lee DJ, Abeyratne A, Carson DA, Corr M. Induction of an antigen-specific, CD1-restricted cytotoxic T lymphocyte response *in vivo*. J Exp Med. 1998;187:433–8.
30. Park SH, Roark JH, Bendelac A. Tissue-specific recognition of mouse CD1 molecules. J Immunol. 1998;160:3128–34.
31. Tangri S, Brossay L, Burdin N, Lee DJ, Corr M, Kronenberg M. Presentation of peptide antigens by mouse CD1 requires endosomal localization and protein antigen processing. Proc Natl Acad Sci USA. 1998;95:14314–19.
32. Schofield L, McConville MJ, Hansen D et al. CD1d-restricted immunoglobulin G formation to GPI-anchored antigens mediated by NKT cells. Science. 1999;283:225–9.
33. Kronenberg M, Gapin L. The unconventional lifestyle of NKT Cells. Nat Rev Immunol. 2002;2:557–68.
34. MacDonald HR. Immunology. T before NK. Science. 2002;296:481–2.
35. Leithäuser F, Krajina T, Trobonjaca Z, Reimann J. Early events in the pathogenesis of a murine transfer colitis. Pathobiology. 2002;70:156–163.
36. Trobonjaca Z, Leithäuser F, Möller P et al. MHC-II-independent CD4$^+$ T cells induce colitis in immunodeficient RAG$^{-/-}$ hosts. J Immunol. 2001;166:3804–12.
37. Shevach EM. CD4$^+$ CD25$^+$ suppressor T cells: more questions than answers. Nat Rev Immunol. 2002;2:389–400.
38. Hori S, Nomura T, Sakaguchi S. Control of regulatory T cell development by the transcription factor Foxp3. Science. 2003;299:1057–61.
39. Bensinger SJ, Bandeira A, Jordan MS, Caton AJ, Laufer TM. Major histocompatibility complex class II-positive cortical epithelium mediates the selection of CD4$^+$ CD25$^+$ immunoregulatory T cells. J Exp Med. 2001;194:427–38.

40. Sakaguchi S, Sakaguchi N, Shimizu J et al. Immunologic tolerance maintained by CD25$^+$ CD4$^+$ regulatory T cells: their common role in controlling autoimmunity, tumor immunity, and transplantation tolerance. Immunol Rev. 2001;182:18–32.

41. McHugh RS, Shevach EM, Margulies DH, Natarajan K. A T cell receptor transgenic model of severe, spontaneous organ-specific autoimmunity. Eur J Immunol. 2001;31:2094–103.

42. Tsuji NM, Mizumachi K, Kurisaki J. Antigen-specific, CD4$^+$ CD25$^+$ regulatory T cell clones induced in Peyer's patches. Int Immunol. 2003;15:525–34.

43. Read S, Malmstrom V, Powrie F. Cytotoxic T lymphocyte-associated antigen 4 plays an essential role in the function of CD25$^+$ CD4$^+$ regulatory cells that control intestinal inflammation. J Exp Med. 2000;192:295–302.

44. Maloy KJ, Powrie F. Regulatory T cells in the control of immune pathology. Nat Immunol. 2001;2:816–22.

45. Maloy KJ, Salaun L, Cahill R, Dougan G, Saunders NJ, Powrie F. CD4$^+$ CD25$^+$ TR cells suppress innate immune pathology through cytokine-dependent mechanisms. J Exp Med. 2003;197:111–19.

46. Mottet C, Uhlig HH, Powrie F. Cure of colitis by CD4$^+$ CD25$^+$ regulatory T cells. J Immunol. 2003;170:3939–43.

47. Sakaguchi S. Control of immune responses by naturally arising CD4$^+$ regulatory T cells that express toll-like receptors. J Exp Med. 2003;197:397–401.

48. Lehmann J, Hühn J, de la Rosa M et al. Expression of the integrin αEβ7 identifies unique subsets of CD25$^+$ as well as CD25$^-$ regulatory T cells. Proc Natl Acad Sci USA. 2002;99:13031–6.

49. Oida T, Zhang X, Goto M et al. CD4$^+$ CD25$^-$ T cells that express latency-associated peptide on the surface suppress CD4$^+$ CD45RB^{high}-induced colitis by a TGF-β-dependent mechanism. J Immunol. 2003;170:2516–22.

50. Groux H, O'Garra A, Bigler M et al. A CD4$^+$ T-cell subset inhibits antigen-specific T-cell responses and prevents colitis. Nature. 1997;389:737–42.

51. Pasare C, Medzhitov R. Toll pathway-dependent blockade of CD4$^+$ CD25$^+$ T cell-mediated suppression by dendritic cells. Science. 2003;299:1033–6.

52. Sakaguchi S. Regulatory T cells: mediating compromises between host and parasite. Nat Immunol. 2003;4:10–11.

53. Das G, Augustine MM, Das J, Bottomly K, Ray P, Ray A. An important regulatory role for CD4$^+$ CD8aa T cells in the intestinal epithelial layer in the prevention of inflammatory bowel disease. Proc Natl Acad Sci USA. 2003;100:5324–9

54. Allez M, Brimnes J, Dotan I, Mayer L. Expansion of CD8$^+$ T cells with regulatory function after interaction with intestinal epithelial cells. Gastroenterology. 2002;123:1516–26.

55. Chen Y, Chou K, Fuchs E, Havran WL, Boismenu R. Protection of the intestinal mucosa by intraepithelial $\gamma\delta$ T cells. Proc Natl Acad Sci USA. 2002;99:14338–43.

56. Kitani A, Chua K, Nakamura K, Strober W. Activated self MHC reactive T cells have the cytokine phenotype of Th3/T regulatory cell 1 T cells. J Immunol. 2000;165:691–702.

57. Kitani A, Fuss IJ, Nakamura K, Schwartz OM, Usui T, Strober W. Treatment of experimental (trinitrobenzene sulfonic acid) colitis by intranasal administration of transforming growth factor (TGF)-b1 plasmid: TGF-b1-mediated suppression of T helper cell type 1 response occurs by interleukin (IL)-10 induction and IL-12 receptor b2 chain downregulation. J Exp Med. 2000;192:41–52.

18
The role of Epstein–Barr virus-induced gene 3 in driving Th2-associated intestinal inflammation

A. KASER, E. E. E. S. NIEUWENHUIS, N. CORAZZA,
H. IIJIMA, M. YOSHIDA, T. NAGAISHI, J. GLICKMAN,
S. WIRTZ, P. GALLE, M. BIRKENBACH, M. NEURATH
and R. S. BLUMBERG

INTRODUCTION

Current ideas of the immunopathogenesis of inflammatory bowel disease (IBD) suggest that decision making by dendritic cells is of central importance to this disease[1,2]. In this model, bacterial antigens, which are translocated across the epithelial barrier either normally or abnormally due to a primary defect in the epithelial barrier, are interpreted by professional antigen-presenting cells, such as dendritic cells, in a pathogenic fashion. Specifically, Crohn's disease, which is believed to be a predominantly T helper 1-mediated disease as supported by a variety of mouse models which reproduce immunopathology, is associated with elevated levels of interleukin-12 (p35/p40)[3,4]. In contrast, in ulcerative colitis, which is viewed as a modified T helper 2 response, there are no significant elevations of IL-12[3,4]. Therefore, the mechanisms by which the dysregulated perception of luminal antigens leads to the development of the immunopathology associated with ulcerative colitis (UC) are unknown.

As mentioned above, IL-12 plays a pivotal role in Th1 immunopathology, especially Crohn's disease (CD)[5]. IL-12 is a covalently linked heterodimer formed of a light chain of 35 kDa (p35) and a heavy chain of 40 kDa (p40)[6] (Table 1). It is derived from phagocytes and dendritic cells (DCs) and forms a link between innate resistance and adaptive immunity, in that it induces the production of IFN-γ and favours the differentiation of T helper 1 (Th1) cells. It exerts its biological functions through the IL-12 receptor, which is composed of IL-12Rβ1 and IL-12Rβ2, and activates the Janus kinase (JAK)-STAT4 (signal transducer and activator of transcription) pathway of signal transduction[6]. As mentioned above, murine models of colitis are dependent on this IL-12-JAK-STAT4 pathway[2,5], and there is a set of data supporting an analogous role of the IL-12 pathway in human CD[4]. Recently, it was demonstrated that IL-12 p40 associates not only with IL-12 p35, but also with another molecule, p19, to form a novel heterodimeric cytokine called IL-23[7] (Table 1). IL-23 binds to and activates a receptor composed of IL-12Rβ1 and a distinct second chain, IL-23R, subsequently inducing largely the same JAK-STAT signalling molecules and transcription factors as IL-12, thus sharing many of the biological functions with IL-12[7]. Another novel member of the emerging IL-12 family has been recently proposed, named IL-27, consisting of a 28 kDa peptide (p28) and Epstein–Barr virus-induced gene 3 (EBI3), with the latter showing homology to IL-12 p40[8] (Table 1). *In vitro*, IL-27 induces proliferation in naive Th cells, and synergizes with IL-12 to produce IFN-γ from naive Th cells, while concomitantly decreasing the production of the Th2 cytokine IL-13[8]. The receptor chain WSX-1/TCCR is required, but not sufficient for inducing biological function of the p28/EBI3 heterodimer[8]. Based on these functions it has been proposed that IL-27 might induce and augment Th1 immune responses. However, the *in-vivo* role of IL-27 has not been characterized so far.

ROLE OF EBI3 IN IBD

It is thus of interest to consider the potential role of Epstein–Barr virus (EBV)-induced gene 3 (EBI3) in the pathogenesis of IBD. EBI3 is a novel haematopoietic receptor family member of humans and rodents that is related to the p40 subunit of IL-12[9]. EBI3 was originally identified due to its induction in human B cells by EBV. The EBI3 gene encodes a 34 kDa glycoprotein that is derived from the human genome, which lacks a membrane-anchoring motif when it is secreted[9]. Thus, EBI3 is a host gene that is induced by EBV. EBI3 has been shown to be expressed by dendritic cells and syncytiotrophoblastic cells of the placenta[10]. Interestingly, EBI3 has also been identified as an epithelial-associated secretory factor that is induced by pathogenic bacterial infections such as those associated

Table 1 IL-12 family of cytokines

	Heterodimeric cytokine	*Receptor binding chain*	*Receptor signalling chain*	*Function*
IL-12	p35-p40	IL-12Rβ1	IL-12Rβ2	Naive → Th1 differentiation
IL-23	p19-p40	IL-12Rβ1	IL-23R	Memory Th1
IL-27	p28-EBI3	WSX-1 (= TCCR)	?	Naive → Th1?
EBI3	EBI3	?	?	Th2 differentiation iNKT: IL-4 & IL-13

with *Salmonella* spp.[11]. EBI3 has been described to associate with itself as a homodimer, with the IL-12 p35 chain to create a novel heterodimer[12], and a novel chain called p28 to create IL-27 as noted above[8]. We have previously shown that EBI3 is expressed at high levels in active UC but not in inactive UC, normal controls or CD subjects[13]. These studies were largely based on a quantitative PCR assay using a competitive template but ultimately confirmed by quantitative PCR assay utilizing real-time PCR[14]. In human UC, immunohistology with an EBI3-specific polyclonal rabbit antibody showed that the EBI3 protein was primarily associated with dendritic cell-like cells in the lamina propria of UC subjects but not either CD subjects or normal controls[13]. These studies suggested that perhaps, like the role of IL-12 in driving Th1 responses in CD, EBI3 might be involved in driving the modified Th2 response that is involved in the pathogenesis of human UC. This seemed, however, to contradict the recent finding that EBI3 or a part of IL-27 promotes Th1 responses[8].

EBI3-DEFICIENT MICE HAVE A MAJOR DEFECT IN Th2 CYTOKINE PRODUCTION

To test this hypothesis, EBI3-deficient mice were generated[15]. The EBI3 gene was disrupted by homologous recombination in 129SvJ embryonic stem cells by replacing the second to fifth exons encoding amino acids 24–28 of the EBI3 protein with the neomycin resistance gene. The mice were ultimately bred and found to be phenotypically normal[15]. Interestingly, the mice bred normally despite the fact that EBI3 has been shown to be expressed at relatively high levels in placenta[10]. EBI3-deficient mice exhibited no gross or histological abnormalities in various organs including liver, kidney, spleen, colon, lung and heart. In addition, the numbers and proportions of $CD4^+$, $CD8^+$ and $B220^+$ lymphocytes were not significantly altered in these mice. Interestingly, EBI3-deficient mice exhibited diminished production of IL-4 by T cells[15]. This diminished production of IL-4 was not due to a primary T-cell defect as IL-4 production could be rescued by differentiating *in vitro* under a Th2-induced environment. Specifically, when splenocytes were obtained from EBI3-deficient, EBI3-heterozygotic and wild-type mice, and stimulated with anti-CD3 and CD28 *in vitro*, EBI3-deficient mice exhibited elevated levels of IFN-γ but significantly diminished levels of IL-4[15]. The heterozygotic mice exhibited a trend towards increased IFN-γ and diminished IL-4, which did not reach statistical significance. However, when splenocytes were differentiated under Th2 conditions in which cells were stimulated with anti-CD3 and anti-CD28 in the presence of anti-IL-12 and anti-IFN-γ with the addition of recombinant IL-4, the EBI3-deficient T cells were able to secrete upon re-stimulation with anti-CD3 and anti-CD28 levels of IL-4 that were similar to the heterozygotic and wild-type animals[15].

Previous studies have suggested that EBI3 might be an antagonist of IL-12[8]. Therefore, this question was further addressed in EBI3-deficient mice. It was first shown that EBI3 was expressed, as defined by semi-quantitative RT-PCR, in $CD8\alpha^+$ and $CD8\alpha^-$ dendritic cells with some enrichment of the EBI3 in the $CD8\alpha^-$ (or DC2)-like DC. When dendritic cells were obtained from wild-type, EBI3 heterozygotic and EBI3-deficient mice, the levels of spontaneous IL-12 production by the EBI3-deficient mice were similar to the levels of IL-12 secreted by the heterozygotic and wild-type mice[15]. Moreover, heterozygotic and EBI3-deficient DCs from EBI3 heterozygotic and knockout mice exhibited similar levels of IL-12 secretion upon stimulation with LPS and IFN-γ as those observed in wild-type animals[15]. Thus, the deficiency of EBI3 does not affect the production of IL-12 as induced by LPS and IFN-γ. These studies suggest that EBI3 is not necessarily an antagonist of IL-12.

EBI3-DEFICIENT DC FAIL TO PROMOTE A Th2 RESPONSE

Interestingly, EBI3-deficient DCs were unable to generate a Th2 response to a model antigen (Nieuwenhuis, Neurath and Blumberg, unpublished observation). This observation was generated by the following series of studies. EBI3-deficient, heterozygotic and wild-type animals were backpacked with a melanoma cell line secreting GM-CSF to increase the numbers of CD11c$^+$ cells that could be isolated from the animals. These CD11c$^+$ cells that were purified from these mice were incubated *in vitro* with the model antigen, keyhole limpet haemocyanin (KLH). These CD11c$^+$ cells that were incubated with KLH were injected into the footpad of wild-type animals and, 7 days later, popliteal T cells isolated and cultivated together with KLH as a recall antigen in the context of wild-type spleen cells as antigen-presenting cells. These T cells were then assessed for their ability to secrete IL-4 and IFN-γ. Dendritic cells from EBI3-deficient and wild-type mice were able to stimulate similar levels of IFN-γ (Nieuwenhuis, Neurath and Blumberg, unpublished observation). DCs from neither EBI3-deficient nor EBI3-heterozygotic mice were able to stimulate IL-4 production from wild-type lymphocytes. In contrast, DCs from wild-type mice, when adoptively transferred into the footpads of wild-type mice, were able to induce a Th2 response as manifest by the production of the Th2 cytokine, IL-4 (Nieuwenhuis, Neurath and Blumberg, unpublished observation).

These aforementioned studies suggested that EBI3 was associated with a Th2 response. This was quite surprising since EBI3 in association with p28 has been previously suggested to be a cytokine that plays an important role in the proliferation of naive T cells and in promoting a Th1 response. Therefore, to further confirm this point, EBI3 transgenic mice were generated in which EBI3 was driven by a ubiquitin promoter. Spleen cells from three different founder lines of the transgenic mice expressing EBI3 under the control of the ubiquitin promoter were shown to secrete increased quantities of IL-4 in response to LPS and SAC in comparison to wild-type FVB/N mice (Wirtz and Neurath, unpublished observation). In addition, when dendritic cells from the EBI3 transgenic animals were pulsed with KLH and adoptively transferred into the footpads of wild-type FVB/N mice, popliteal T cells from these mice receiving the DC expressing the EBI3 transgene were shown to promote high levels of IL-4 production by T cells (Wirtz and Neurath, unpublished observation). These studies confirm that, in contrast to EBI3-deficient mice, which have DC that display inability to drive a Th2 response, DC from EBI3-transgenic mice were able to induce higher levels of IL-4 production (Wirtz and Neurath, unpublished observation).

EBI3-DEFICIENT MICE ARE PROTECTED FROM OXAZOLONE COLITIS

Previous studies have shown that oxazolone colitis is a model that contains a significant Th2 component[16]. Therefore, to determine whether this inability to drive Th2 cytokine responses had an immunopathological consequence, EBI3-deficient mice were examined for the development of oxazolone colitis in comparison with trinitrobenzene sulphonic acid colitis in $129 \times B6 \ F_1$ mice. EBI3-deficient mice were observed to be protected from the development of oxazolone colitis but not TNBS colitis, which is primarily a Th1-mediated colitis model[15]. Interestingly, EBI3 heterozygotic mice were similarly protected from the development of the colitis, suggesting that the level of EBI3 might have a threshold effect in generating immunopathology and possibly Th2 responses. This clinical protection, as defined by weight loss in the EBI3-deficient mice, was also associated with decreased pathological injury to oxazolone in the context of EBI3 deficiency. Moreover, as observed clinically, EBI3 heterozygotic mice were protected to a similar extent as EBI3-deficient mice[15]. Similarly, the pathological score of colitis-associated injury in the TNBS colitis model was severe in the wild-type animals with few differences observed in either the EBI3 heterozygotic or EBI3-deficient mice. This protection from oxazolone colitis in the absence of EBI3 was also associated with decreased IL-4 production by lamina propria lymphocytes in the EBI3-deficient mice in comparison to the wild-type mice and decreased nuclear translocation of GATA3 in the EBI3-deficient mice during the course of oxazolone colitis[15]. There was also a trend towards slightly increased IFN-γ production in the EBI3-deficient mice consistent with a role of EBI3 in driving Th2-associated inflammation.

EBI3-DEFICIENT MICE HAVE A DEFECT IN iNKT CELL NUMBER AND FUNCTION

Since previous studies have shown that oxazolone-induced colitis is CD1d and invariant NK-T-cell dependent, since oxazolone colitis is diminished when CD1d is deleted or blocked with a mAb or not present in the context of deletion of invariant NK-T cells through analysis of an NK-T cell-deficient model[17], it was of interest to examine invariant NK-T cells in EBI3-deficient mice. Therefore, liver mononuclear cells and splenocytes were obtained from wild-type mice, EBI3-heterozygotic mice and EBI3-deficient mice and examined by flow cytometry with an α-galactosylceramide-loaded CD1d tetramer after gating on $CD3^+$ cells. Whereas there was no difference in the numbers of $CD4^+$ and $CD8^+$ cells in the EBI3-deficient and heterozygotic mice, the proportion of CD1d tetramer-positive cells that were also $CD3^+$ in the EBI3-deficient mice was significantly decreased in the liver and spleen in comparison to the wild-type mice[15]. These studies suggested that the loss of EBI3 was associated with a diminution in invariant NK-T cells.

It was therefore of interest to determine whether this quantitative decrease in invariant NK-T cells was also associated with a qualitative alteration in the function of invariant NK-T cells in EBI3-deficient mice, so the following studies were performed. Liver mononuclear cells were obtained from wild-type and EBI3-deficient mice. These liver mononuclear cells were co-cultivated with either a CD1d-negative B cell line, C1R, or a CD1d-transfected C1R cell line. In the presence of α-galactosylceramide it was observed that wild-type and EBI3-deficient mice were induced to secrete similar levels of IFN-γ. In contrast, EBI3-deficient mononuclear cells secreted significantly less IL-4 in contrast to the wild-type liver mononuclear cells[15]. Moreover, when α-galactosylceramide was injected by tail vein into EBI3-deficient or wild-type mice, the levels of IL-4 in the serum at 4, 24 and 48 h in the EBI3-deficient mice were noted to be significantly diminished in the EBI3-deficient in comparison to the wild-type mice. The levels of IFN-γ were slightly decreased at early time points (4 h) in the EBI3-deficient mice but by 24 and 48 h the levels of IFN-γ in the knockout and wild-type animals were similar[15]. This study suggested that perhaps EBI3 deficiency was associated with a major quantitative defect in invariant NK-T cell numbers that was associated with a diminution in the production of IFN-γ that was ultimately superseded by production of IFN-γ from cells such as natural killer cells, which are known to be regulated by NK-T cells. In comparison, there was a profound quantitative and qualitative defect in invariant NK-T cells with respect to their ability to secrete Th2 cytokines.

SUMMARY AND DISCUSSION

Overall, these experiments unambigously revealed that EBI3 is involved in the augmentation of Th2 immune responses *in vivo*[15], rather than Th1 induction as might have been anticipated by the *in-vitro* function of the p28/EBI3 heterodimer IL-27 as reported by Pflanz et al.[8] While induction of proliferation in naive T cells has been ascribed to IL-27, the normal numbers of T cells in EBI3$^{-/-}$ mice as compared to wild-type animals suggest that EBI3 might be dispensable for T cell homeostasis with the important exception of invariant NKT cells (see below).

At what stage EBI3 interacts with conventional T cells to drive Th2 development is still an open question. Preliminary results suggest that adoptive transfer of antigen-primed DCs to EBI3$^{-/-}$ mice might be sufficient to drive an antigen-specific Th2 response in EBI3$^{-/-}$ mice, suggesting that EBI3 derived from DCs could directly act on conventional T cells. A model might be proposed wherein DCs secrete either IL-12 or EBI3 (with a presumptive binding partner to be determined) and direct Th1 and Th2 responses, respectively (Figure 1). The nature of the antigen processed and presented by DCs might influence this decision-making as to what direction (i.e. IL-12 or EBI3) to take. This might have important implications for the understanding of colitis, as luminal content with its microbially diverse flora could itself shape the pathogenic immune response in either direction, and this is well in line with diverse pattern-recognition receptors expressed on antigen-presenting cells shaping the DCs' response[18]. Well in accordance with this view is the fact that rectal administration of a Th1-inducing hapten, namely TNBS, induces colitis, which is not abrogated or influenced in EBI3-deficient mice[15].

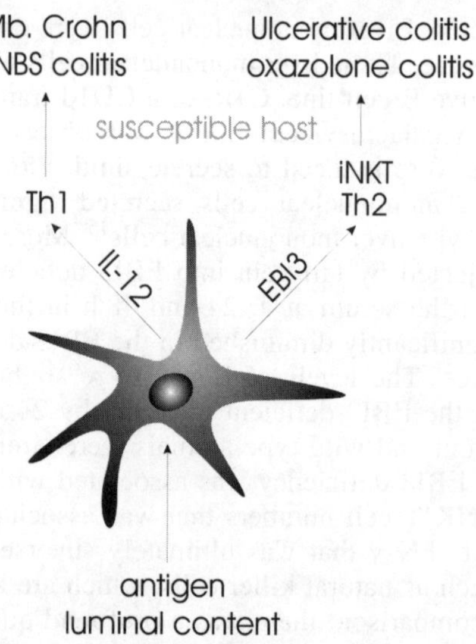

Figure 1 Immunopathology in inflammatory bowel disease

The second – and interrelated – aspect of EBI3 deficiency is its association with a decrease in iNKT cell number as well as function. Mice rendered deficient in iNKT cells, either by the absence of the non-polymorphic restricting CD1d antigen or the invariant Jα281 TCR, are protected from oxazolone colitis[17], as are EBI3$^{-/-}$ mice[15]. The number of iNKT cells in EBI3-deficient mice is about 40% of that in wild-type mice[15], and might by itself not account for the almost complete protection from colitis. As noted, it is associated with a severe impairment of IL-4 secretion upon stimulation with a cognate CD1d-restricted antigen, αGalCer. This impairment in early IL-4 secretion from iNKT cells might substantially add to the diminished Th2 response[15]. In contrast to its effect on IL-4 secretion, IFN-γ secretion is only mildly affected at early time-points, and not affected at later ones. This might be related to compensation for IFN-γ production by other cell types, for example the NK cell, and might also explain the non-impaired development of Th1-associated TNBS colitis in EBI3$^{-/-}$ mice[15].

Furthermore, it remains to be determined at what stage EBI3 interacts with the developmental pathway of iNKT cells. Some other cytokines (IL-15), receptors (IL-2R, GM-CSF-R, γ^c chain), and transcription factors (Ets1, Irf1) have been linked to impaired development of iNKT cells[19], but their and EBI3's exact role in the development of iNKT are largely not understood to date.

In conclusion, it is intriguing to note that IL-12 and EBI3, both derived from DCs, support the development and opposite outcomes of T-cell differentiation, namely Th1 and Th2 (Figure 1). While Th2 differentiation has long been considered a default pathway of T helper cell differentiation, these data lend strong support on the notion that Th2 development might be as instructed by EBI3 as is Th1 development by IL-12. EBI3's increased expression in ulcerative colitis, and more importantly the abrogation of oxazolone colitis, in EBI3$^{-/-}$ mice lends further support to the appreciation of this cytokine as a central mediator of 'Th2'-mediated disease, and might possibly open the door to therapeutic intervention.

References

1. Blumberg RS, Saubermann LJ, Strober W. Animal models of mucosal inflammation and their relation to human inflammatory bowel disease. Curr Opin Immunol. 1999;11:648–56.
2. Strober W, Fuss IJ, Blumberg RS. The immunology of mucosal models of inflammation. Annu Rev Immunol. 2002;20:495–549.
3. Podolsky DK. Inflammatory bowel disease. N Engl J Med. 2002;347:417–29.
4. Monteleone I, Vavassori P, Biancone L, Monteleone G, Pallone F. Immunoregulation in the gut: success and failures in human disease. Gut. 2002;50(Suppl. 3):III60–4.
5. Neurath MF, Fuss I, Kelsall BL, Stuber E, Strober W. Antibodies to interleukin 12 abrogate established experimental colitis in mice. J Exp Med. 1995;182:1281–90.
6. Trinchieri G. Interleukin-12 and the regulation of innate resistance and adaptive immunity. Nat Rev Immunol. 2003;3:133–46.
7. Oppmann B, Lesley R, Blom B et al. Novel p19 protein engages IL-12p40 to form a cytokine, IL-23, with biological activities similar as well as distinct from IL-12. Immunity. 2000;13: 715–25.
8. Pflanz S, Timans JC, Cheung J et al. IL-27, a heterodimeric cytokine composed of EBI3 and p28 protein, induces proliferation of naive CD4(+) T cells. Immunity. 2002;16:779–90.
9. Devergne O, Hummel M, Koeppen H et al. A novel interleukin-12 p40-related protein induced by latent Epstein–Barr virus infection in B lymphocytes. J Virol. 1996;70:1143–53.
10. Devergne O, Coulomb-L'Hermine A, Capel F, Moussa M, Capron F. Expression of Epstein–Barr virus-induced gene 3, an interleukin-12 p40-related molecule, throughout human pregnancy: involvement of syncytiotrophoblasts and extravillous trophoblasts. Am J Pathol. 2001;159: 1763–76.
11. Eckmann L, Smith JR, Housley MP, Dwinell MB, Kagnoff MF. Analysis by high density cDNA arrays of altered gene expression in human intestinal epithelial cells in response to infection with the invasive enteric bacteria *Salmonella*. J Biol Chem. 2000;275:14084–94.
12. Devergne O, Birkenbach M, Kieff E. Epstein–Barr virus-induced gene 3 and the p35 subunit of interleukin 12 form a novel heterodimeric hematopoietin. Proc Natl Acad Sci USA. 1997;94: 12041–6.
13. Christ AD, Stevens AC, Koeppen H et al. An interleukin 12-related cytokine is up-regulated in ulcerative colitis but not in Crohn's disease. Gastroenterology. 1998;115:307–13.
14. Omata F, Birkenbach M, Matsuzaki S, Christ AD, Blumberg RS. The expression of IL-12 p40 and its homologue, Epstein–Barr virus-induced gene 3, in inflammatory bowel disease. Inflamm Bowel Dis. 2001;7:215–20.
15. Nieuwenhuis EE, Neurath MF, Corazza N et al. Disruption of T helper 2-immune responses in Epstein–Barr virus-induced gene 3-deficient mice. Proc Natl Acad Sci USA. 2002;99:16951–6.
16. Boirivant M, Fuss IJ, Chu A, Strober W. Oxazolone colitis: a murine model of T helper cell type 2 colitis treatable with antibodies to interleukin 4. J Exp Med. 1998;188:1929–39.
17. Heller F, Fuss IJ, Nieuwenhuis EE, Blumberg RS, Strober W. Oxazolone colitis, a Th2 colitis model resembling ulcerative colitis, is mediated by IL-13-producing NK-T cells. Immunity. 2002;17:629–38.
18. Kaisho T, Akira S. Regulation of dendritic cell function through Toll-like receptors. Curr Mol Med. 2003;3:373–85.
19. Kronenberg M, Gapin L. The unconventional lifestyle of NKT cells. Nat Rev Immunol. 2002;2:557–68.

19
Effector mechanisms governing experimental mucosal inflammation and human inflammatory bowel disease; new targets for anticytokine therapy

I. J. FUSS, P. J. MANNON and W. STROBER

INTRODUCTION: Th1 AND Th2 MODELS OF EXPERIMENTAL COLITIS

Some of the most important recent advances in our understanding of inflammatory bowel disease (IBD) (Crohn's disease and ulcerative colitis, CD and UC respectively) have come from the study of the many murine models of mucosal inflammation resembling these diseases[1]. Perhaps the key finding to emerge from these studies is that in most if not all cases the mucosal inflammation can be shown to be due to either an excessive Th1 T cell response or an excessive Th2 T cell response, with the former characterized by increased IL-12, IFN-γ and TNF-α production and the latter by increased IL-4 production. This is nicely shown in the parallel models of colitis induced by the administration of haptenating agents such as trinitrobenzene sulphonic acid (TNBS) or oxazolone[2,3]. Thus, in TNBS-colitis-susceptible mouse strains (SJL/J or C57Bl/10 mice) one sees a dense transmural inflammation associated with an almost 'pure' Th1 response dominated by IL-12 and other Th1 cytokine production (see Figure 1). In addition, one sees a complete prevention of inflammation or a reversal of established inflammation by administration of anti-IL-12 (p40 chain) antibody, an agent that may oppose the activity of both IL-12 and IL-23, the two major initiating cytokines of the Th1 response. Conversely, in oxazolone colitis (also induced in the above mouse strains) one sees a relatively superficial inflammation marked by epithelial cell disruption associated with an equally pure Th2 response, in this case initially dominated by IL-4 production and reversed by

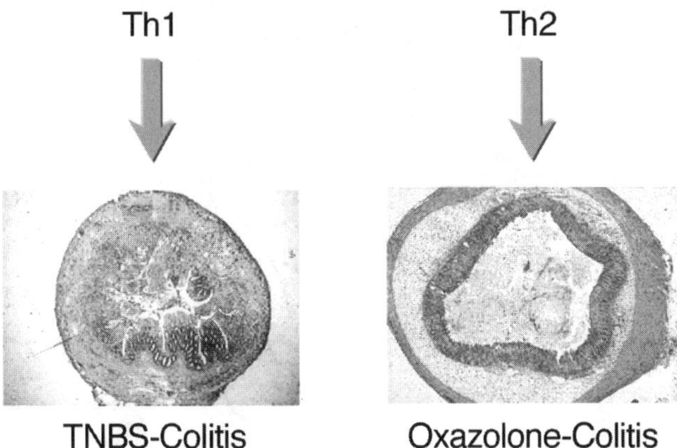

Figure 1 Th1 and Th2 experimental colitides. Two haptenating agents, TNBS and oxazolone, elicit very different forms of experimental colitis in SJL/J and C57BL/10 mice following their intrarectal administration in ethanol (the latter an agent that decreases epithelial barrier function). TNBS causes an IL-12-induced Th1 immune response that results in a transmural inflammation resembling Crohn's disease. Oxazolone causes an IL-4-induced Th2 immune response that rapidly 'morphs' into an IL-13-mediated inflammation resembling ulcerative colitis

administration of anti-IL-4 antibodies (see Figure 1). Recently, we have shown, using a more chronic form of oxazolone colitis, that the initial IL-4 response is rapidly superseded by an IL-13 response and that the inflammation can also be reversed by inhibitors of IL-13 such as IL-13Rα2-Fc, a decoy IL-13 receptor that binds to IL-13 and prevents its signalling[4]. In addition, we have shown that the cell producing IL-13 in oxazolone colitis is an NKT cell, i.e. a cell that bears a T cell receptor (TCR) along with NK markers. Thus, mice administered antibodies that eliminate NKT cells (anti-NK1.1 antibodies) or interfere with the presentation of antigen to NKT cells (anti-CD1d antibodies) prevent the development of oxazolone colitis. Similarly, knockout mice lacking CD1d or having a defective T cell receptor specific for NKT cells are also resistant to the development of oxazolone colitis. Finally, we have shown that the NKT cells producing IL-13 in oxazolone colitis bear a TCR that is found in the vast majority of NKT cells, that is the so-called invariant TCR receptor containing (in the mouse) the Vα14 α-chain variable region marker that reacts with a 'generic' NKT cell antigen known as α-galactosyl-ceramide, and the latter glycolipid antigen induces NKT cells from mice with oxazolone colitis to produce IL-13. It is interesting to speculate that, while the tissue damage in TNBS colitis is due to the elaboration of TNF-α and other proinflammatory Th1 cytokines, in oxazolone colitis it may be due to direct toxic effects of IL-13 and/or cytotoxic NKT cells (acting directly) or indirectly on epithelial cells (see Figure 2).

The histopathological features of TNBS colitis and oxazolone colitis bear a strong resemblance to CD and UC, as do other models of Th1 and Th2 immune responses respectively. It is thus of great interest to determine if the two forms of

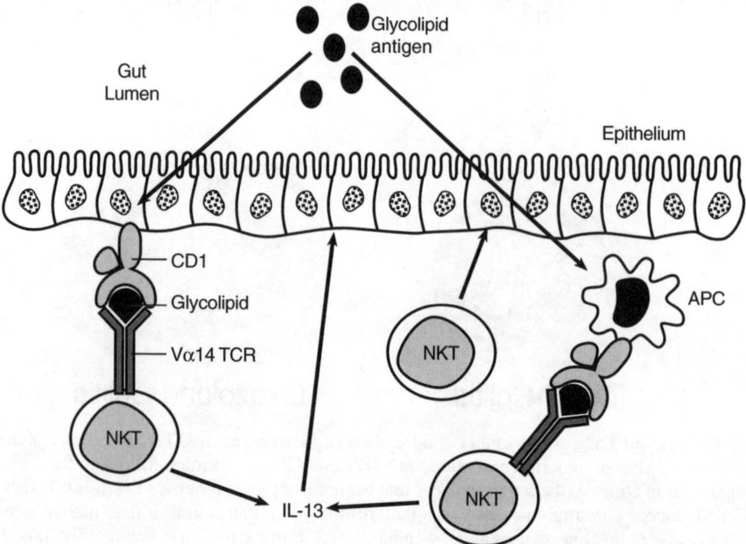

Figure 2 Immunopathogenesis of oxazolone colitis. In this Th2 experimental colitis, NKT cells undergo stimulation and expansion by a glycolipid in the mucosal milieu. The latter are presented to NKT cells by CD1d molecules and the resulting stimulation leads to the production of IL-13. Epithelial cells are subject to damage either as a result of exposure to IL-13 or to the NKT cells that recognize epithelial cells as targets. A similar mechanism may underlie the pathogenesis of ulcerative colitis

human IBD also conform to the Th1/Th2 paradigm. This question is not a trivial one, since many students of IBD are still uncertain that CD is a Th1 T cell-mediated inflammation or that UC is a Th2 T cell-mediated inflammation. Thus, it is well worth analysing the available evidence to demonstrate whether human IBD can be organized immunologically in the same way as in the murine models.

EFFECTOR CELLS MEDIATING CD

Turning our attention first to CD, we can point to a large body of compelling evidence that this form of IBD is in fact associated with a Th1 response. First, when inflamed intestinal tissue from patients with IBD is subjected to immuno-histological study, it is found that such tissue from CD patients is replete with macrophages producing IL-12, whereas tissue from UC patients is not[5]. These *in-situ* studies of IL-12 are corroborated by studies of IL-12 production by macrophages that are isolated from inflamed intestinal tissues. In this case gut mucosal macrophages from CD patients produce increased IL-12 compared to control patients, whereas macrophages from UC patients produce decreased IL-12 compared to control patients[6].

Second, the above evidence of increased IL-12 production in CD is reaffirmed by data showing that CD is associated with increased IL-12 signalling. In particular it has been demonstrated that nuclear extracts of T cells from CD lesions contain Th1-related transcription factors that are detected by electrophoretic mobility shift assays (EMSAs). T cells from CD patients, but not UC patients, contain activated (intranuclear) Stat4 and T-bet, the former a factor that is activated directly by IL-12 and the latter a factor activated indirectly by IL-12 via the production of IFN-γ and stimulation of cells via Stat1[7]. A final piece of evidence that IL-12 signalling is a feature of CD but not UC arises from the fact that cells isolated from CD tissues bear the IL-12Rβ2 chain, the signalling chain of the IL-12 receptor that is up-regulated during exposure to IL-12[8].

It should be noted that the above evidence of increased IL-12 signalling in CD but not in UC does not explain the observation that lamina propria cells from both CD and UC patients can produce IFN-γ upon stimulation, albeit in different amounts. The fact is that the IFN-γ production in UC is not associated with a level of IL-12 signalling that can be easily discerned, but appears to be the result of low-level IL-12 signalling that may be the result of 'background', non-pathological stimulation of cells by antigens in the normal mucosal microflora. That this type of stimulation is not associated with disease is widely presumed to be due to the capacity of the normal mucosal immune system to mount counter-regulatory responses characterized the production of IL-10 and TGF-β[9].

Third and last, stimulation of either purified (CD4+) T cells extracted from IBD tissues or T cell lines derived from such cells with polyclonal stimulants reveals that cells from CD patients produce substantially more IFN-γ than do cells from control patients, whereas cells from UC patients produce the same amount as controls[10]. Furthermore, peripheral blood CD45RO cells from CD patients, i.e. cells with a mature phenotype that enter the circulation from affected intestinal sites, also overproduce IFN-γ. These data complete the circle in that they show that the increased IL-12 production by CD inflammatory cells is accompanied by the production of Th1 cytokines, notably IFN-γ.

The data supporting the presence of a Th1 response in CD (but not in UC) provide evidence that CD is associated with a Th1 response; nevertheless, the data fall short of proving that CD is caused by a dysregulated Th1 response. In the TNBS colitis model (as well as in other Th1 murine models of IBD) this proof was provided by studies (already mentioned above) that administration of anti-IL-12 prevented and treated the colitis (reviewed in ref. 1). Recently we have performed a similar experiment in humans in the course of testing the therapeutic effect of a monoclonal human anti-IL-12 antibody in CD (P. Mannon, I. Fuss, and W. Strober, unpublished observations). These data will be reported in full elsewhere. Suffice to say here that, at a certain dose and administration regimen, anti-IL-12 treatment was highly effective in treatment of patients with CD, even patients with long-standing, highly active disease. Moreover, in a subset of patients in whom the immunological effect of the antibody was determined, this response was accompanied by a dramatic fall in IL-12 and IFN-γ production by cells extracted from biopsy tissue of patients taken after therapy (as compared to production by cells extracted from tissue before therapy). When administered to mice with colitis, anti-IL-12 induces apoptosis of Th1 cells; thus the mechanism of the therapy may contribute to its cytotoxic potential[11]. Whether a similar mechanism underlies anti-IL-12 therapy in humans remains to be seen.

So far in this discussion of the immunological basis of CD we have been focusing on IL-12, a cytokine long thought to be the only cytokine capable of initiating a fully-fledged Th1 response. In recent years, however, it has become evident that a second Th1-inducing cytokine, termed IL-23, may also be an important player in the Th1 response (see Figure 3A). Evidence for this possibility comes from a recent publication showing that, in another Th1 model of inflammation,

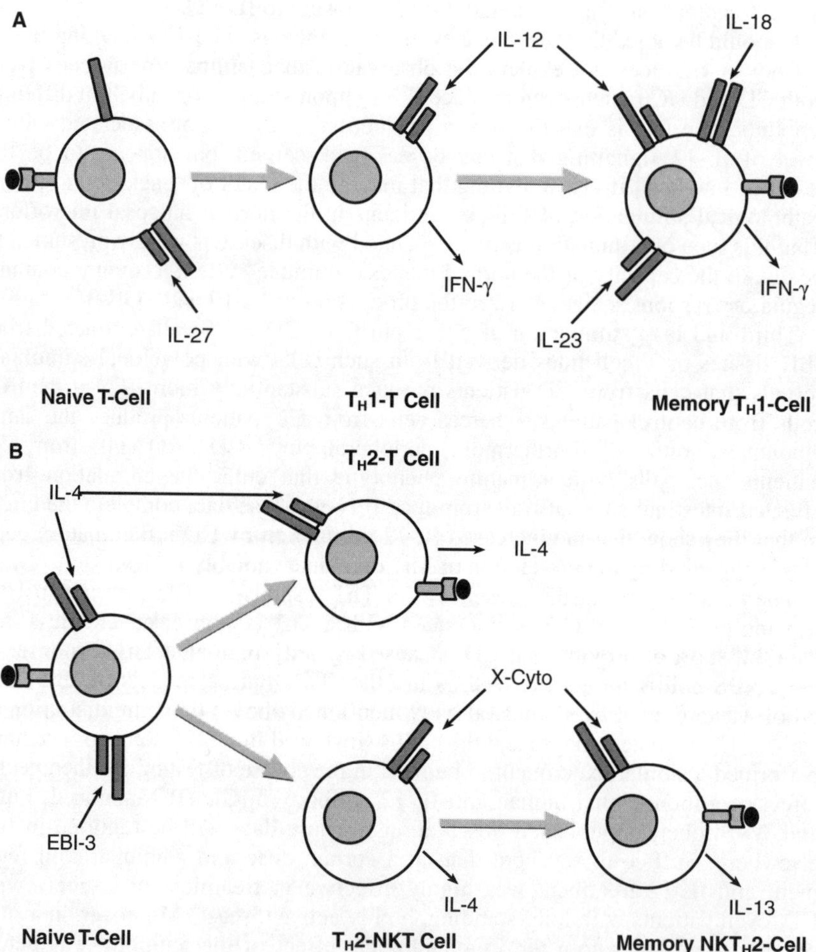

Figure 3   The possible role of EBI3 in the induction of Th1 and Th2 responses. **A:** When associated with the p28 chain to form IL-27, EBI3 acts on early (naive) T cells via a unique receptor (containing the 'WSX' chain) to induce the Th1 factor, T-bet. This activity may channel T cell differentiation towards a Th1 response. **B:** When linked to an alternative chain that could be p19 (the chain associated with IL-23), EBI3 favours NKT cell differentiation into Th2 cells that support oxazolone colitis; thus in the absence of EBI3 one sees poor Th2 responses and resistance to the development of oxazolone colitis. (X-Cyto refers to an unknown cytokine which may function to differentiate cells from IL-4-producing cells to IL-13-producing cells)

experimental autoimmune encephalomyelitis (a murine model of human multiple sclerosis), blockade of IL-23 response prevents development of disease[12]. IL-23 is similar to IL-12 in that the two share an identical chain, the p40 chain. However, whereas in IL-12 p40 is linked to a second chain known as p35, in IL-23 p40 is linked to another second chain, known as p19[13]. The limited data available concerning the role of IL-23 in the Th1 response show that this cytokine activates a more mature cell population than does IL-12; thus it is possible that, whereas IL-12 is important at an early stage of the Th1 response, IL-23 is necessary to sustain that response[14]. So far we have little information concerning the levels of IL-23 in IBD, but it seems likely that this cytokine will also be found to play a role in disease pathogenesis. It should be noted, however, that the antibodies that have proved effective in either experimental or human Th1 colitides have been anti-IL-12 (p40) antibodies that would address both IL-12 and IL-23. Whether anti-IL-12 (p35) or anti-IL-23 (p19) antibodies (or indeed, antibodies to receptors of these cytokines) can be used in the treatment of CD remains to be seen.

EFFECTOR CELLS MEDIATING UC

Turning our attention to the T cell response in UC, we should first note that, while there is abundant evidence that in CD T cells extracted from the lamina propria produce increased amounts of the 'signature' Th1 cytokine, IFN-γ, in UC the corresponding T cells do not produce increased amounts of the signature Th2 cytokine, IL-4[10]. These cells produced decreased amounts of IL-4 compared to cells from controls. Despite this inconsistency there is considerable data suggesting that UC is a Th2-mediated inflammation, arising both from existing and emerging reports.

The first point to mention in this respect is the fact that UC, to a far greater extent than CD, is characterized by the production of various autoantibodies such as antineutrophil cytoplasmic antibody (ANCA) and antitropomyosin[15]. This association can be attributable to the presence of an underlying Th2 response, inasmuch as it is well known that the production of Th2 cytokines such as IL-4 and IL-5 provide more efficient help for B cell production of antibodies than do Th1 cytokines such as IFN-γ. Along these lines it is known that immunoglobulin classes produced in UC and CD differ from one another in a manner explainable by the kind of cytokines characteristic of Th1 and Th2 responses. IgG1 and IgG4 immunoglobulins, 'Th2 immunoglobulins' are produced *in vivo* and *in vitro* by patients with UC, whereas IgG2 antibody, 'a Th1 immunoglobulin', is produced under the same conditions by patients with CD[15].

To this evidence of a Th2 response in UC one can add the fact that, while IL-4 production is not increased in this disease, production of another Th2 cytokine, IL-5, is increased[10]. In addition, it has recently been shown that production of a newly identified cytokine with potential Th2 function, Epstein–Barr virus-induced gene 3 (EBI3) is increased in UC but not in CD[16]. As discussed at greater length below, EBI3 production is necessary for the development of oxazolone colitis, and thus at least one function of this molecule is to play some role in Th2 responses.

Yet another piece of evidence that UC is mediated by a Th2 response flows from the fact that oxazolone colitis, the Th2-mediated experimental colitis discussed above, bears a histopathological resemblance to UC[3,4]. Recently we have conducted studies to formally determine if indeed the immunological findings in human UC are similar to those in murine oxazolone colitis. Suffice to say at this point that one does indeed find that cells from patients with UC exhibit increased IL-13 production as compared to cells from CD patients or controls (I. Fuss, F. Heller, M. Boirivant et al., CD1d-restricted (NKT) cells that produce IL-13 characterize an atypical Th2 response in ulcerative colitis (submitted)). Thus, these findings are pointing in the direction that UC is indeed mediated by a type of Th2 response.

DOWNSTREAM EFFECTOR CYTOKINES IN IBD

While, as emphasized above, the emerging evidence that IL-12/IL-23 or IL-4/IL-13 are the key cytokines in the initiation of the inflammation seen in CD and UC respectively, other important cytokines that are not necessarily associated with either the Th1 or Th2 immune response, such as IL-15, IL-16 and IL-18, have also been shown to be over-produced in these diseases[17–19]. Nevertheless, if we rely on the evidence from the murine models showing that most experimental mucosal inflammation is reversed by antibodies to IL-12 (anti-p40) or anti-IL-4/IL-13, then it becomes less likely that these other cytokines play a decisive role in disease pathogenesis (although they may certainly contribute to inflammation).

Within this context it should also be noted that Th1 and Th2 cytokines act on macrophages and other cells to induce proinflammatory cytokines such as TNF-α, IL-1β, and IL-6, which may in fact be the immediate effectors of inflammation. An additional fact is that, while the increase in the primary Th1 and Th2 cytokines in IBD is surprisingly modest (on the order of 3–5-fold), the increases in these more downstream cytokines are quite robust (on the order of 10–20-fold)[20,21]. This argues that even small perturbations in the production of primary cytokines can lead to inflammation as a result of a poorly understood multiplier effect, and that these cytokines are, of necessity, under tight control.

NEWLY EMERGING CYTOKINES THAT MAY INITIATE OR REGULATE Th1/Th2 RESPONSES

In the past few years several new cytokines have been described that appear to play specialized roles in the shaping of the overall Th1 response, and we need to begin to consider the possibility that these cytokines also enter into the pathological picture of IBD. One or more of such cytokines are those that contain EBI3 as a constituent chain[13]. EBI3 is a molecule that was initially shown to be produced by EB virus-transformed B cells and that was subsequently found to have homology with the p40 chain of IL-12[22,23]. Thus, like IL-23 mentioned above, cytokines containing EBI3 can be considered part of the IL-12 family of cytokines.

In one line of study it was shown that EBI3 is bound to a newly discovered and novel p28 chain that is related to the p35 chain of IL-12, thus creating an additional link between EBI3 and IL-12[24]. The heterodimer thus formed has been named IL-27, and has been shown to be a Th1-class cytokine in that it induces IFN-γ rather than IL-4 production. In addition, it was shown that IL-27 tends to act on naive rather than memory T cells, and thus appears to be a cytokine acting relatively early in the Th1 response[24]. This latter view is corroborated by studies showing that IL-27 acts through a novel receptor containing a chain known as 'WSX', whose absence in WSX knockout mice leads to delayed but ultimately adequate Th1 responses to *Leishmania* infection, suggesting that, while this cytokine 'jump-starts' the Th1 response, the expected Th1 response can still occur in its absence[25]. Further evidence that IL-27 is a Th1-type cytokine comes from very recent studies showing that signalling via WSX leads to T-bet expression, i.e. expression of an important intracellular factor necessary for Th1 differentiation[26].

In a second and somewhat contrary line of study, it was shown that EBI3 is linked to another chain, perhaps the p19 chain otherwise associated with IL-23, and in this form is an important element in the generation of Th2 responses (see Figure 3B). The data that support the latter possibility are from a recent study showing that EBI3 knockout mice produce significantly less IL-4 and somewhat more IFN-γ than wild-type mice[27]. More relevant to IBD is the fact that these knockout mice have a reduced number of NKT cells, and the latter cells from these mice produced decreased amounts of IL-4 under appropriate stimulation. In addition, EBI3 knockout mice were resistant to the induction of oxazolone colitis, but not to the induction of TNBS colitis. Taken together, these results indicate that EBI3, in association with a chain other than p28, acts as a Th2 cytokine rather than as a Th1 cytokine. Furthermore, they imply that elevations in EBI3 in UC, mentioned above, are fully compatible with the idea that UC is a Th2 disease.

In the face of the discovery that EBI3 may form the basis of two new cytokines that separately affect the Th1 and Th2 responses, we now need to seriously consider the possibility that defects in the expression of EBI3 proteins may play a role in IBD pathogenesis. This applies particularly to UC, since the data indicate that EBI3 has a critical role in the development of Th2 responses mediated by NKT cells, i.e. the responses that, on the basis of the oxazolone-colitis model, may be key factors in the development of UC.

CONCLUSION: THE STURDINESS OF THE Th1/Th2 PARADIGM

The message that emerges from the data provided by both murine models of inflammation and human IBD is that very diverse genetic abnormalities of mucosal immune function resolve themselves into dominant activity of either the Th1 or Th2 T cell effector pathways. This conclusion has important theoretical implications for the understanding of the mechanism of IBD, as well as practical implications for its therapy. The fact is that, if the pathogenesis of IBD is ultimately 'channelled' into one of two effector cell pathways, we can focus the treatment of these diseases on the cytokines controlling these mechanisms. Since Th1 responses ultimately depend on the elaboration of the IL-12 family of cytokines (which now includes IL-12, IL-23 and IL-27) then these molecules and their respective receptors become a primary therapeutic target of anticytokine therapy in CD. This idea is realized by the therapeutic success of anti-IL-12 (p40) in CD, as briefly discussed above. Conversely, since Th2 responses ultimately depend on IL-4 production, then this molecule, or a molecule immediately downstream or upstream of IL-4, IL-13 and/or an EBI3-associated cytokine or their respective receptors, becomes a primary therapeutic target of anticytokine therapy in UC. We await further clinical studies to validate these basic principles.

References

1. Strober W, Fuss IJ, Blumberg RS. The immunology of mucosal models of inflammation. Annu Rev Immunol. 2002;20:495–549.
2. Neurath MF, Fuss IJ, Kelsall BL, Stüber E, Strober W. Antibodies to interleukin-12 abrogate established experimental colitis in mice. J Exp Med. 1995;182:1281–90.
3. Boirivant M, Fuss IJ, Chu A, Strober W. Oxazalone colitis: a murine model of T helper cell type 2 colitis treatable with antibodies to interleukin 4. J Exp Med. 1998;188:129–39.
4. Heller F, Fuss IJ, Nieuwenhuis EE, Blumberg RS, Strober W. Oxazalone colitis, a Th2 colitis model resembling ulcerative colitis, is mediated by IL-13-producing NK-T cells. Immunity. 2002;17:629–38.
5. Parronchi P, Romagnani P, Annunziato F et al. Type 1 T-helper cell predominance and IL-12 expression in the gut of patients with Crohn's disease. Am J Pathol. 1997;150:823–32.
6. Monteleone G, Biancone L, Marasco R et al. Interleukin 12 is expressed and actively released by Crohn's disease intestinal lamina propria mononuclear cells. Gastroenterology. 1997;112:1169–78.
7. Neurath MF, Weigmann B, Finotto S et al. The transcription factor T-bet regulates mucosal T cell activation in experimental colitis and Crohn's disease. J Exp Med. 2002;195:1129–43.
8. Parello T, Monteleone G, Cucchiara S et al. Up-regulation of the IL-12 receptor beta 2 chain in Crohn's disease. J Immunol. 2000;165:7234–9.
9. Kullberg MC, Jankovic D, Gorelick PL et al. Bacteria-triggered CD4$^+$ T regulatory cells suppress *Helicobacter hepaticus*-induced colitis. J Exp Med. 2002;196:505–15.
10. Fuss IJ, Neurath M, Boirivant M et al. Disparate CD4$^+$ lamina propria (LP) lymphokine secretion profiles in inflammatory bowel disease. Crohn's disease LP cells manifest increased secretion of IFN-γ, whereas ulcerative colitis LP cells manifest increased secretion of IL-5. J Immunol. 1996;157:1261–70.
11. Fuss IJ, Marth T, Neurath MF, Pearlstein GR, Jain A, Strober W. Anti-interleukin 12 treatment regulates apoptosis of Th1 T cells in experimental colitis in mice. Gastroenterology. 1999;117:1078–88.
12. Cua DJ, Sherlock J, Chen Y et al. Interleukin-23 rather than interleukin-12 is the critical cytokine for autoimmune inflammation of the brain. Nature. 2003;421:744–8.
13. Brombacher F, Kastelein RA, Alber G. Novel IL-12 family members shed light on the orchestration of Th1 responses. Trends Immunol. 2003;24:207–12.
14. Frucht DM. IL-23: a cytokine that acts on memory T cells. Sci STKE. 2002;114:PE1.
15. Podolsky DK. Inflammatory bowel disease. N Engl J Med. 2002;347:417–29.
16. Christ AD, Stevens AC, Koeppen H et al. An interleukin-12 related cytokine is upregulated in ulcerative colitis but not in Crohn's disease. Gastroenterology. 1998;115:307–13.
17. Liu Z, Geboes K, Colpaert S, D'Haens GR, Ruteerts P, Ceuppens JL. IL-15 is highly expressed in inflammatory bowel disease and regulates local T cell-dependent cytokine production. J Immunol. 2000;164:3608–15.
18. Seegert D, Rosenstiel P, Pfahler H, Pfefferkorn P, Nikolaus S, Schreiber S. Increased expression of IL-16 in inflammatory bowel disease. Gut. 2001;48:326–32.
19. Pages F, Lazar V, Berger A et al. Analysis of interleukin-18, interleukin-1 converting enzyme (ICE) and interleukin-18-related cytokines in Crohn's disease lesions. Eur Cytokine Netw. 2001;12:97–104.
20. Breese EJ, Michie CA, Nicholls SW et al. Tumor necrosis factor alpha-producing cells in the intestinal mucosa of children with inflammatory bowel disease. Gastroenterology. 1994;106:1455–66.

21. Reinecker HC, Steffen M, Witthoeft T et al. Enhanced secretion of tumor necrosis factor-alpha, IL-6, and IL-1 beta by isolated lamina propria mononuclear cells from patients with ulcerative colitis and Crohn's disease. Clin Exp Immunol. 1993;94:174–81.
22. Devergne O, Hummel M, Koeppen H et al. A novel interleukin-12 p40-related protein induced by latent Epstein–Barr virus infection in B lymphocytes. J Virol. 1996;70:1143–53.
23. Devergne O, Birkenbach M, Kieff E. Epstein–Barr virus-induced gene 3 and the p35 subunit of interleukin 12 form a novel heterodimeric hematopoietin. Proc Natl Acad Sci USA. 1997;94:12041–6.
24. Pflanz S, Timans JC, Cheung J et al. IL-27, a heterodimeric cytokine composed of EB13 and p28 protein, induces proliferation of naïve CD4$^+$ T cells. Immunity. 2002;16:779–90.
25. Yoshida H, Hamano S, Senaldi G et al. WSX-1 is required for the initiation of Th1 responses and resistance to *L. major* infection. Immunity. 2001;15:569–78.
26. Takeda A, Hamano S, Yamanaka A et al. Cutting edge: role of IL-27/WSX-1 signaling for induction of T-bet through activation of STAT1 during initial Th1 commitment. J Immunol. 2003;170:4886–90.
27. Niewenhuis ES, Neurath MF, Corazza N et al. Disruption of T helper 2-immune responses in Epstein–Barr virus-induced gene 3-deficient mice. Proc Natl Acad Sci USA. 2002;99:16951–6.

20
Why and how should we target tumour necrosis factor-α and interleukin-18?

B. SIEGMUND

INTRODUCTION

While the entire aetiology and pathogenesis of inflammatory bowel disease (IBD) remain unresolved, understanding has improved extensively over recent years. In parallel to the better understanding of the immunological disbalance in the mucosa, strategies targeting specific mediators in contrast to broad immuno-suppressive therapy as applied for decades are currently under investigation. The first successfully targeted specific mediator has been tumour necrosis factor-α (TNF-α)[1]. As initially demonstrated in the study by Targan and colleagues, neutralization of TNF-α by the chimeric antibody infliximab is resulting in a clinical, histological and endoscopic amelioration of disease[1]. The efficacy of infliximab treatment has been confirmed by follow-up studies in recent years, and will not form the focus of this chapter. However, one can state that infliximab treatment is efficacious for a defined subgroup of patients with Crohn's disease.

Since infliximab was primarily shown to result in therapeutic amelioration in rheumatoid arthritis (RA), other anti-TNF-α strategies shown to be effective in RA were investigated in Crohn's disease; for instance, etanercept, the TNF-α-receptor type II:Fc construct, which is highly effective in RA[2]. Surprisingly, etanercept failed to present clinical efficacy in Crohn's disease[3]; therefore, the first part of this chapter will focus on the differences between infliximab and etanercept, and the experimental evidence providing a possible explanation for this mystery. More important, at the end of this part a conclusion for future anti-TNF-α strategies will be drawn.

In the second part the focus will be on a cytokine whose function has not yet been investigated in clinical trials, namely the interferon-γ-inducing factor interleukin-18 (IL-18). IL-18 belongs to the IL-1 superfamily and seems to be of particular interest because of its strong synergism with IL-12, thereby supporting a T helper cell type 1 (Th1) polarization.

Experimental data *in vitro* and *in vivo* will be discussed, suggesting a pivotal role for IL-18 in the inflammatory process of IBD. In addition, different strategies will be presented taking advantage of the unique biology and activation mechanism of this cytokine.

SPECIFIC CYTOKINE TARGETING

Tumour necrosis factor-α

Targeting tumour necrosis factor-α (TNF-α) was initially investigated by Targan and colleagues, who could demonstrate the efficacy of the chimeric anti-TNF-α antibody infliximab in a multicentre, double-blind, placebo-controlled trial over 12 weeks in patients with moderate-to-severe, treatment-resistant Crohn's disease[1]. Since then numerous studies have been able to confirm the efficacy for a defined subgroup of patients with Crohn's disease[4]. Infliximab was initially found to be efficacious in the treatment of RA[5]. In addition to infliximab, other anti-TNF-α strategies were investigated, and shown to result in clinical amelioration in RA[2]. Since infliximab as well as etanercept presented with equal efficacy in RA, and infliximab was also shown to be efficacious in Crohn's disease, etanercept was subsequently investigated in the treatment of Crohn's disease.

Mystery of etanercept failure in the treatment of Crohn's disease

Etanercept is a construct of two identical extracellular chains of the soluble TNF-RII (also known as the p75 receptor) linked to the Fc domain of IgG1. It has been demonstrated to be highly effective in the treatment of RA[2]; hence it was first obvious to assume that etanercept administration would result in clinical amelioration in Crohn's disease patients. Sandborn and colleagues[3] performed an 8-week placebo-controlled trial in 43 patients with moderate-to-severe active Crohn's disease. Etanercept was injected twice weekly at a concentration of 25 mg, the concentration which has been shown to be of therapeutic impact in patients with RA[2]. After 4 weeks 39% of etanercept-treated versus 45% of placebo-treated patients presented with a clinical response[2]. The authors concluded at this point that administration is safe but not efficacious, and that higher doses may be required to attain a response in patients with active Crohn's disease. However, one might speculate whether or not the low dose or a different mechanism is responsible for the observed differences between etanercept and infliximab.

Infliximab versus etanercept

To understand the differences between infliximab and etanercept one has to pay attention to the biology of TNF-α and the different ways of neutralization by either agent. As shown in Figure 1 there are two TNF-α receptors, the type 1

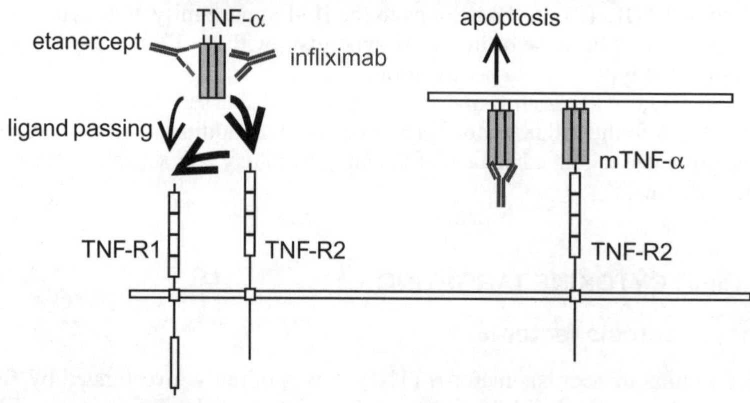

Figure 1 Biology of TNF-α, neutralization by either infliximab or etanercept. Soluble TNF-α binds primarily to the TNF-R2, subsequently ligand passing occurs and TNF-α is transferred to the TNF-R1, thereby activating intracellular signalling pathways. Activation of the intracellular signalling pathways of the TNF-R2 occurs after binding to the membrane-bound form of TNF-α (mTNF-α). Etanercept neutralizes soluble TNF-α while it exerts no effect on mTNF-α. In contrast, infliximab neutralizes soluble TNF-α; in addition it binds with a high affinity to the membrane-bound form, thereby inducing apoptosis

(TNF-R1) and the type 2 (TNF-R2) receptor, respectively. Soluble TNF-α binds to the TNF-R2 and then, due to ligand passing, TNF-α is transferred to the TNF-R1, resulting in activation of the intracellular signalling pathway. In addition to soluble TNF-α there is the so-called membrane-bound TNF-α (mTNF-α) which binds primarily to the TNF-R2, thereby resulting in the activation of the intracellular signalling pathway. The question arises as to where, in this system, infliximab and etanercept interact.

As shown in Figure 1, infliximab neutralizes soluble TNF-α; however, in addition, it binds to mTNF-α. The binding to the membrane-bound form has been shown by several groups to result in an induction of apoptosis. The mechanism has not been completely resolved; however, complement activation participates in this process[6]. In addition, apoptosis occurs through a caspase-dependent and Fas-Fas ligand-independent pathway[7]. In contrast, etanercept equally neutralizes the soluble TNF-α; however, due to a short binding affinity it does not bind sufficiently to mTNF-α, and is thereby incapable of inducing apoptosis. Since apoptosis induction seems to be crucial in order to achieve clinical improvement this might in fact represent the significant difference between the two therapeutic strategies.

TNF receptor type II

Additional experimental data suggest an important role for TNF-R2 in the inflammatory process of experimental colitis, as well as Crohn's disease. For instance, the TNF-R2 has been demonstrated to be up-regulated in peripheral blood mononuclear cells as well as in lamina propria lymphocytes of patients with Crohn's disease[8]. Furthermore, in the CD4CD62L transfer model of experimental colitis, mice receiving CD4CD62L cells from the TNF-R2 transgenic mice develop more severe colitis compared to mice receiving CD4CD62L cells from wild-type mice[8], thus emphasizing the significance of the TNF-R2 in the intestinal inflammatory process.

Small molecules suppressing TNF-α

A variety of small molecules have been shown to suppress TNF-α *in vitro* as well as *in vivo*, and have also been proven to result in amelioration in experimental colitis. However, looking at the data discussed above, one has to question whether or not the anti-TNF-α effect is responsible for the observed efficacy, or whether this is due to a secondary effect. The conclusion at this point should be that there are numerous small molecules currently under clinical investigation with an anti-inflammatory potency, and one should avoid subsuming those under the name anti-TNF-α therapy.

Conclusions for future anti-TNF-α therapy

The precise mechanism by which infliximab induces apoptosis and exerts its efficacy is not yet completely resolved. Concluding from the experimental data available, the interaction of the TNF-R2 and mTNF-α, and not the soluble TNF-α, seems to represent the target for future therapy.

Interleukin-18

While anti-TNF-α therapy has been well established for a distinct subgroup of patients with Crohn's disease, neutralization of IL-18 has not yet been investigated in humans. In the following paragraphs the experimental data available will be presented, suggesting a pivotal role for IL-18 in IBD, in particular Crohn's disease.

Biology of IL-18

Monocytes/macrophages are the best-studied source of IL-18[9]. Most of the information on the production of IL-18 is derived from mice preconditioned with *Propionibacterium acnes* and subsequently challenged with lipopolysaccharide, the original model used to isolate and clone this cytokine[10]. IL-18 acts via an IL-18 receptor complex. The IL-18 receptor complex consists of two non-identical chains: a ligand-binding chain termed IL-18Rα and a non-ligand-binding chain termed IL-18Rβ[11–13]. IL-18 does not directly induce IFN-γ and other Th1 cytokines[14], but acts together with IL-2 or IL-12 as a costimulant. The synergism between IL-12 and IL-18 and the subsequent effects on the immune system are illustrated in Figure 2.

Clinical evidence

Several studies provide strong direct and indirect evidence for a significant role of IL-18 in intestinal inflammation. Consistent with an increased Th1 response in Crohn's disease, several groups could independently demonstrate a significant

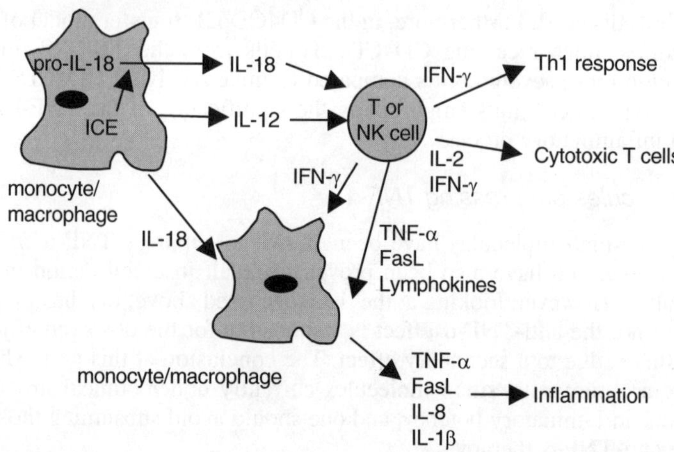

Figure 2 Biological activities of IL-18 and cell activation. Starting at the upper left, monocytic/macrophagic cells use ICE to cleave inactive pro-IL-18 into active IL-18, which is then secreted from the cell. The same cells also release IL-12 by an ICE-independent mechanism. The combination of IL-18 and IL-12 causes T lymphocytes and natural killer (NK) cells to produce IFN-γ, which (1) acts on macrophages to increase ICE expression and further activates the macrophage and (2) activates CD4[+] T lymphocytes as part of the Th1 response. The IL-18/IL-12-stimulated T cell or NK cell releases several lymphokines, TNF-α, and/or Fas ligand (FasL). In turn, these cytokines stimulate macrophages to release TNF-α, FasL, IL-8, and IL-1β, which result in increased inflammation. The IL-18/IL-12-stimulated T lymphocyte or NK cell also releases IFN-γ and IL-2, which results in the generation of cytotoxic T cells

up-regulation of IL-18 expression in the inflamed lesions of the intestine, mostly localized to macrophages and epithelial cells[15,16]. This is of particular interest mainly because no up-regulation of IL-18 was observed in patients with active ulcerative colitis or in healthy controls. While increased IL-18 expression is providing early evidence for a possible role in disease, in order to prove that IL-18 participates in the inflammatory process of intestinal inflammation it needs to be demonstrated that neutralization of IL-18 results in amelioration of disease severity.

IL-18 and intestinal inflammation

Several studies provide strong direct and indirect evidence for a significant role of IL-18 in intestinal inflammation. Nakamura and colleagues confirmed *in vivo* the synergistic effect of IL-12 and IL-18, originally described *in vitro*[17], by concomitant injection of both cytokines or either one alone[18]. While mice injected with IL-18 alone did not present with macroscopic changes, IL-12-injected mice showed significant weight loss and colitis. However, the combined administration of both cytokines resulted in severe colitis and high mortality. Chikano and colleagues confirmed this *in-vivo* synergism and showed, in addition, that the intestinal inflammation occurs in an IFN-γ-dependent but TNF-α-, NO- and Fas ligand-independent manner[19]. Consistent with an increased Th1 response in Crohn's disease, several groups could independently demonstrate a significant up-regulation of IL-18 expression in the inflamed lesions of the intestine, mostly localized to macrophages and epithelial cells[15,16]. Interestingly, no increase in IL-18 expression could be observed in inflamed lesions from patients with ulcerative colitis, which is partly characterized by an increase of Th2 cytokines[16].

In the recent literature four studies using different animal models of colitis, and different ways of IL-18 blockade, approach the question of whether neutralization of IL-18 protects from experimental colitis. An overview is provided in Table 1, and the studies are summarized in subsequent paragraphs. Our group examined the role of IL-18 blockade in the model of dextran sulphate sodium (DSS)-induced colitis[20]. In this model colitis is induced chemically, and is associated with up-regulation of proinflammatory cytokines[21]. DSS-induced colitis can be induced in *severe combined immunodeficiency* mice and is hence not T-cell-dependent[22]. However, during the course of DSS-induced colitis, T cells at the site of inflammation become activated and participate in the inflammatory process[23]. In this model an anti-IL-18 antiserum was administered to achieve IL-18 blockade. IL-18 expression could be localized to the epithelial cells and was significantly reduced in anti-IL-18-treated mice. Blockade of IL-18 was accompanied by a significant reduction in the release of other proinflammatory cytokines. In addition, histological signs of inflammation were significantly decreased by anti-IL-18 blockade.

Kanai and colleagues investigated the model of trinitrobenzene sulphonic acid (TNBS)-induced colitis and focused in particular on the role of IL-18 produced by macrophages[24]. It is hypothesized that the ethanol used as vehicle in the rectal administration of TNBS disrupts the mucosal epithelial barrier, enabling this hapten to bind covalently to proteins of colonic epithelial cells and modify cell-surface proteins. Fragments of these altered cells can be taken up by macrophages, and associated presentation of antigen to T cells by macrophages and dendritic cells results in a Th1-dominated colitis. Earlier studies showed that administration of neutralizing IL-12 antibodies, and thereby blockade of the Th1 pathway, is protective[25]. In mice treated with anti-IL-18 antibody, as well as in IL-18 knockout mice, TNBS was unable to induce significant colitis. Increase in IL-18 synthesis in this model could be localized to macrophages. Administration of an antibody directed against macrophages conjugated to the ribosome-inactivating protein saporin also resulted in protection against TNBS-induced colitis.

Ten Hove and colleagues also examined the model of TNBS-induced colitis; however, they applied a different strategy to neutralize IL-18[26]. In this study the naturally occurring IL-18 antagonist IL-18 binding protein (IL-18BP) was administered[27]. The human IL-18BP gene encodes for four different isoforms (*a–d*) generated by alternative mRNA splicing[28]. These isoforms vary in their ability to bind IL-18; only human IL-18BP isoform *a* (hIL-18BPa) and *c* have a neutralizing ability, and recombinant hIL-18BP*a* neutralizes murine IL-18. In this study, mice were treated with recombinant hIL-18BPa during the course of TNBS-induced colitis. Blockade of IL-18 by the recombinant hIL-18BP*a* resulted in a reduced clinical score accompanied by reduction of TNF-α, IL-6 and IL-1β in the colon homogenate, while IFN-γ, IL-10 and IL-4 remained unchanged.

Finally, Wirtz and colleagues neutralized IL-18 by local administration of an adenovirus expressing IL-18 antisense mRNA in the T-cell-dependent transfer

Table 1 Blockade of IL-18 in experimental colitis in mice

Animal model of colitis	IL-18 blocking strategy	Study results	References
Dextran sulphate sodium	Anti-IL-18 antiserum	IL-18 expression localized to intestinal epithelial cells; colitis aggravation accompanied by IL-18 increase; histological amelioration of colitis by anti-IL-18 treatment; significant decrease in IFN-γ, IL-18 and TNF-α in the colon after anti-IL-18 treatment	20
Trinitrobenzene sulphonic acid	Anti-IL-18 antibody	IL-18 expression localized to macrophages; anti-Mac1-saporin antibody as well as neutralizing antibody against IL-18 resulted in a dramatic histological attenuation of colitis; TNBS cannot induce significant colitis in the IL-18 knockout mice; reduction in IFN-γ in IL-18 knockout, anti-IL-18 or anti-Mac1-saporin-treated mice	24
Trinitrobenzene sulphonic acid	IL-18 binding protein	Significantly less histological signs of inflammation after hIL-18BP$_a$ treatment; significant reduction in TNF-α, IL-1β and IL-6, but no decrease in IFN-γ, IL-10 and IL-4 in colon homogenates	26
CD62L$^+$CD4$^+$ transfer model	Local administration of adenovirus expressing IL-18 antisense mRNA	IL-18 expression localized to intestinal epithelial and some mononuclear cells in the lamina propria; significant decrease in inflammation after treatment as evaluated histologically and endoscopically; attenuation of IL-18 synthesis in lamina propria mononuclear cells after treatment	29

model of colitis[29]. This model is based on the transfer of CD62L$^+$CD4$^+$ T cells in *severe combined immunodeficiency* mice, resulting, after 6–12 weeks, in chronic colitis, which is histologically similar to Crohn's disease in humans[30]. In this study a significant IL-18 reduction in adenovirus expressing IL-18 antisense mRNA-treated mice, accompanied by a decrease in endoscopically and histologically evaluated inflammation, as well as in IFN-γ production, could be observed.

Interestingly, when comparing these four studies, the administration of the neutralizing antibody, the antiserum or the adenovirus expressing IL-18 antisense mRNA and the IL-18 knockout mice seems to result in a more dramatic amelioration than the administration of recombinant hIL-18BP*a*. In particular, in the IL-18 knockout mice, as well as in the studies with the neutralizing anti-IL-18 antibody/antiserum, or after local administration of the adenovirus expressing IL-18 antisense mRNA, a significant reduction in colonic IFN-γ concentrations was observed. However, no suppression could be measured in mice after recombinant hIL-18BPa treatment[20,24,26,29]. These differences are of significance and may indicate that, although in theory all strategies described aim at the neutralization of IL-18, the IL-18BP might exert additional biological functions which are currently unknown, and require further investigations in the future.

Cleavage of IL-18 by the IL-1β converting enzyme

Posttranslational, enzymatic processing is a critical step in the modulation of the activity of several cytokines. The genes for some cytokines do not encode for a typical signal sequence common to the vast number of secretory, structural, and membrane-bound proteins. IL-1β and IL-18 are examples of cytokines lacking a leader peptide[31–33]. These cytokines gain access to the extracellular environment via secretory mechanisms that are linked to their processing. The relationship between the unprocessed IL-1β and IL-18 and the mature form of both cytokines is essential to identify the pleiotropic functions of these molecules. Both pro-IL-1β and pro-IL-18 are biologically inactive and require activation by the IL-1β converting enzyme (ICE)[9] (Figure 3).

ICE IN IBD

An early study on ICE in the context of IBD, by McAlindon and colleagues, led to an important observation[34]. Exposure of normal colonic macrophages to lipopolysaccharide induced production of precursor IL-1β, because the cells failed to activate ICE. In contrast, colonic macrophages from patients with IBD were able to activate ICE and hence release mature IL-1β in a manner similar to circulating monocytes. This is consistent with IBD macrophages being recently recruited from the circulating monocyte population. Recent studies from our group examined the acute and chronic model of DSS-induced colitis in ICE knockout mice[35]. In particular, during chronic administration of DSS over 4 weeks, ICE knockout mice presented with almost complete absence of colitis. This significant amelioration was accompanied by reduced cell activation in the draining mesenteric lymph nodes and a significant reduction of the proinflammatory cytokines IL-18, IFN-γ and IL-1β in the colon.

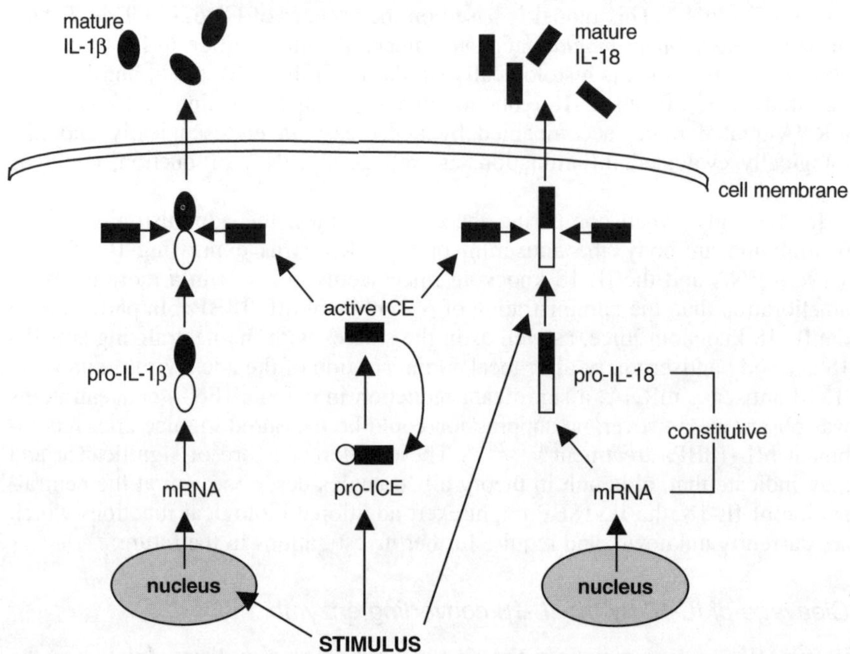

Figure 3 Synthesis, ICE processing, and secretion of IL-1β and IL-18. A human monocyte is shown. After cell stimulation, mRNA for pro-IL-1β is induced and enters the cytosol. Pro-ICE is cleaved into active ICE by members of the caspase family including ICE itself. Pro-IL-1β is found diffusely in the cytosol and is cleaved by active ICE into mature IL-1β which is secreted from the cell. Pro-IL-18 is expressed constitutively, as is the IL-18 mRNA. After stimulation of the monocyte, pro-IL-18 is cleaved by activated ICE and released

Several ICE inhibitors are available for experimental use *in vivo* or *in vitro*. Pralnacasan, an orally active inhibitor of human ICE, has been administered to healthy volunteers in phase I trials. The phase I and phase II clinical programmes have confirmed that pralnacasan is well absorbed from oral solutions and tablet formulations, and achieves plasma levels sufficient to inhibit production of IL-1β in an *ex-vivo* assay. The preliminary safety profile from these studies in healthy volunteers and RA patients is excellent[36]. Pralnacasan is currently in phase II trials in RA; no toxic side-effects have been observed[37]. Pralnacasan has also been administered to mice during acute DSS-induced colitis, resulting in significant amelioration of disease activity[38].

Conclusions for future anti-IL-18 therapies

The experimental data discussed suggest that targeting IL-18 might result in clinical amelioration in patients with Crohn's disease; however, a clinical trial is required to provide the answer. Compared to currently used strategies to suppress specific cytokines, which mostly implicate antibody therapy, the possibility of having an orally available drug whose half-life can be easily controlled is highly intriguing.

CONCLUSIONS

In summary, TNF-α and IL-18 represent very specific targets in the complex system of the mucosal immune regulation. Future clinical studies are needed, to evaluate whether neutralization of a sole mediator is superior to the treatment with 'classic' immunosuppressive agents.

References

1. Targan SR, Hanauer SB, van Deventer SJ et al. A short-term study of chimeric monoclonal antibody cA2 to tumor necrosis factor alpha for Crohn's disease. Crohn's Disease cA2 Study Group. N Engl J Med. 1997;337:1029–35.
2. Moreland LW, Schiff MH, Baumgartner SW et al. Etanercept therapy in rheumatoid arthritis. A randomized, controlled trial. Ann Intern Med. 1999;130:478–86.
3. Sandborn WJ, Hanauer SB, Katz S et al. Etanercept for active Crohn's disease: a randomized, double-blind, placebo-controlled trial. Gastroenterology. 2001;121:1088–94.
4. Hanauer SB, Feagan BG, Lichtenstein GR et al. Maintenance infliximab for Crohn's disease: the ACCENT I randomised trial. Lancet. 2002;359:1541–9.
5. Elliott MJ, Maini RN, Feldmann M et al. Treatment of rheumatoid arthritis with chimeric monoclonal antibodies to tumor necrosis factor-alpha. Arthritis Rheum. 1993;36:1681–90.
6. Scallon BJ, Moore MA, Trinh H, Knight DM, Ghrayeb J. Chimeric anti-TNF-alpha monoclonal antibody cA2 binds recombinant transmembrane TNF-alpha and activates immune effector functions. Cytokine. 1995;7:251–9.
7. Lügering A, Schmidt M, Lügering N, Pauels H-G, Domschke W, Kucharzik T. Infliximab induces apoptosis in monocytes from patients with chronic active Crohn's disease by using a caspase-dependent pathway. Gastroenterology. 2001;121:1145–57.
8. Holtmann MH, Douni E, Schütz M et al. Tumor necrosis factor-receptor 2 is up-regulated on lamina propria T cells in Crohn's disease and promotes experimental colitis *in vivo*. Eur J Immunol. 2002;32:3142–51.
9. Dinarello CA. IL-18: TH1-inducing, proinflammatory cytokine and new member of the IL-1 family. J Allergy Clin Immunol. 1999;103:11–24.
10. Okamura H, Tsutsi H, Komatsu T et al. Cloning of a new cytokine that induces IFN-gamma production by T cells. Nature. 1995;378:88–91.
11. Born TL, Thomassen E, Bird TA, Sims JE. Cloning of a novel receptor subunit, AcPL, required for interleukin-18 signaling. J Biol Chem. 1998;273:29445–50.
12. Parnet P, Garka KE, Bonnert TP, Dower SK, Sims JE. IL-1Rrp is a novel receptor like molecule similar to the type I interleukin-1 receptor and its homologues T1/ST2 and IL-1R AcP. J Biol Chem. 1996;271:3967–70.
13. Torigoe K, Ushio S, Okura T et al. Purification and characterization of the human interleukin-18 receptor. J Biol Chem. 1997;272:25737–42.
14. Ushio S, Namba M, Okura T et al. Cloning of the cDNA for human IFN-gamma-inducing factor, expression in *Escherichia coli*, and studies on the biologic activities of the protein. J Immunol. 1996;156:4274–9.
15. Monteleone G, Trapasso F, Parrello T et al. Bioactive IL-18 expression is up-regulated in Crohn's disease. J Immunol. 1999;163:143–7.
16. Pizarro TT, Michie MH, Bentz M et al. IL-18, a novel immunoregulatory cytokine, is up-regulated in Crohn's disease: expression and localization in intestinal mucosal cells. J Immunol. 1999;162:6829–35.
17. Barbulescu K, Becker C, Schlaak JF, Schmitt E, Meyer zum Büschenfelde KH, Neurath MF. IL-12 and IL-18 differentially regulate the transcriptional activity of the human IFN-gamma promoter in primary CD4+ T lymphocytes. J Immunol. 1998;160:3642–7.
18. Nakamura S, Otani T, Ijiri Y, Motoda R, Kurimoto M, Orita K. IFN-gamma-dependent and -independent mechanisms in adverse effects caused by concomitant administration of IL-18 and IL-12. J Immunol. 2000;164:3330–6.
19. Chikano S, Sawada K, Shimoyama T et al. IL-18 and IL-12 induce intestinal inflammation and fatty liver in mice in an IFN-gamma dependent manner. Gut. 2000;47:779–86.

20. Siegmund B, Fantuzzi G, Rieder F et al. Neutralization of interleukin-18 reduces severity in murine colitis and intestinal IFN-gamma and TNF-alpha production. Am J Physiol Regul Integr Comp Physiol. 2001;281:R1264–73.

21. Dieleman LA, Ridwan BU, Tennyson GS, Beagley KW, Bucy RP, Elson CO. Dextran sulfate sodium-induced colitis occurs in severe combined immunodeficient mice. Gastroenterology. 1994;107:1643–52.

22. Dieleman LA, Palmen MJ, Akol H et al. Chronic experimental colitis induced by dextran sulphate sodium (DSS) is characterized by Th1 and Th2 cytokines. Clin Exp Immunol. 1998;114:385–91.

23. Saubermann LJ, Beck P, De Jong YP et al. Activation of natural killer T cells by alpha-galactosylceramide in the presence of CD1d provides protection against colitis in mice. Gastroenterology. 2000;119:119–28.

24. Kanai T, Watanabe M, Okazawa A et al. Macrophage-derived IL-18-mediated intestinal inflammation in the murine model of Crohn's disease. Gastroenterology. 2001;121:875–88.

25. Neurath MF, Fuss I, Kelsall BL, Stuber E, Strober W. Antibodies to interleukin 12 abrogate established experimental colitis in mice. J Exp Med. 1995;182:1281–90.

26. Ten Hove T, Corbaz A, Amitai H et al. Blockade of endogenous IL-18 ameliorates TNBS-induced colitis by decreasing local TNF-alpha production in mice. Gastroenterology. 2001;121:1372–9.

27. Novick D, Kim SH, Fantuzzi G, Reznikov LL, Dinarello CA, Rubinstein M. Interleukin-18 binding protein: a novel modulator of the Th1 cytokine response. Immunity. 1999;10:127–36.

28. Kim SH, Eisenstein M, Reznikov L et al. Structural requirements of six naturally occurring isoforms of the IL-18 binding protein to inhibit IL-18. Proc Natl Acad Sci USA. 2000;97:1190–5.

29. Wirtz S, Becker C, Blumberg R, Galle PR, Neurath MF. Treatment of T cell-dependent experimental colitis in SCID mice by local administration of an adenovirus expressing IL-18 antisense mRNA. J Immunol. 2002;168:411–20.

30. Atreya R, Mudter J, Finotto S et al. Blockade of interleukin 6 trans signaling suppresses T-cell resistance against apoptosis in chronic intestinal inflammation: evidence in Crohn disease and experimental colitis in vivo. Nat Med. 2000;6:583–8.

31. Dinarello CA. Biologic basis for interleukin-1 in disease. Blood. 1996;87:2095–147.

32. Gu Y, Kuida K, Tsutsui H et al. Activation of interferon-gamma inducing factor mediated by interleukin-1beta converting enzyme. Science. 1997;275:206–9.

33. Zhang Y, Center DM, Wu DM et al. Processing and activation of pro-interleukin-16 by caspase-3. J Biol Chem. 1998;273:1144–9.

34. McAlindon ME, Hawkey CJ, Mahida YR. Expression of interleukin 1 beta and interleukin 1 beta converting enzyme by intestinal macrophages in health and inflammatory bowel disease. Gut. 1998;42:214–19.

35. Siegmund B, Lehr HA, Fantuzzi G, Dinarello CA. IL-1 beta-converting enzyme (caspase-1) in intestinal inflammation. Proc Natl Acad Sci USA. 2001;98:13249–54.

36. Siegmund B, Zeitz M. Pralnacasan Vertex Pharmaceuticals. I Drugs. 2003;6:154–58.

37. Randle JC, Harding MW, Ku G, Schönharting M, Kurrle R. ICE/Caspase-1 inhibitors as novel anti-inflammatory drugs. Expert Opin Investig Drugs. 2001;10:1207–9.

38. Loher F, Bauer C, Schmall K et al. The ICE inhibitor, pralnacasan, reduces DSS-induced murine colitis and Th1-cell activation. Gastroenterology. 2002;122(Suppl. 1 A1–688):T971 (abstract).

21
Why and how should we target CD44?

B. M. WITTIG

DYSREGULATED IMMUNE RESPONSE IN CHRONIC INFLAMMATORY BOWEL DISEASE

Mice and humans are normally tolerant to their own gut flora, and a breakdown of tolerance is associated with the development of chronic intestinal inflammation[1]. In the pathogenesis of chronic inflammatory bowel disease, such as Crohn's disease or ulcerative colitis, dysregulated activation and proliferation of CD4-positive T cells in the intestinal mucosa is a key component[2,3]. Crohn's disease is characterized as a Th1-directed immune response with increased CD4-positive T cell production of IFN-γ and activated macrophages that secret TNF-α and IL-12[4]. In T-cell activation the initial signal is delivered by the strength of the T-cell receptor signal or antigen density. The second signal is provided by engagement of one or more T-cell surface receptors with their ligands on antigen-presenting cells. In the normal individual harmless intraluminal antigens fail to induce this costimulatory activity in antigen-presenting cells. In inflammatory bowel disease, costimulatory molecules are up-regulated in lamina propria mononuclear cells. Therefore, one cause of inflammatory bowel disease might be a factor that induces aberrant costimulation and thus causes breakdown of oral tolerance.

CD44 AS A CELL ADHESION MOLECULE AND A SIGNALLING RECEPTOR

One of the lymphocyte activation markers, supposed to work as a costimulatory molecule, is the transmembrane glycoprotein CD44. The role of CD44 as a hyaluronan receptor has been known for many years and defines CD44 as a cell adhesion molecule[5]. However, there is also substantial evidence that CD44 is a potent signalling receptor. Early studies using anti-CD44 monoclonal antibodies to trigger the receptor established CD44 as a costimulatory molecule on T cells[6-9]. For example, stimulation through CD44 has been reported to enhance T-cell proliferation and IL-2 production independently of CD28[6,7,9,10]. Furthermore, it has been shown that ligation of the costimulatory molecule CD40 rapidly up-regulates CD44 expression on T cells[10]. In addition to T cells, stimulation through CD44 enhances macrophage production of proinflammatory mediators, including IL-12, IL-1β, and TNF-α[11,12]. In the past decade it has been reported that anti-CD44 antibodies have potent anti-inflammatory activity *in vivo*[13-15], most probably resulting from an antibody-mediated (anti-panCD44 antibody IM7) shedding of CD44 from leucocytes, thus preventing cell recruitment and activation[16]. Although IM7 has been taken into consideration for clinical immunotherapy in autoimmune disease and cancer, recent data have pointed out harmful side-effects, such as systemic shock[17]. This might also be due to the broad expression of the standard form of CD44 on various cells of epithelial and haematopoietic origin. Alternative splicing of at least 10 exons of the extracellular region of CD44, encoding variant extracellular regions, generates a large number of isoforms[18]. Expression of these so-called variant isoforms is strictly controlled[19] and confined to specific states of lymphocyte activation, haematopoiesis and tumour progression[20-23].

CD44v7 IS ESSENTIAL FOR A Th1-TYPE IMMUNE RESPONSE

In the mouse model for experimental colitis, CD44v6 and v7 containing isoforms are little expressed on resting lymphocytes in the spleen, lymph nodes, peripheral blood or Peyer's patches[20,24]. After *in-vitro* stimulation via a T-cell mitogen or a nominal antigen, however, there is an up-regulation of CD44v6 and v7 isoforms. Expression patterns of these splice variants define the molecules as activation markers in gut-associated lymphoid tissue. In experimental colitis CD44v7 expression is strongly up-regulated on mononuclear cells of intestinal inflammatory lesions in Th1-polarized inflammation. Unlike *in-vitro* stimulation, expression of CD44v7 is not transient, but persistent[25]. Based on these data it was demonstrated that administration of a monoclonal antibody against CD44v7[26], cures TNBS (2,4,6-trinitrobenzene sulphonic acid)-induced colitis in mice. The colitis induced by the haptenizing agent TNBS has been described as Th1-cytokine-driven inflammation[27]. In this model, after an initial increase of the proinflammatory cytokine IFN-γ, the therapeutic effect of anti-CD44v7 antibody treatment was accompanied by an increased production of IL-10 and a decreased production of IL-12 in lamina propria lymphocytes as well as systemically[28]. Furthermore, co-administration of a neutralizing antibody to IL-10 (2A5.7) completely abrogated the therapeutic effect of anti-CD44v7 antibody in TNBS colitis, which indicates the central role of IL-10 in CD44v7 regulation. It appears that the CD44v7-specific antibody functions by regulating an overshooting Th1 reaction in chronic inflammation[29]. To further define the role of CD44v6 and v7 in colitis, mice bearing a targeted deletion of exons v6 and v7 of CD44 – without affecting the expression of the other exons – were generated. Under normal conditions these mice have no altered phenotype or changes in the distribution of cell subpopulations in the lymphatic systems. In the TNBS-induced colitis mice with deletion of CD44v7 alone and v6/v7 are protected from severe inflammation and wasting disease. Adoptive transfer of bone-marrow cells clearly identifies expression of CD44v7 on haematopoietic cells, and not on intestinal epithelia, to be necessary to establish intestinal inflammation[25]. Moreover, crossing CD44v6/v7 mutants with IL-10-deleted mice, which develop a chronic enterocolitis[30], protects mice against experimental colitis for an observation period of more than 1 year[25].

CD44v7 PROMOTES EFFECTOR LYMPHOCYTE SURVIVAL

Why and at which stage is the region encoded by CD44v6 and v7 important in intestinal inflammation? According to the expression profile and proliferation studies, CD44v7 functions as a costimulatory molecule and might be a receptor molecule on antigen-presenting cells for an as-yet-unidentified ligand. The absence of intrinsic catalytic activity in the cytoplasmic tail of CD44 suggests a lack of direct signal transfer through the molecule. The ability of the costimulatory molecule CD40 to modulate an immune response towards cell proliferation and to delay activation-induced cell death[31–33] may depend on the availability of additional co-receptors or ligands that are transiently up-regulated during T-cell activation. We have shown in the animal model that CD40 ligation rapidly induces CD44v7 expression[25]. The role of CD44 in apoptosis is controversially discussed[34–37]. However, this co-receptor function might explain how CD44 variant isoforms influence cell signalling. In our studies, in experimental colitis analysis of cell death in the inflamed lesions revealed that mononuclear cells in the CD44v7- and CD44v6/v7-deleted infiltrates had higher rates of apoptosis as compared to those from wild-type mice. The increase in apoptotic markers is restricted to inflamed lesions in CD44v7 (and v6/v7) null mice, indicating that blockade of CD44v7 may be a highly specific therapeutic approach in inflammatory bowel disease[25]. Finally, the apparent influence of CD44v7 on IL-10 production needs to be pointed out. In the mouse model IL-10 becomes significantly up-regulated by the curative treatment with anti-CD44v7[28]. In a clinical study an increased number of IL-10-producing peripheral blood mononuclear cells in patients with inflammatory bowel disease has been described after *in-vitro* culture with anti-CD44v7[38]. Interestingly, anti-CD44v7 stimulates T cells as well as B cells and monocytes to produce IL-10[38]. In line with these findings is the observation that cells induced to undergo apoptosis produce a significant amount of IL-10 protein[39,40]. Thus, apoptosis of immune effector cells can redirect an ongoing immune response to minimize dysregulated immune reactions, e.g. a Th1-cytokine response, and thus prevent tissue damage[41–43].

IS CD44v7 ALSO IMPORTANT IN HUMAN AUTOIMMUNE DISEASE?

Recent data in murine models of experimental autoimmune encephalomyelitis and rheumatoid arthritis unequivocally demonstrate that not the standard region of CD44, whose expression is unaffected by the mutation, but rather the region

Table 1 CD44v7 expression on lamina propria mononuclear cells (LPMC). Cell staining with the anti-CD44v7 antibody (vFF9) (BenderMedSystems/ Vienna). Flow cytometric analysis on a FACSCalibur (Becton Dickinson)

	Percentage CD44v7-positive LPMC median (range)
Crohn's disease	32 (18–42), $n = 12$
Ulcerative colitis	17 (6–22), $n = 9$
Controls	13 (7–1), $n = 15$

encoded by exon v7, is causally involved in autoimmune or chronic inflammation (reviewed in ref. 34). So far there are no compelling data on the relevance of CD44 in human autoimmune disease. Although both CD44v6 and CD44v7 are up-regulated upon mitogenic stimuli *in vitro*, we find an increased expression of only CD44v7, but not CD44v6, in peripheral blood and inflamed mucosa of patients with Crohn's disease, but not with ulcerative colitis (Table 1)[38,44]. Since deletion of CD44v7 protects mice from colitis by induction of apoptosis of activated T cells and macrophages, blockade of CD44v7 might be a new approach to re-induce cell death of activated cells in chronic inflammatory conditions in humans. Indeed, preliminary data demonstrate that, in patients with Crohn's disease, blockade of CD44v7 with a monoclonal antibody induces apoptosis in lamina propria mononuclear cells of inflamed mucosa, but not in non-inflamed mucosa of Crohn's disease or control tissue. This effect is not detected in the lamina propria of patients with active ulcerative colitis or acute diverticulitis. Since apoptosis induction might restore immunological tolerance in intestinal mucosa, neutralizing CD44v7 might provide a promising therapeutic approach in inflammatory bowel disease.

THE EMERGING ROLE OF CD44 VARIANTS AS OSTEOPONTIN RECEPTORS

A gene product that may play an important role in the development of type-1 immunity is the T cell cytokine-like protein osteopontin, also known as Eta-1 (early lymphocyte activation-1). Osteopontin regulates two early cytokine checkpoints, IL-10 and IL-12 production, that decide on the development of a Th1- or Th2-type immune response. It has been shown that osteopontin can enhance T-cell-dependent IL-12 production from human peripheral blood mononuclear cells, in part via its ability to regulate the expression of IFN-γ and CD40-ligand by T cells, thus promoting an early Th1 response. Mice deficient in osteopontin gene expression have a severely impaired Th1 cytokine immune response, and do not develop sarcoid-type granulomas[45]. Osteopontin is widely expressed by a variety of inflammatory cells, including T cells and NK cells, and it is produced by macrophages upon antigenic challenge. Osteopontin ligates CD44 variant isoforms v6 and v7, which might represent an essential early step in the pathway

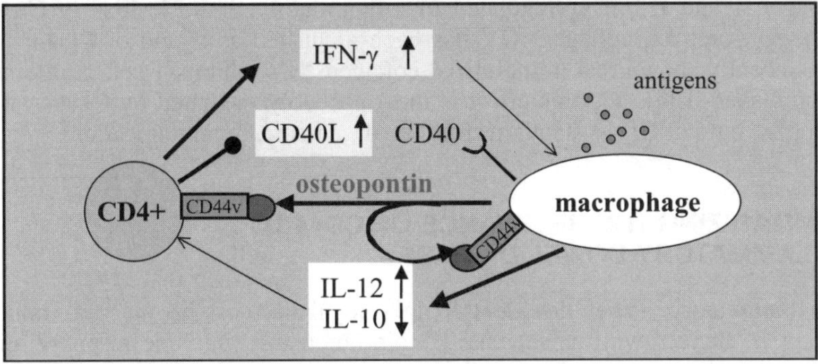

Figure 1   Model of the role of osteopontin in cellular immunity. Osteopontin is produced by macrophages upon antigenic challenge and stimulates macrophages to produce IL-12 and decrease IL-10 production. Interaction of osteopontin with its ligand CD44v6/7 costimulates activated T cells to express CD40 ligand (CD40L) and IFN-γ which further induces CD44v7 expression on T cells and macrophages in a positive feedback loop

that leads to a Th1-type immune response[46]. The interaction of CD44v6 and CD44v7 with osteopontin has been implicated in either maintaining or reconfiguring the integrity of inflamed tissue. The regulation of macrophage cytokine production by osteopontin depends on engagement of the CD44 receptor and can be blocked by antibodies to CD44. Further, CD44 antibodies inhibited the ability of osteopontin to promote the survival of mouse bone-marrow cells[47]. Our data on experimental colitis in mice are compatible with an osteopontin function in suppression of apoptosis in inflammatory conditions as well as cytokine regulation. Futhermore, inhibition of the osteopontin function in human mononuclear cells using a synthetic osteopontin peptide induces decreased cell proliferation, inhibition of IFN-γ production and an increase of IL-10 in both mononuclear cells of the peripheral blood and the lamina propria. Most interestingly, incubation with the peptide induces apoptosis in activated peripheral blood but not lamina propria mononuclear cells, indicating differences in CD44-dependent cell survival in these two tissues (Häder et al., unpublished results)[48].

Other functions of CD44, e.g. interaction with hyaluronan, could also account for its involvement in inflammation. CD44 itself plays a role in the assembly and organization of hyaluronan-rich matrices, and therefore has the potential to contribute to matrix remodelling[49,50]. While CD44 is the major cellular receptor of hyaluronan polymers, components of the extracellular matrix and a substrate for CD44-mediated cell adhesion, hyaluronan fragments are signalling molecules, which activate the immune system at the site of inflammation. These hyaluronan fragments are themselves capable of activating NFκB and are present at abnormally high levels in chronic inflammatory conditions. It can be suggested that binding of matrix components, e.g. hyaluronan fragments, via CD44 variant isoforms might mediate a specific activation signal in chronic inflammation. Besides the CD44 standard molecule, fragmented hyaluronic acid or collagen II and collagen XIV are putative ligands of the variant CD44 isoforms that may contribute to the immune-modulating activities of CD44 in chronic inflammation.

Collagen I and II are up-regulated in inflammatory tissue lesions in Crohn's disease. Moreover, collagen XIV has been identified as ligand of CD44[51]. We have recently shown that immobilized collagen XIV inhibits T-cell proliferation (unpublished data), and this effect is most probably mediated by CD44 variant isoforms, but not CD44-standard (Rühl et al., personal communication).

SUMMARIZING THE RELEVANCE OF CD44 TO INFLAMMATORY BOWEL DISEASE

In inflammatory bowel disease the tight regulation of the mucosal immune system is altered, with an increased proinflammatory immune response and a defective immune regulation. In Crohn's disease there is evidence of mucosal T-cell resistance to apoptosis that might contribute to the perpetuation of the inflammatory process. Obstruction of CD44v7 isoforms can antagonize Th1-cytokine-dependent immune pathology in animal models, identifying CD44v7 as an attractive target for the treatment of inflammatory diseases also. Although neutralizing antibodies to different antigens have been used successfully in a restricted number of clinical settings to date, small-molecule inhibitors that target either the receptor or the ligand-binding sites could provide a more feasible approach to the long-term treatment of chronic inflammatory bowel disease.

References

1. Duchmann R, Schmitt E, Knolle P, Meyer zum Büschenfelde KH, Neurath M. Tolerance towards resident intestinal flora in mice is abrogated in experimental colitis and restored by treatment with interleukin-10 or antibodies to interleukin-12. Eur J Immunol. 1996;26:934–8.
2. Zeitz M. Immunoregulatory abnormalities in inflammatory bowel disease. Eur J Gastroenterol Hepatol. 1990;2:246–50.
3. Strober W, Ludviksson BR, Fuss IJ. The pathogenesis of mucosal inflammation in murine models of inflammatory bowel disease and Crohn's disease. Ann Intern Med. 1998;128:848–56.
4. Fuss IJ, Neurath N, Boirivant M et al. Disparate CD4$^+$ lamina propria lymphokine secretion profiles in inflammatory bowel disease. Crohn's disease LP cells manifest increased secretion of IFN-gamma, whereas ulcerative colitis LP cells manifest increased secretion of IL-5. J Immunol. 1996;157:1261–70.
5. Jalkanen S, Bargatze RF, Herron LR, Butcher EC. A lymphoid cell surface glycoprotein involved in endothelial cell recognition and lymphocyte homing in man. Eur J Immunol. 1986;16:1195–202.
6. Huet S, Groux H, Caillou B, Valentin H, Prieur M, Bernard A. CD44 contributes to T cell activation. J Immunol. 1989;143:798–804.
7. Shimizu Y, Van Seventer GA, Siraganian R, Wahl L, Shaw S. Dual role of the CD44 molecule in T cell adhesion and activation. J Immunol. 1989;143:2457–63.
8. Rothman BL, Blue ML, Kelley KA, Wunderlich D, Mierz DV, Aune TM. Human T cell activation by OKT3 is inhibited by a monoclonal antibody to CD44. J Immunol. 1991;147:2493–9.
9. Denning SM, Le PT, Singer KH, Haynes BF. Antibodies against the CD44 p80, lymphocytes homing receptor molecule augment human peripheral blood T cell activation. J Immunol. 1990;144:7–15.
10. Guo Y, Wu Y, Shinde S, Sy M, Arruffo A, Liu Y. Identification of a costimulatory molecule rapidly induced by CD40L as CD44H. J Exp Med. 1996;184:955–61.
11. Hodge-Dufour J, Noble P, Horton M et al. Induction of IL-12 and chemokines by hyaluronan requires adhesion-dependent priming of resident but not elicited macrophages. J Immunol. 1997;159:2492–501.

12. Levesque MC, Haynes BF. TNF-a and IL-4 regulation of hyaluronan binding to monocyte CD44 involves posttranslational modification of CD44. Cell Immunol. 1999;193:209–14.

13. Camp RL, Scheynius A, Johansson C, Puré E. CD44 is necessary for optimal contact allergic responses but is not required for normal leukocyte extravasation. J Exp Med. 1993;178:497–507.

14. Verdrengh M, Holmdahl R, Tarkowski A. Administration of antibodies to hyaluronan receptor (CD44) delays the start and ameliorates the severity of collagen II arthritis. Scand J Immunol. 1995;42:353–8.

15. Mikecz K, Brennan FR, Kim JH, Glant TT. Anti-CD44 treatment abrogates tissue oedema and leukocyte infiltration in murine arthritis. Nature Med. 1995;1:558–63.

16. McKee CM, Penno MB, Cowman M, Bao C, Noble PW. Hyaluronan (HA) fragments induce chemokine gene expression in alveolar macrophages. The role of HA size and CD44. J Clin Invest. 1996;98:2403–13.

17. Tanaka Y, Makiyama Y, Mitsui Y. Anti-CD44 monoclonal antibody (IM7) induces murine systemic shock mediated by platelet activating factor. J Autoimmun. 2002;18:9–15.

18. Ponta H, Wainwright D, Herrlich P. The CD44 protein family. Int J Biochem Cell Biol. 1998;30:299–305.

19. König H, Ponta H, Herrlich P. Coupling of signal transduction to alternative pre-mRNA splicing by a composite splice regulator. EMBO J. 1998;17:2904–13.

20. Arch R, Wirth K, Hofmann M et al. Participation in normal immune responses of a metastasis-inducing splice variant CD44. Science. 1992;257:682–5.

21. Günthert U, Hofman M, Rudy S et al. A new variant of glycoprotein CD44 confers metastatic potential to rat carcinoma cells. Cell. 1991;65:13–24.

22. Günthert U, Schwärzler C, Wittig B et al. Functional involvement of CD44, a family of cell adhesion molecules, in immune response, tumor progression and haematopoesis. Adv Exp Med Biol. 1998;451:43–9.

23. Stauder R, Günthert U. CD44 isoforms: impact on lymphocyte activation and differentiation. Immunologist. 1995;3:78–83.

24. Wittig B, Seiter S, Föger N, Schwärzler C, Günthert U, Zöller M. Functional activity of murine CD44 variant isoforms in allergic and delayed type hypersensitivity. Immunol Lett. 1997;57:217–23.

25. Wittig BM, Johansson B, Zöller M, Schwärzler C, Günthert U. Abrogation of experimental colitis correlates with increased apoptosis in mice deficient for CD44v7. J Exp Med. 2000;191:2053–63.

26. Schwärzler C, Oliferenko S, Günthert U. Variant isoforms of CD44 are required in early thymocyte development. Eur J Immunol. 2001;10:2997–3005.

27. Neurath M, Fuss I, Kelsall BL, Stüber E, Strober W. Antibodies to interleukin 12 abrogate established experimental colitis in mice. J Exp Med. 1995;182:1281–90.

28. Wittig B, Schwärzler C, Föhr N, Günthert U, Zoller M. Curative treatment of an experimentally induced colitis by a CD44 variant v7-specific antibody. J Immunol. 1998;161:1069–73.

29. Wittig BM, Zöller M, Zeitz M, Stallmach A. IL-10 regulates the therapeutic effect of anti-CD44v7 antibody in experimental colitis. Z Gastroenterol. 1999;37:P164.

30. Kühn R, Löhler J, Rennick D, Rajewski K, Müller W. Interleukin-10-deficient mice develop chronic enterocolitis. Cell. 1993;75:263–74.

31. Björck P, Banchereau J, Flores-Romo L. CD40 ligation counteracts Fas-induced apoptosis of human dendritic cells. Int Immunol. 1997;9:365–72.

32. Blair PJ, Riley JL, Harlan DM et al. CD40 ligand (CD154) triggers a short-term CD4+ T cell activation response that results in secretion of immunmodulatory cytokines and apoptosis. J Exp Med. 2000;191:651–60.

33. Maxwell JR, Campbell JD, Kim CH, Vella AT. CD40 activation boosts T cell immunity *in vivo* by enhancing T cell clonal expansion and delaying peripheral T cell deletion. J Immunol. 1999;162:2024–34.

34. Günthert U, Johansson B. CD44 – a protein family involved in autoimmune diseases and apoptosis. Immunologist. 2000;8:106–109.

35. Ayroldi E, Cannarile L, Migliorati G, Bartoli A, Nicoletti I, Riccardi C. CD44 (Pgp-1) inhibits CD3 and dexamethasone-induced apoptosis. Blood. 1995;86:2672–8.

36. Fujita Y, Kitagawa M, Nakamura S et al. CD44 signaling through focal adhesion kinase and its anti-apoptotic effect. FEBS Lett. 2002;528:101–8.

37. Föger N, Marhaba R, Zöller M. CD44 supports T cell proliferation and apoptosis by apposition of protein kinases. Eur J Immunol. 2000;30:2888–99.
38. Wittig B, Seiter S, Schmidt DS, Zuber M, Neurath M, Zöller M. Selective upregulation of CD44 variant isoforms on peripheral blood leukocytes in patients with chronic inflammatory bowel disease and other systemic autoimmune diseases. Lab Invest. 1999;79:747–59.
39. Gao Y, Herndon JM, Zhang H, Griffith TS, Ferguson TA. Anti-inflammatory effects of CD95 ligand (FasL)-induced apoptosis. J Exp Med. 1998;188:887–96.
40. Nishigori C, Yarosh DB, Ullrich SE et al. Evidence that DNA damage triggers interleukin 10 cytokine production in UV-irradiated murine keratinocytes. Proc Natl Acad Sci USA. 1996;93:10354–9.
41. Neurath MF, Finotto S, Fuss I, Boirivant M, Galle PR, Strober W. Regulation of T-cell apoptosis in inflammatory bowel disease: to die or not to die, that is the question. Trends Immunol. 2001;22:21–6.
42. Schmidt M, Lügering N, Pauels HG, Schulze-Osthoff K, Domschke W, Kucharzik T. IL-10 induces apoptosis in human monocytes involving the CD95 receptor/ligand pathway. Eur J Immunol. 2000;30:1769–77.
43. Daigle I, Rückert B, Schnetzler G, Simon HU. Induction of the IL-10 gene via the Fas receptor in monocytes – an anti-inflammatory mechanism in the absence of apoptosis. Eur J Immunol. 2000;30:2991–7.
44. Pfister K, Wittig BM, Mueller-Molaian I, Remberger K, Zeitz M, Stallmach A. Decreased CD44v6 expression in lamina propria lymphocytes of patients with inflammatory bowel disease. Exp Mol Pathol. 2001;71:186–93.
45. Ashkar S, Weber GF, Panoutsakopoulou V et al. Eta-1 (osteopontin): an early component of type-1 (cell mediated) immunity. Science. 2000;287:860–4.
46. O'Regan AW, Nau GJ, Chupp GL, Berman JS. Osteopontin (Eta-1) in cell-mediated immunity: teaching an old dog new tricks. Trends Immunol. 2000;121:475–8.
47. Denhardt DT, Noda M. Osteopontin expression and function: role in bone remodeling. J Cell Biochem Suppl. 1998;30–31:92–102.
48. Lin YH, Yang-Yen HF. The osteopontin-CD44 survival signal involves activation of the phosphatidylinositol 3-kinase/Akt signaling pathway. J Biol Chem. 2001;276:46024–30.
49. Puré E, Cuff CA. A crucial role for CD44 in inflammation. Trends Mol Med. 2001;7:213–21.
50. Lisignoli G, Grassi F, Zini N et al. Anti-Fas induced apoptosis in chondrocytes reduced by hyaluronan. Arthritis Rheum. 2001;44:1800–7.
51. Ehnis T, Dieterich W, Bauer M, Lampe B, Schuppan D. A chondroitin/dermatan sulfate form of CD44 is a receptor for collagen XIV (undulin). Exp Cell Res. 1996;229:388–97.

Section V
Modulation of mucosal immune responses by targeting signal transduction pathways

22
New insights into the molecular mechanisms of action of azathioprine

M. F. NEURATH

INTRODUCTION

Azathioprine and its metabolite 6-mercaptopurine (6-MP) were discovered by Gertrude B. Elion and George Hitchings (Winners of the 1988 Nobel Prize in Medicine)[1]. These drugs are important immunosuppressive agents used in gastroenterology and transplant medicine. They have been widely used as immunosuppressive and anti-inflammatory agents in organ transplantation (e.g. kidney and liver transplantation) and the treatment of chronic inflammatory diseases. For instance, azathioprine and its metabolite 6-MP have been used in multiple sclerosis[2], rheumatoid arthritis[3], systemic lupus erythematosus[4], primary biliary cirrhosis[5] and inflammatory bowel diseases (IBD)[6–11]. With regard to the latter indication azathioprine and 6-MP have been suggested as gold standard for IBD treatment and have been in clinical use for more than four decades[11]. In addition to the excellent efficacy of azathioprine there is little long-term toxicity associated with azathioprine therapy[10]. However, the precise mechanism of action of azathioprine is still unknown, although inhibition of purine nucleotide biosynthesis with suppression of DNA and RNA synthesis (Figure 1) and downregulation of B- and T-cell function have been suggested as major therapeutic mechanisms[12–16]. However, such mechanism of action based on random incorporation into DNA and RNA would primarily affect tissues with rapid turnover and cell division (such as intestinal epithelial cells), and this is in contrast to the clinical findings on suppression of lymphocyte function in azathioprine-treated patients. Furthermore, azathioprine and 6-MP have recently been shown to require very high dosages to suppress proliferation of primary T cells *in vitro*[17] that are outside the clinically relevant dosages in IBD patients. Taken together, these data make it very unlikely that the classical model on azathioprine action

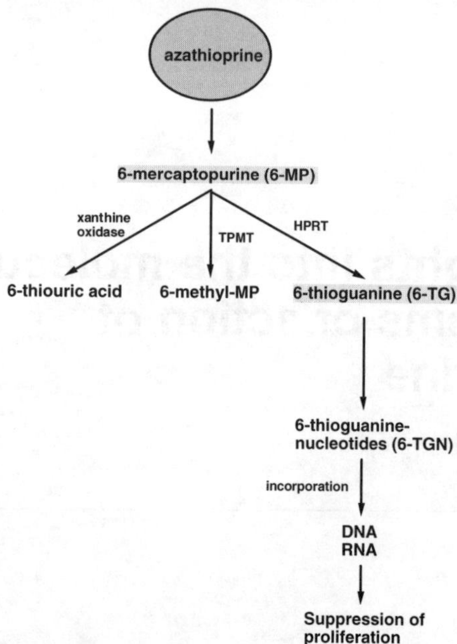

Figure 1 Old concept on azathioprine action: azathioprine and its metabolites are randomly incorporated into DNA and RNA, thereby blocking cell proliferation

based on random incorporation of 6-thioguanine nucleotides (6-TGN) is in fact operative *in vivo* in IBD patients (Figure 1). Consistent with this concept, Gertrude B. Elion stated that a knowledge of the biochemical loci of action of 6-MP in the inhibition of nucleic acid synthesis is not sufficient to explain the effects of thiopurines on the immune system[1].

This chapter will first discuss biochemical and pharmacological findings on azathioprine and then discuss the implications of recent findings on a specific molecular target of azathioprine in T lymphocytes. It has been known for a long time that the azathioprine molecule is composed of two moieties: mercapto-purine and an imidazole derivative[1,13,18]. After oral administration the prodrug azathioprine undergoes conversion to 6-MP by non-enzymatic attack by sulph-hydryl containing compounds such as glutathione or cysteine[13,19]. 6-MP is then enzymatically converted by hypoxanthine phosphoribosyl transferase (HPRT) to 6-thioguanine (6-TG). Interestingly, it has been suggested for a long time that the 6-TG generated by the HPRT pathway most likely mediate the immunosup-pressive properties of 6-MP[13]. In particular, lymphocytes have been shown to enzymatically convert 6-MP to 6-TG[20]. However, the conversion of 6-TG into 6-TGN with random incorporation into DNA and RNA could not explain the excellent therapeutic efficacy of azathioprine on T cells with little toxic effects, as discussed above.

IBD consists of two major forms: Crohn's disease and ulcerative colitis. While the latter disease is restricted to the colon, Crohn's disease is a major form of

IBD that can occur anywhere in the alimentary tract[21]. Although the precise pathogenesis of IBD is still unknown, recent data suggest that genetic factors (e.g. NOD2 mutations in Crohn's disease), environmental factors (e.g. luminal bacterial antigens) and an activation of the mucosal immune system play a major pathogenic role[21–29]. Furthermore, in the chronic phase of this disease, cytokines produced by macrophages and T lymphocytes in the lamina propria have been shown to play a key pathogenic role[30–32]. In particular, it has recently been demonstrated that proinflammatory cytokines such as TNF, IL-6 and IL-12 may cause T-cell resistance against apoptosis in Crohn's disease that leads to inappropriate lymphocyte accumulation in the gut and disease perpetuation[30,33–35].

Interestingly, it has been shown that Crohn's disease patients treated with azathioprine for only a few weeks did not respond to therapy, suggesting that this drug requires prolonged periods of time to achieve clinical responses *in vivo*[36,37]. Furthermore, a meta-analysis by Pearson et al. demonstrated that the odds ratio of response to azathioprine in this disease increased with the cumulative dose administered[36]. Since azathioprine has been considered as gold standard of immunosuppressive therapy in IBD[10,38,39], it was of interest to determine the molecular mechanism of action of this drug.

Although it was clear that azathioprine-generated thioguanine nucleotides were unlikely to mediate immunosuppression in T cells *in vivo*, there was good evidence to suggest that the active metabolites would be based on 6-TG[13]. Interestingly, Tiede et al.[40] recently showed that 6-TG, as well as azathioprine and 6-MP, are able to induce T-cell apoptosis (Figures 2 and 3). Further analysis showed that this apoptosis required prolonged periods of time, occurred at relevant dosages and was mediated by activation of caspase-9, suggesting a mitochondrial pathway of apoptosis[40]. In addition, a marked induction of apoptosis in the lamina propria was noted in azathioprine-treated patients, and azathioprine responsiveness in IBD patients correlated with the presence of apoptotic cells in the lamina propria. Finally, Tiede et al. showed that the small GTPase Rac1 is the molecular target for the azathioprine metabolite 6-thioguanine triphosphate (6-ThioGTP) (Figure 2). Azathioprine thus appears to induce immunosuppression by inhibiting Rac1 activation in T cells that is specifically linked to T-cell costimulation via CD28. In summary these data defined a unique and unexpected role for azathioprine and its metabolites in the control of T-cell apoptosis by modulation of Rac1 activation upon CD28 costimulation. Specific blockade of Rac1 activation is achieved by azathioprine-generated 6-ThioGTP that binds to Rac1 instead of GTP. Consecutively, the activation of Rac1 target genes such as MEK, NFκB and bcl-xL is suppressed by azathioprine, leading to a mitochondrial caspase-9-dependent pathway of apoptosis. Azathioprine thus converts a costimulatory signal into an apoptotic signal by modulating Rac1 activity. These findings explain the beneficial immunosuppressive effects of azathioprine, and have important implications for the design of novel specific therapies for organ transplantation and autoimmune diseases.

Since azathioprine specifically targets a protein of the Rac family, it is of interest to summarize some data on the function of Rac family members. Rac proteins have been shown to play a major role in T-cell development, differentiation and proliferation, as demonstrated by the fact that Rac2-deficient mice have a profound Th1 T-cell defect[41–43]. Whereas dominant positive Rac mutations

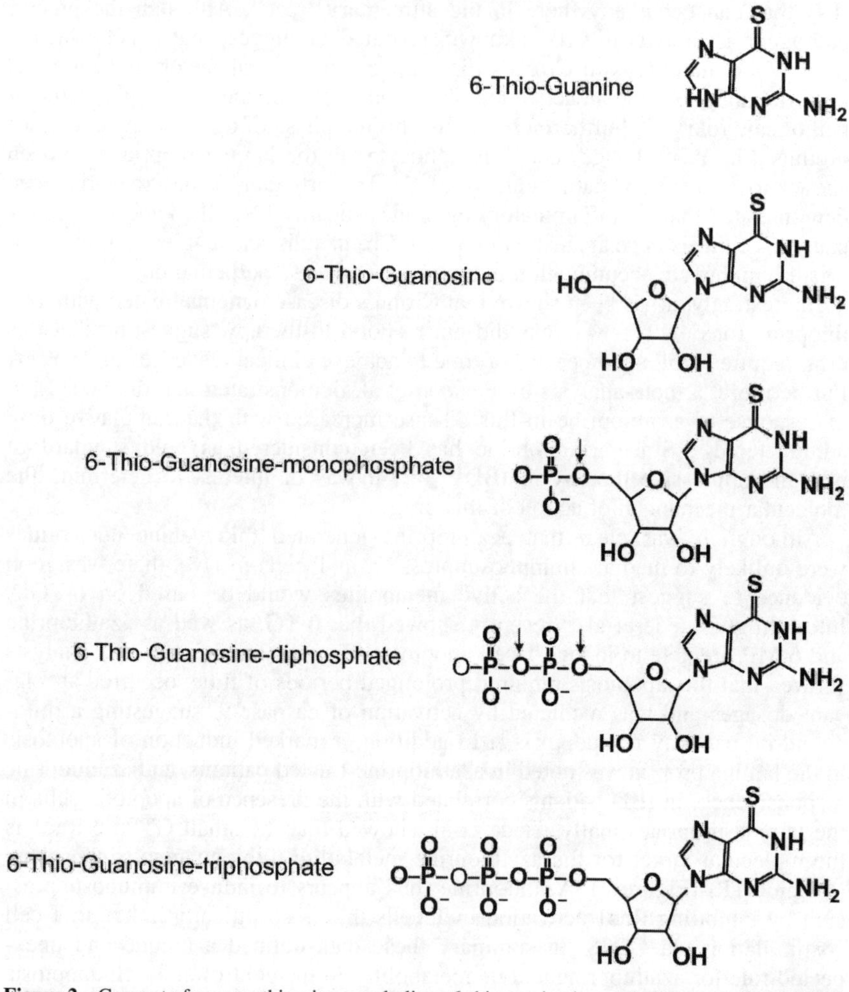

6-Thio-Guanine

6-Thio-Guanosine

6-Thio-Guanosine-monophosphate

6-Thio-Guanosine-diphosphate

6-Thio-Guanosine-triphosphate

Figure 2 Concept of new azathioprine metabolites; 6-thioguanine is metabolized into 6-Thio-GTP

have been associated with increased cell proliferation and tumorigenesis, functionally inactive Rac2 mutations are associated with immunodeficiencies in humans[44]. With regard to Rac1, it has been shown that this protein is important for thymic selection of T cells and their activation in the periphery via the CD28 signalling pathway, that is important for the initial activation of T cells and for their viability and responsiveness during a persistent immune response[41,45]. It is thus reasonable to assume that azathioprine-induced suppression of CD28 signalling events may be particularly important for the mechanism of action of this drug, as it is frequently used in chronic inflammatory diseases in which repeated antigen-specific stimulation of effector T cells occurs and in which elimination of effector T cells is needed[33,46].

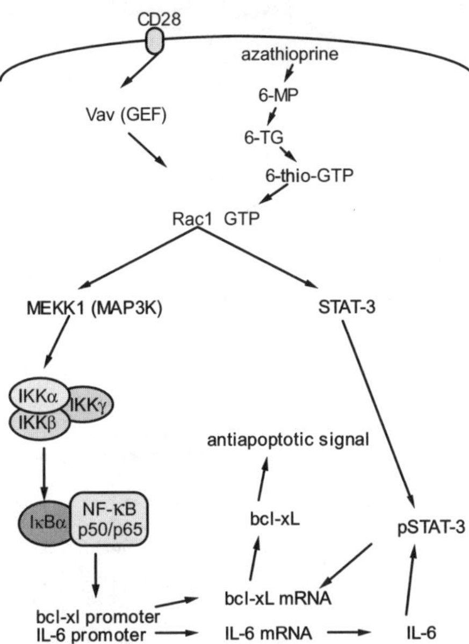

Figure 3 A new molecular model for azathioprine-mediated immunosuppression. In normal peripheral T cells CD28 costimulation leads to vav activation causing replacement of the Rac1 bound GDP by GTP[47] and thus leading to Rac1 activation. Activated Rac1 leads to activation of the IκB/NFκB pathway and STAT-3 activation that both result in enhanced bcl-xL levels. NF-κB induces IL-6 production that further induces STAT-3 activation. Augmented bcl-xL levels provide an important antiapoptotic signal in primary T cells. Azathioprine and its metabolites 6-MP and 6-TG specifically target Rac1 activation by the generation of 6-Thio-GTP that binds to Rac1 instead of the normal GTP following CD28 costimulation. Blockade of Rac1 activation leads to a mitochondrial pathway of T-cell apoptosis

Taken together, azathioprine and its metabolite 6-MP are immunosuppressive drugs that are used in organ transplantation and autoimmune and chronic inflammatory diseases such as IBD (Crohn's disease, ulcerative colitis). In IBD azathioprine and 6-MP have been successfully used since 1962, and these drugs are currently considered as gold standard for maintenance of remission in IBD patients. However, their molecular mechanism of action has been unknown. The data by Tiede and co-workers have identified a unique and unexpected role for azathioprine and its metabolites in the control of T-cell apoptosis by modulation of Rac1 activation upon CD28 costimulation. These workers also found that azathioprine and its metabolites induced apoptosis of blood and lamina propria T cells from patients with Crohn's disease and control patients. Apoptosis induction required costimulation with CD28 and was mediated by specific blockade of Rac1 activation via binding of azathioprine-generated 6-Thio-GTP to Rac1 instead of GTP (Figure 4). Azathioprine was shown to convert a costimulatory signal into an apoptotic signal by modulating Rac1 activity. These findings explain the immunosuppressive effects of azathioprine in IBD patients, define a

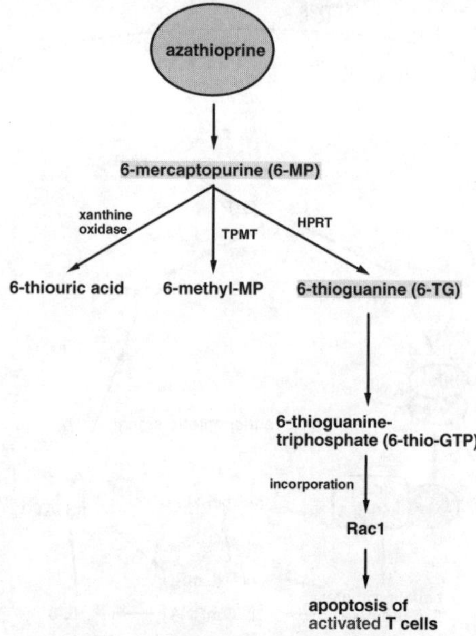

Figure 4 A new concept on azathioprine action: azathioprine blocks the Rac1/MEK kinase pathway and therefore selectively eliminates costimulated and activated T effector cells

novel concept of azathioprine action (Figure 4) and suggest that 6-Thio-GTP derivates may be useful as potent immunosuppressive agents in IBD patients in the near future.

Acknowledgements

The research of M.F.N. was supported by grants from the Deutsche Forschungsgemeinschaft (Ne 490/4-1, Sonderforschungsbereich 548, 432, 490) and the Gerhard Hess program of the Deutsche Forschungsgemeinschaft (Ne 490/3–1). M.F.N. is a recipient of a Fullbright scholarship for advanced scientists.

References

1. Elion GB. The George Hitchings and Gertrude Elion Lecture. The pharmacology of azathioprine. Ann NY Acad Sci. 1993;685:400–7.
2. Huglus DG. Double-masked trial of azathioprine in multiple sclerosis. Lancet. 1988;2:179–86.
3. DeSilva M, Hazleman BL. Long-term azathioprine in rheumatoid arthritis. A double-blind study. Ann Rheum Dis. 1981;40:560–8.
4. Ginzler E, Sharon E, Diamond H, Kaplan D. Long term maintenance therapy with azathioprine in systemic lupus erythematosus. Arthritis Rheum. 1975;18:27–35.
5. Christensen E, Neuberger J, Crowe DG et al. Beneficial effect of azathioprine and prediction of prognosis in primary biliary cirrhosis. Final results of an international trial. Gastroenterology. 1985;89:1084–91.

6. Candy S, Wright J, Gerber M, Adams G, Gerig M, Goodman R. A controlled double blind study of azathioprine in the management of Crohn's disease. Gut. 1995;37:674–8.

7. Bouhnik Y, Lemann M, Mary JY et al. Long-term follow-up of patients with Crohn's disease treated with azathioprine or 6-mercaptopurine. Lancet. 1996;347:215–19.

8. D'Haens G, Geboes K, Ponette E, Penninckx F, Rutgeerts P. Healing of severe recurrent ileitis with azathioprine therapy in patients with Crohn's disease. Gastroenterology. 1997; 112:1475–81.

9. Lewis JD, Schwartz JS, Lichtenstein GR. Azathioprine for maintenance of remission in Crohn's disease: benefits outweigh the risk of lymphoma. Gastroenterology. 2000;118:1018–24.

10. Present DH, Korelitz BI, Wisch N, Glass JL, Sachar DB, Pasternack BS. Treatment of Crohn's disease with 6-mercaptopurine: a long-term randomized, double-blind study. N Engl J Med. 1980;302:981–7.

11. Bean RHD. The treatment of chronic active ulcerative colitis with 6-mercaptopurine. Med J Aust. 1962;2:592–3.

12. Dimitriu A, Fauci AS. Activation of human B lymphocytes. XI. Differential effects of azathioprine on B lymphocytes and lymphocyte subpopulations regulating B cell function. J Immunol. 1978;121:2335–9.

13. Lennard L. The clinical pharmacology of 6-mercaptopurine. Eur J Clin Pharmacol. 1992;43:329–35.

14. Röllinghoff M, Schrader J, Wagner H. Effect of azathioprine and cytosine arabinoside on humoral and cellular immunity in vitro. Clin Exp Immunol. 1973;15:261–9.

15. Abdou NI, Zweiman B, Casella SR. Effects of azathioprine therapy on bone marrow-dependent and thymus-dependent cells in man. Clin Exp Immunol. 1973;13:55–64.

16. Bach MA, Bach JF. Activities of immunosuppressive agents *in vitro*. II. Different timing of azathioprine and methotrexate in inhibition and stimulation of mixed lymphocyte reaction. Clin Exp Immunol. 1972;11:89–98.

17. Quemeneur L, Gerland LM, Flacher M, Ffrench M, Revillard JP, Genestier L. Differential control of cell cycle, proliferation, and survival of primary T lymphocytes by purine and pyrimidine nucleotides. J Immunol. 2003;170:4986–95.

18. Hoffmann M, Rychlewski J, Chrzanowska M, Hermann T. Mechanism of activation of an immunosuppressive drug: azathioprine. Quantum chemical study on the reaction of azathioprine with cysteine. J Am Chem Soc. 2001;123:6404–9.

19. Kroplin T, Iven H. Methylation of 6-mercaptopurine and 6-thioguanine by thiopurine S-methyltransferase. A comparison of activity in red blood cell samples of 199 blood donors. Eur J Clin Pharmacol. 2000;56:343–5.

20. vanOs EC, Zins BJ, Sandborn WJ et al. Azathioprine pharmacokinetics after intravenous, oral, delayed release oral and rectal foam administration. Gut. 1996;39:63–8.

21. Podolsky DK. Inflammatory bowel disease. N Engl J Med. 1991;325:928–37

22. Beutler B. Autoimmunity and apoptosis: the Crohn's connection. Immunity. 2001;15:5–14.

23. Neurath MF, Finotto S, Glimcher LH. The role of Th1/Th2 polarization in mucosal immunity. Nature Med. 2002;8:567–73.

24. MacDonald TT, Monteleone G, Pender SLF. Recent developments in the immunology of inflammatory bowel disease. Scand J Immunol. 2000;51:2–9.

25. Shanahan F. Crohn's disease. Lancet. 2002;359:62–9.

26. Hugot JP, Chamaillard M, Zouali H et al. Association of NOD2 leucine-rich repeat variants with susceptibility to Crohn's disease. Nature. 2001;411:599–603.

27. Ogura Y, Bonen DK, Inohara N et al. A frameshift mutation in NOD2 associated with susceptibility to Crohn's disease. Nature. 2001;411:603–6.

28. Targan SR, Hanauer SB, Deventer SJV et al. A short-term study of chimeric monoclonal antibody cA2 to tumor necrosis factor alpha for Crohn's disease. N Engl J Med. 1997;337:1029–35.

29. Elson CO, Sartor RB, Tennyson GS, Riddell RH. Experimental models of inflammatory bowel disease. Gastroenterology. 1995;109:1344–67.

30. Atreya R, Mudter J, Finotto S et al. Blockade of IL-6 trans-signaling suppresses T cell resistance against apoptosis in chronic intestinal inflammation: evidence in Crohn's disease and experimental colitis *in vivo*. Nature Med. 2000;6:583–8.

31. Breese E, Braegger CP, Corrigan CJ, Walker-Smith JA, MacDonald TT. Interleukin-2 and interferon-gamma secreting T cells in normal and diseased human intestinal mucosa. Immunology. 1993;78:127–31.

32. Plevy SE, Landers CJ, Prehn J et al. A role for TNF-alpha and mucosal T helper-1 cytokines in the pathogenesis of Crohn's disease. J Immunol. 1997;159:6276–82.

33. Boirivant M, Marini M, Di-Felice G et al. Lamina propria T cells in Crohn's disease and other gastrointestinal inflammation show defective CD2 pathway-induced apoptosis. Gastroenterology. 1999;116:557–65.

34. Deventer SJv. Transmembrane TNF-alpha, induction of apoptosis, and the efficacy of TNF-targeting therapies in Crohn's disease. Gastroenterology. 2001;121:1242–6.

35. Hove Tt, Montfrans Cv, Peppelenbosch MP, Deventer SJv. Infliximab treatment induces apoptosis of lamina propria T lymphocytes in Crohn's disease. Gut. 2002;50:206–11.

36. Pearson DC, May GR, Fick GH, Sutherland LR. Azathioprine and 6-mercaptopurine in Crohn disease. A meta-analysis. Ann Intern Med. 1995;123:132–42.

37. Ewe K, Press A, Singe CC, Stufler M, Hommel G, Büschenfelde KHMz. Azathioprine combined with prednisolone or monotherapy with prednisone in active Crohn's disease. Gastroenterology. 1993;105:367–76.

38. Sandborn WJ, Tremaine WJ, Wolf DC et al. Lack of effect of intravenous administration on time to respond to azathioprine for steroid-treated Crohn's disease. Gastroenterology. 1999; 117:527–35.

39. Neurath MF, Stange E. Evidenzbasierte Immunsuppression bei chronisch entzündlichen Darmerkrankungen. Deutsches Ärzteblatt. 2000;97:1977–83.

40. Tiede I, Fritz G, Strand S et al. CD28-dependent Rac1 activation is the molecular target of azathiopurine in primary human CD4+ T lymphocytes. J Clin Invest. 2003;111:1133–45.

41. Li B, Yu H, Zheng W-P et al. Role of the guanosine triphosphate Rac2 in T helper 1 cell differentiation. Science. 2000;42:2219–22.

42. Gomez M, Tybulewicz V, Cantrell DA. Control of pre T cell proliferation and differentiation by the GTPase Rac1. Nat Immunol. 2000;1:348–52.

43. Joneson T, Bar-Sagi D. Suppression of Ras-induced apoptosis by the Rac GTPase. Mol Cell Biol. 1999;19:5892–901.

44. Williams DA, Tao W, Yang F et al. Dominant negative mutation of the hematopoietic-specific Rho GTPase, Rac2, is associated with a human phagocyte immunodeficiency. Blood. 2000;71:1646–54.

45. Noel PJ, Boise LH, Green JM, Thompson CB. CD28 costimulation prevents cell death during primary T cell activation. J Immunol. 1996;157:636–47.

46. Neurath MF, Finotto S, Fuss I, Boirivant M, Galle PR, Strober W. Regulation of T-cell apoptosis in inflammatory bowel disease: to die or not to die, that is the mucosal question. Trends Immunol. 2001;22:21–6.

47. Kaga S, Ragg S, Rogers KA, Ochi A. Activation of p21-CDC42/Rac-activated kinases by CD28 signaling: p21-activated kinase (PAK) and MEK kinase 1 (MEKK1) may mediate the interplay between CD3 and CD28 signals. J Immunol. 1998;160:4182–9.

23
Targeting NFκB by use of antisense oligonucleotides in patients with inflammatory bowel disease

S. PETTERSSON and R. LÖFBERG

INTRODUCTION

The aetiology of IBD remains largely unknown, even though certain factors that may trigger or reactivate disease into the active stage have been identified (for example NSAIDs, severe stress-like infections, etc.). The active stage of IBD is associated with an activation of NFκB, a known key regulator of the inflammatory response[1]. The functional importance of NFκB in acute and chronic inflammation is based on its ability to regulate the promoters of a variety of genes whose products, such as proinflammatory cytokines, cell surface receptors, adhesion molecules and acute-phase proteins, are critical for inflammatory processes. A number of reports have shown that NFκB is essential to maintain the chronic inflammatory process. Most notably the signals that can activate NFκB are considerable, and an array of pathogenic stimuli or immune response mediators clearly targets NFκB in order to execute their function in the build-up of an innate and adaptive immune response.

NFκB components are defined in part by their ability to bind a specific DNA sequence. One of the more important NFκB factors is the p65 subunit, which mediates transcriptional activation of a cascade of genes linked to the control of cell proliferation and differentiation. In addition several reports from animal models and human tissue sampling support the observation that the p65 subunit is one of the more important players in acute and chronic inflammation. As a consequence of these observations the p65 subunit has become an attractive target for intervention in anti-inflammatory strategies.

It is well known that several drugs already in use today as potent anti-inflammatory drugs for IBD exert their action, at least partly, by effects at the NFκB level. Corticosteroids decrease NFκB activity, and other drugs,

"

e.g. aminosalicylates and butyrate, may also have anti-NFκB effects but to a lesser extent. Although the precise molecular mechanism of action is still far from resolved, current drugs one way or another converge into and inhibit or perpetuate the function of NFκB.

NFκB INTERVENTION WITH ANTISENSE OLIGONUCLEOTIDES

Several new approaches to specifically decrease or inhibit NFκB activity have been discussed. One of the most promising is the use of antisense oligonucleotides (ASON). Antisense agents are synthetic segments of nucleic acid residues and are designed to specifically recognize and inhibit the target mRNA. ASON technology has already been extensively evaluated for parenteral use in IBD conditions (ISIS2302 vs. ICAM-1), showing acceptable toxicity but poor efficacy. In this context ASON against NFκB may be a more appropriate target. Several preclinical studies have been performed to assess the potential role of ASONs directed towards NFκB as a potent anti-inflammatory treatment. In 1996 it was reported that a single installation of a p65 ASON, administered directly into the lumen of colon, abrogated clinical signs of active experimental colitis induced in two separate murine models (TNBS and IL-10 knockout mice)[2]. In this study we could demonstrate that protein and mRNA analysis showed a reduction in p65 levels only in those mice receiving the ASON. As a result of reduced levels of functional NFκB, a significant down-regulation of proinflammatory genes (TNF-α, IL-1, IL-6), known to be directly activated by NFκB was observed. Interestingly, the single application of the ASON was more efficacious than corticosteroids in induction of healing[2]. Most notably this study and additional experiments did not show any significant toxicity when the ASON was applied topically. It was assumed that apparently sufficient amounts of the ASON reached the cells involved in the inflammatory process in the gut.

Additional studies in experimental murine colitis using the DSS model have, since then, confirmed the original observations[3,4]. In both these reports it was observed that p65 ASON resulted in a significant improvement in the disease activity index, which was paralleled by a drop in IL-1, IL-6 and TNF-α concentrations, as well as a significant improvement in the histological score. Encouraged by these findings it was of interest to assess whether a similar type of positive result could also be obtained when applied in humans with IBD. Here we describe, in brief, our results obtained from a single pilot study performed in Sweden.

RESULTS

In an explorative, placebo-controlled, double-blind study, NFκB p65 phosphorothionated ASON was administered to patients (11 total) with mild or moderately active ulcerative colitis or Crohn's disease who had responded poorly to treatment with systemic or topical glucocorticoid steroids. A single rectal administration was delivered at two dose levels, 3 mg and 30 mg. Whereas four patients received the 3-mg dose, three patients received the 30-mg dose. Four patients received placebo. Treatment compliance was excellent in all patients. All patients could maintain or hold the enema preparation for at least 2 h. No significant early leakage was observed. Importantly, no significant changes in vital signs were recorded and no serious adverse events occurred.

The ASON was well tolerated and no serious adverse event occurred. Efficacy was based on clinical and endoscopic evaluation after 1 week; 71% (five out of seven) of the patients who received active treatment were considered responders as compared to 25% (one of four) of the patients who received placebo. Efficacy also correlated with a decrease in p65 immunohistochemistry staining in rectal biopsies after 1 week (Figure 1). Histological improvement paralleled clinical response and was significantly better in the ASON groups. Two patients with ulcerative colitis, who received ASON treatment, responded promptly and a dramatic improvement was observed. These two patients soon stopped taking steroids and have been in long-term remission for more than 3 years.

DISCUSSION

This is the first study evaluating an ASON targeting NFκB p65 subunit in a human chronic disease, i.e. IBD. As stated above, no technical problems were observed and tolerability and compliance was excellent. Moreover, no side-effects related to the study drug were seen or reported. Overall clinical response to a single topical rectally administered dose was substantial and 71% of those patients receiving active compound responded vs. 25% of those allocated to placebo after 7 days. Despite the low numbers of patients we feel that our observation is of potential interest as a new possible component in the current drug arsenal to attenuate or stop the chronic inflammatory process in IBD. Of profound interest is the two patients treated with ASON who attained long-term remission, in both cases in excess of more than 30 months.

Currently it is not known whether repeated doses of ASON may be more efficacious than a single administration. In the future it would be interesting to conduct a repeat dose study in patients. Furthermore, the virtual absence of severe adverse events raises several interesting questions concerning the distribution of the compound. One possibility may be low systemic uptake of the ASON. This may be explained by the large size of the molecule, i.e. the ASON used is about 19 times the size of a standard small molecule. In addition, experimental models have demonstrated limited toxicity even after high doses of systemically administered ASON, and in this clinical study no adverse events were attributable to the active compound.

The down-regulation of NFκB p65 activity in mucosal sections (Figure 1) was accompanied by a significant improvement of histologically assessed inflammatory changes. This indicates a high degree of specificity of the compound, a prerequisite of ASON to be successful.

Interestingly, treatment with another ASON directed towards ICAM-1 has not shown consistent efficacy in IBD conditions. The underlying reason for this discrepancy can be discussed, but in terms of hierarchy it is well documented that the transcription factor NFκB is acting upstream of ICAM-1. It is not surprising, therefore, that abrogation of the p65 subunit will result in abortion of a larger

(a)

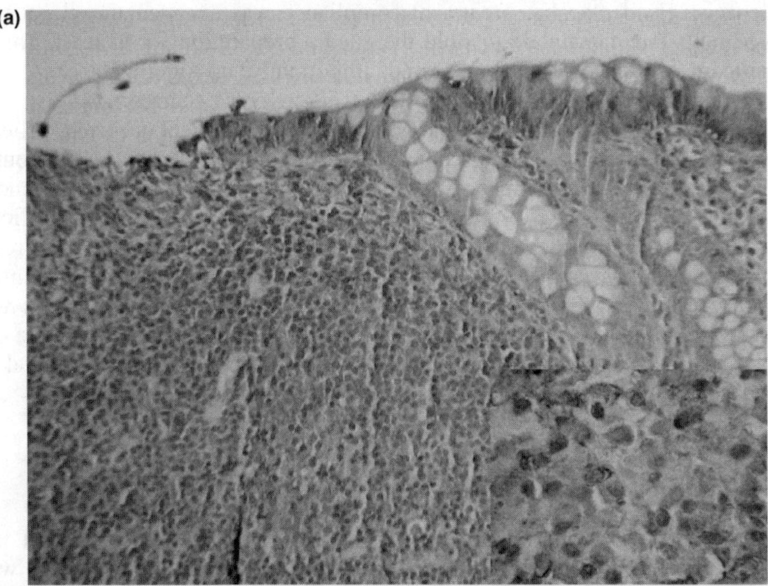

(b)

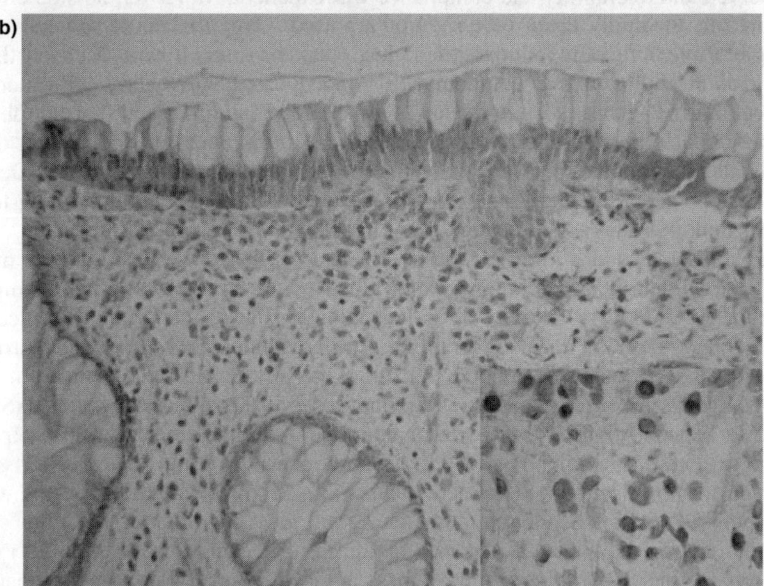

Figure 1 Immunohistology. Biopsies from a patient with ulcerative colitis; before and after administration of p65-ASON. Detection of the p65 protein by the use of specific antibodies directed against the human p65 subunit of NFκB. (**a**) Biopsy prior to treatment. As can be seen, there is profound infiltration of inflammatory cells, many of them with high levels of p65 staining. Additional findings are loss of crypts and disrupted epithelial border. (**b**) Biopsy taken 7 days after ASON treatment. As can be seen, there is a profound reduction of inflammatory cells combined with a strong reduction of strong p65 positive cells. In addition, there is an almost normalized epithelial cell border with intermittent or low basal p65 levels

number of inflammatory-related proteins compared to the single abrogation of ICAM-1. In summary, a rectal single dose of ASON directed against the NFκB p65 subunit can be safely administered to patients with active IBD. Patients receiving active ASON seem to respond favourably to this compound; two of them in an extraordinary way. Further studies are currently under way to explore the potential efficacy of this ASON for the treatment of colitis. A larger, Scandinavian multi-centre, placebo-controlled phase II study is currently being carried out with this human ON (Kappaproct, Index Pharmaceuticals, Sweden).

Acknowledgements

We are grateful for support and funding from Vetenskaprådet, Sweden (S.P., R.L.) and Centre for Strategic Research (S.P.), Juhlins foundation (R.L.).

References

1. Li Q, Verma IV. NF-κB regulation in the immune system. Nature Rev. 2002;2:725–34.
2. Neurath MF, Pettersson S, zum Büschenfelde K-H, Strober W. Local administration of antisense phosphorothioate oligonucleotides to the p65 subunit of NFκB abrogates established experimental colitis in mice. Nature Med. 1996;2:998–1004.
3. Spiik AK, Ridderstad A, Axelsson LG, Midtvedt T, Bjork L, Pettersson S. Related articles, links abstract abrogated lymphocyte infiltration and lowered CD14 in dextran sulfate induced colitis in mice treated with p65 antisense oligonucleotides. Int J Colorectal Dis. 2002;17:223–32.
4. Murano M, Maemura K, Hirata I et al. Therapeutic effect of intracolonically administered nuclear factor kappa B (p65) antisense oligonucleotide on mouse dextran sulphate sodium (DSS)-induced colitis. Clin Exp Immunol. 2000;120:51–8.

24
Biologics in clinical studies on inflammatory bowel diseases: problems

J. SCHÖLMERICH

INTRODUCTION

During the past 20 years an enormous increase in knowledge regarding the aetiology and pathophysiology of inflammatory bowel disease has taken place. In particular numerous mediators have been found which are involved in the inflammatory cascade in the gut, and have meanwhile been used as a target for innovative therapeutic strategies. However, thus far the success of this enterprise has been limited; the only really successful drug which has found its way into the standard armamentarium is infliximab, a chimeric TNF-α antibody.

In this chapter I will briefly discuss four points:

1. The question of how large the population in need for new treatments is.
2. Whether it is a good idea to target single mediators.
3. Whether Crohn's disease (CD) and ulcerative colitis (UC) are diseases or maybe syndromes consisting of many different phenotypes based on different genotypes as clinical evidence would suggest. If so the studies should probably reflect these subgroups.
4. The problem of 'professional study patients' will be discussed. Finally I will take a look at what possible alternatives could be.

PATIENT POPULATION IN NEED

Those data which are available demonstrate that the life expectancy of patients with inflammatory bowel disease (IBD) is almost normal, in contrast to 50 years ago when it was 80% for the next 10 years[1-3]. Social integration is preserved in more than 90%, as evidenced by the ability to work, to go to school and to participate in leisure activities[2]. Active disease and acute flares can be treated effectively in most cases[4]. When looking at population-based data it becomes evident

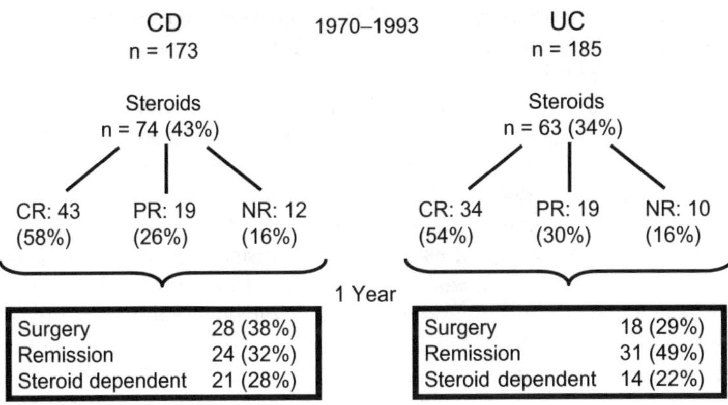

Figure 1   Steroids for IBD – population-related data[4]

that less than half of all patients with CD, and even less (34%) of those with UC, ever receive steroids. Of those about 45% have only partial remission or no response. This means that the practical number which is in need of an alternative treatment may be much lower than many researchers or investigators have come to believe (Figure 1).

However, a number of problems remain, which indicate that we still have a need for improved and new treatments. There is a group of patients who need surgery or are refractory to conventional treatment, and even more patients become steroid-dependent[4,5]. The side-effects of steroids and other drugs are not to be forgotten. They are feared by patients and by physicians, and probably rightfully so. In particular long-term treatment with steroids should for several reasons be avoided. When doing so a high relapse rate, at least in CD, is predictable, while for UC 5-ASA is obviously effective for remission maintenance in most cases. Ultimately we still have no mucosal healing with conventional treatments, at least not in CD, which means that the disease is chronic and will not terminate during a lifetime. Thus, mucosal healing, and in addition a normal life quality, due to successful remission maintenance are predominant goals of current efforts to improve our treatment strategies.

TARGETING SINGLE MEDIATORS – A USEFUL STRATEGY?

When looking at our current understanding of the pathophysiology of IBD in a simplified way (Figure 2) it is evident that many cell types, and a huge number of mediators such as chemokines, cytokines, and effector molecules, are involved. This could be compared to an orchestra with many different instruments. It is rather obvious that inhibiting a single instrument will not silence the orchestra. Thus, until now all attempts to inhibit a single mediator or effector molecule have been unsuccessful, as for example seen by leukotriene synthesis inhibitors, interleukin 1 receptor antagonists and others. This is also evident in

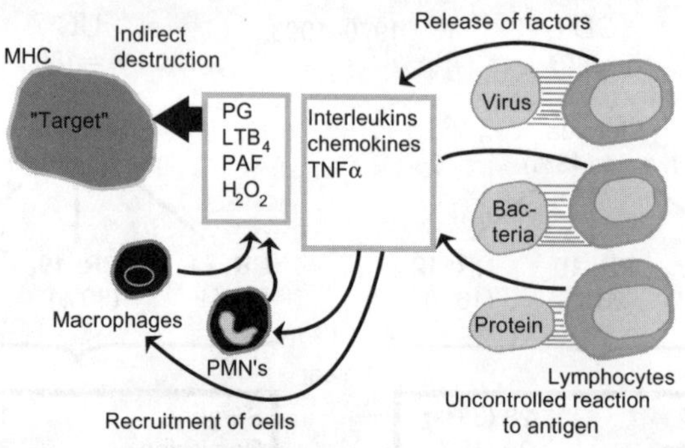

Figure 2 Principles of pathophysiology of IBD

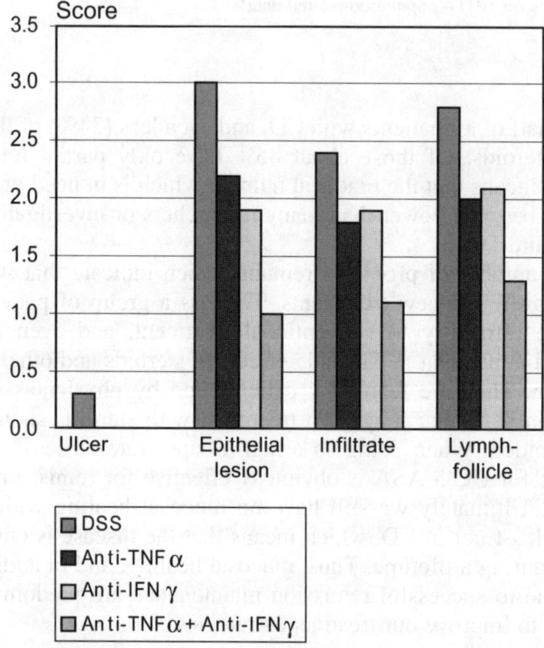

Figure 3 Chronic DSS-colitis – anti-TNF-α and anti-IFN-γ – effects[6]

animal experiments, from which it can be seen that inhibiting a single mediator somehow improves the experimental colitis, but that combining two is better than each of them alone (Figure 3)[6].

It has been argued that the undeniable effects of infliximab – a chimeric TNF-α antibody – prove that inhibiting a single mediator may be a useful approach. This could be compared to inhibiting the 'conductor' of the orchestra. However, recent experiences using other anti-TNF strategies indicate that infliximab obviously works in a different way. It seems to induce apoptosis of immune cells – lymphocytes and macrophages[7,8]. The soluble TNF receptor etanercept, which does not induce apoptosis, has no significant effect in CD (Figure 4)[9]. This is in sharp contrast to data with infliximab (Table 1)[10–14]. It remains to be seen if this holds true for all anti-TNF approaches, for example other antibodies[15,16] or other soluble receptors such as TNF receptor P55[17]. In any case the apoptosis-inducing effect of infliximab to some extent explains its possible problem regarding the lack of resistance to infections[18]. Furthermore it remains to be seen if infliximab will have an effect in UC. Up to now no defect of apoptosis has been described in UC, in contrast to CD[19]; thus far controlled studies with infliximab in UC have not been positive[20].

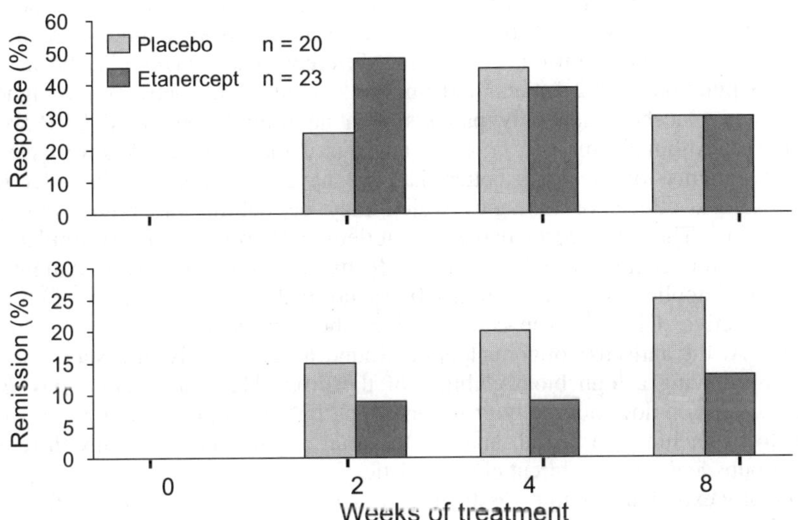

Figure 4 Clinical response and remission with etanercept in moderate to severe active Crohn's disease[9]

Table 1 Long-term effects of infliximab – Accent I[13]

	Responder to first infusion (week 2; 335/573 patients)			
54 weeks	*Remission (%)*	*Remission steroid-free (%)*	*Response (%)*	*Time to LOR (weeks)*
Placebo	13.6	8.9	17.0	19
5 mg	28.3*	24.1*	43.0*	38*
10 mg	38.4*	32.1*	53.0*	>54*

32% infections, 3.8% serious, four deaths (two sepsis, one lymphoma); 49% new ANA (>1:160), 26% anti-DS DNS AB (≥1:10); 54% steroids, 24% immunomodulators, 50% 5-ASA! LOR = loss of response; * significant vs. placebo.

At the moment it appears that, in order to be effective, biologics may need to be pluripotent, i.e. acting on several cell types or on several mediators and signal transduction pathways.

TREATING SYNDROMES, NOT TWO DISEASES?

Recent evidence from clinical trials suggests that some of the biologics studied are effective in subgroups of patients. It has long been recognized that at least CD is probably a collection of different genotypes also presenting as different phenotypes. This is evident from daily clinical experience when looking at a short stricturing CD in the ileocaecal region and comparing that with extensive colonic involvement, or in particular extensive perianal disease. In a similar way it may be possible to distinguish patients having an elevated acute-phase reaction from those who do not. A recent study with an anti-TNF antibody fragment which did not find a difference of three different doses versus placebo in the total population of 292 patients did find a clear difference between the highest dose and placebo when only patients with an initially increased CRP were analysed. Although this is a *post-hoc* analysis it may indicate that we have to select patients for the trials better than we have done thus far, in order not to overlook effects of biologics which may be helpful in clinical practice (Table 2)[21]. The evidence available for interleukin-10 indicates a very similar situation. While enemas have been rather effective in a small number of patients[22], parenteral application of interleukin-10 was not really helpful in active or chronically active CD[23,24]. The study using the anti-adhesion approach with anti-ICAM 1 antisense oligonucleotides found an effect only in a subgroup of patients having a high bioavailability of the drug. This was again a *post-hoc* analysis which does not really prove an effect, but may indicate that a subgroup has to be included in a trial, and not the total population with many different subgroups and many different characteristics[25].

Finally experience with the $\alpha_4\beta_7$ integrin antibodies in CD and UC indicates a similar situation. While this promising approach was clearly effective in UC (Table 3)[26] this was not the case in CD (Table 4)[27]. Thus it may be helpful to test new approaches in a small group of mixed patients, as recently done for example with NFκB P65 antisense (Table 5)[28], and then try to select the right patient group out of the two syndromes in order to prove efficacy at least for that group.

Table 2   CDP 870 an anti-TNF antibody fragment in 'active' Crohn's disease[21] (292 patients)

| | Dosing weeks 0, 4, 8 | | | |
	Placebo	*100 mg*	*200 mg*	*400 mg*
Clinical response week 12 (%) (CDAI ↓ >100)	35.6	36.5	36.1	44.4
Clinical remission with initial CRP ⩾ 10 mg/L	10.7	35.5	32.1	41.9*

* significant vs. placebo.

Table 3 $\alpha_4\beta_7$ integrin antibodies for ulcerative colitis[26]

	Dosing days 1 and 29, 181 patients		
	Placebo	0.5 mg/kg	2.0 mg/kg
Clinical remission, day 43(%)	15	33*	34*
Normal mucosa (%)	8	29*	14
Response (%)	33	66*	57*

* significant vs. placebo.

Table 4 $\alpha_4\beta_7$ integrin antibodies for Crohn's disease[27]

	Dosing days 1 and 29		
Day 57	Placebo (n = 58)	0.5 mg/kg (n = 62)	2.0 mg/kg (n = 65)
Clinical remission (%)	20.7	29.5	36.9*
Response (%)	41.4	49.2	53.1

* significant vs. placebo.

Table 5 NFκB P65 antisense oligonucleotide for active distal IBD[28]

	11 patients (5 UC, 6 CD)	
	7 Oligo	4 Placebo
Improvement day 7	5/7	1/4

Two steroid-refractory patients with long-lasting steroid-free remission.

'PROFESSIONAL STUDY PATIENTS' – A PROBLEM?

Some of the more recent trials have found an incredibly high placebo response in patients otherwise steroid-dependent or even steroid-refractory. This is exemplified by a study using anti-IFN-γ antibodies (Table 6)[29] but was also seen in studies on IFN-β in steroid-treated active CD or UC[30], or with keratinocyte growth factor (Table 7)[31]. The only explanation available seems to be that patients undergoing consecutive trials over a period of years, and experiencing improvement in one of the trials, have a tendency to report improvement in later trials. It is unclear up to now if this is a real explanation of otherwise surprising placebo effects.

Table 6 Anti-interferon γ AB (Huzaf) in Crohn's disease[29]

	Placebo (n = 10)	Huzaf (mg/kg)		
		0.1 (n = 6)	1.0 (n = 14)	4.0 (n = 15)
CDAI ↓ > 100 (%)	**60**	17	42	57
Remission (%)	**40**	0	25	50
SE ('influenza') (%)	0	3	6	9

Table 7 Keratinocyte growth factor (Repifermin) in ulcerative colitis[31]

4 weeks	Placebo (n = 28)	Repifermin (μg/kg)				
		1	5	10	25	50
Remission (%)	11	11	9	0	0	0
Response (%)	36	46	18	33	42	29

88 patients with moderate UC

WHICH OTHER ALTERNATIVES DO WE HAVE?

Looking at the current status of the development of 'biological treatments' it is obvious that no magic bullet has yet been found. Infliximab is indeed effective in CD, although only in a not-yet-predictable subgroup and with some limitations regarding long-term use. Biological activity has been found for a couple of other substances such as anti-α_4 integrin[32] or anti-$\alpha_4\beta_7$ integrin[26], and some other principles (Table 8); however, most of the tested principles have been disappointing. It remains to be seen if inhibiting MAP kinases[33] or interleukin-12[34] will show better results[35]. It is therefore of great interest to look for alternative approaches which may also be called biologic. For example, modulation of the interaction between luminal bacteria and the mucosa may be a different approach which could be called the 'microbiological strategy'. The fact that the first gene detected, in which a mutation causes part of the Crohn's syndrome, namely the NOD2/CARD15 gene[36–38], is involved in the recognition of bacterial products, peptidoglycans, by macrophages, and probably other cells of the mucosa, points in this direction (Figure 5). New approaches modulating the bacterial–mucosal interaction, such as cytosine guanosine motifs of bacterial DNA[39,40] or gene-modified lactococci releasing interleukin-10[41], have been found effective in animal studies and are currently being tested in humans. Probiotics have been proven successful in some indications such as remission maintenance of UC (Table 9)[42] or pouchitis[43], but not in others. Probably the best probiotics for different indications also need to be defined in the future. It remains to be seen where this approach will lead.

Table 8 'Biologic treatments' for IBD – state of development, May 2003

Substance		CD		UC
IL-1 RA		(−)		?
TNF-AB	⟶	+		(−)
RNF-R 75 and 55		−		?
MAP kinase inhibitor		?		?
NFκB p65 antisense		(+)		(+)
Anti-CD4	⟶	+		?
Anti-IL-12		(−)		?
Anti-INF-γ		−		?
Anti-IL-2 R		(+)		?
IL-10		(+)		?
Anti-α$_4$ integrin	⟶	(+)		?
Anti-α$_4$β$_7$ integrin		(−)	⟶	(+)
Anti ICAM-1		−		?
EGF		?		(+)
KGF		?		−
INF-α		(−)		−
INF-β		(−)	⟶	(+)
GCSF/GMCSF	⟶	(+)		?
Growth hormone	⟶	(+)		?
DHEA	⟶	(+)		(+)
IL-11		(−)		?

Table 9 *E. coli* Nissle versus mesalazine for remission maintenance in ulcerative colitis[42]

1 Year	E. coli	5-ASA	p*
Relapse (PP/%) ($n = 110/112$)	36.4	33.0	0.004
Relapse (ITT/%) ($n = 162/165$)	45.1	36.4	0.017
AE (%)	29.6	29.1	

* Tested for equivalence.

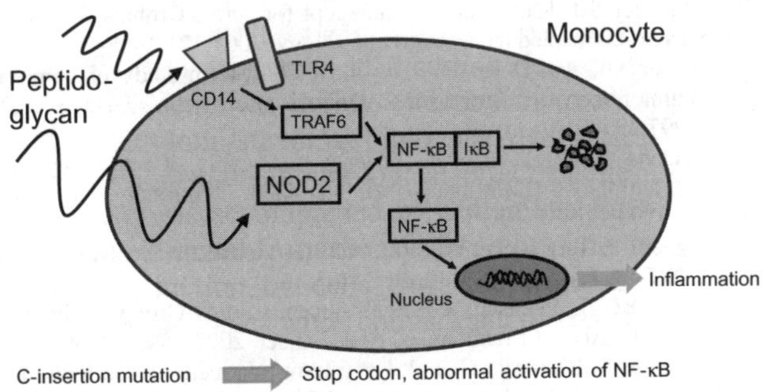

Figure 5 Identification of the first IBD-gene – NOD2/CARD15

SUMMARY

There is obviously some need for new treatments, although the size of the problem seems to have been overestimated by many investigators and companies producing biologics. A huge variety of 'biologics' work in different experimental models; not every approach works in each model. Biological effects are proven in humans for few principles which may work by affecting several cell types and several mediators. Clinically relevant effects have been found for only a small number, in particular infliximab. However, long-term risks and effects are still not completely defined. Many approaches are not really effective in a clinically relevant order of magnitude. However, market forces still dominate the selection of substances for development. Since not too many patients are available for these trials 'professional study patients' may be a real problem for future developments. Several alternatives, in particular approaches targeting the microbiota in the gut, deserve study, but seem to attract less interest due to their low profit expectations.

References

1. Softley A, Clamp SE, Watkinson G, Bouchier IA, Myren J, de Dombal FT. The natural history of inflammatory bowel disease: has there been a change in the last 20 years? Scand J Gastroenterol Suppl. 1988;144:20–3.
2. Langholz E, Munkholm P, Davidsen M, Binder V. Course of ulcerative colitis: analysis of changes in disease activity over years. Gastroenterology. 1994;107:3–11.
3. Ekbom A, Helmick CG, Zack M, Holmberg L, Adami HO. Survival and causes of death in patients with inflammatory bowel disease: a population-based study. Gastroenterology. 1992;103:954–60.
4. Faubion WA Jr, Loftus EV Jr, Harmsen WS, Zinsmeister AR, Sandborn WJ. The natural history of corticosteroid therapy for inflammatory bowel disease: a population-based study. Gastroenterology. 2001;121:255–60.
5. Munkholm P, Langholz E, Davidsen M, Binder V. Frequency of glucocorticoid resistance and dependency in Crohn's disease. Gut. 1994;35:360–2.
6. Kojouharoff G, Hans W, Obermeier F et al. Neutralization of tumour necrosis factor (TNF) but not of IL-1 reduces inflammation in chronic dextran sulphate sodium-induced colitis in mice. Clin Exp Immunol. 1997;107:353–8.
7. Van den Brande JM, Braat H, van den Brink GR et al. Infliximab but not etanercept induces apoptosis in lamina propria T-lymphocytes from patients with Crohn's disease. Gastroenterology. 2003;124:1774–85.
8. Lugering A, Schmidt M, Lugering N, Pauels HG, Domschke W, Kucharzik T. Infliximab induces apoptosis in monocytes from patients with chronic active Crohn's disease by using a caspase-dependent pathway. Gastroenterology. 2001;121:1145–57.
9. Sandborn WJ, Hanauer SB, Katz S et al. Etanercept for active Crohn's disease: a randomized, double-blind, placebo-controlled trial. Gastroenterology. 2001;121:1088–94.
10. Targan SR, Hanauer SB, van Deventer SJ et al. A short-term study of chimeric monoclonal antibody cA2 to tumor necrosis factor a for Crohn's disease. Crohn's Disease cA2 Study Group. N Engl J Med. 1997;337:1029–35.
11. Rutgeerts P, D'Haens G, Targan S et al. Efficacy and safety of retreatment with anti-tumor necrosis factor antibody (Infliximab) to maintain remission in Crohn's disease. Gastroenterology. 1999:117:761–9.
12. Present DH, Rutgeerts P, Targan S et al. Infliximab for the treatment of fistulas in patients with Crohn's disease. N Engl J Med. 1999;340:1398–405.
13. Hanauer SB, Feagan BG, Lichtenstein GR et al. Accent I Study Group. Maintenance infliximab for Crohn's disease: the Accent I randomised trial. Lancet. 2002;359:1541–9.
14. Sands B, Van Deventer S, Bernstein C et al. Long-term treatment of fistulizing Crohn's disease: response to infliximab in the Accent II trial through 54 weeks. Gastroenterology. 2002;122:A81–2.

15. Sandborn WJ, Feagan BG, Hanauer SB et al. CDP571 Crohn's Disease Study Group. An engineered human antibody to TNF (CDP571) for active Crohn's disease: a randomized double-blind placebo-controlled trial. Gastroenterology. 2001;120:1330–8.

16. Feagan BG, Sandborn WJ, Baker JP et al. A randomized, double-blind, placebo-controlled, multi-center trial of the engineered human antibody to TNF (CDP571) for steroid sparing and maintenance of remission in patients with steroid-dependent Crohn's disease. Gastroenterology. 2000;118:A655.

17. Rutgeerts P, Lemmens L, Van Assche G, Noman M, Borghini-Fuhrer I, Goedkoop RJ. Treatment of active Crohn's disease with onercept (recombinant human soluble p55 tumour necrosis factor receptor): results of a randomized, open-label, pilot study. Aliment Pharmacol Ther. 2003;17:185–92.

18. Echtenacher B, Falk W, Männel DN, Krammer PH. Requirement of endogenous tumor necrosis factor/cachectin for recovery from experimental peritonitis. J Immunol. 1990;145:3762–6.

19. Ina K, Itoh J, Fukushima K et al. Resistance of Crohn's disease T cells to multiple apoptotic signals is associated with a Bcl-2/Bax mucosal imbalance. J Immunol. 1999;163:1081–90.

20. Probert CSJ, Hearing SD, Schreiber S et al. Infliximab in moderately severe glucocorticoid resistant ulcerative colitis: a randomised controlled trial. Gut. 2003;52:998–1002.

21. Schreiber S, Rutgeerts P, Fedorak R, Khaliq-Kareemi M, Kamm MA, Patel J and the CDP870 Crohn's Disease Study Group. CDP870, a humanized anti-TNF antibody fragment, induces clinical response with remission in patients with active Crohn's disease (CD). Gastroenterology. 2003;124:A–61.

22. Schreiber S, Heinig T, Thile HG, Raedler A. Immunoregulatory role of interleukin 10 in patients with inflammatory bowel disease. Gastroenterology. 1995;108:1434–44.

23. Fedorak RN, Gangl A, Elson CO et al. The Interleukin 10 Inflammatory Bowel Disease Cooperative Study Group. Recombinant human interleukin 10 in the treatment of patients with mild to moderately active Crohn's disease. Gastroenterology. 2000;119:1473–82.

24. Schreiber S, Fedorak RN, Nielsen OH et al. Safety and efficacy of recombinant human interleukin 10 in chronic active Crohn's disease. Crohn's Disease IL-10 Cooperative Study Group. Gastroenterology. 2000;119:1461–72.

25. Yacyshyn BR, Chey WY, Goff J et al. ISIS 2302-CS9. Double blind, placebo controlled trial of the remission inducing and steroid sparing properties of an ICAM-1 antisense oligodeoxynucleotide, alicaforsen (ISIS 2302), in active steroid dependent Crohn's disease. Gut. 2002,51.30–6.

26. Feagan B, Greenberg G, Wild G et al. A randomized controlled trial of a humanized α4β7 antibody in ulcerative colitis. AGA Late-Breaking Abstract Symposium 2003.

27. Feagan BG, Greenberg G, Wild G et al. Efficacy and safety of a humanized α4β7 antibody in active Crohn's disease. Gastroenterology. 2003;124:A25–6.

28. Lötberg R, Neurath M, Ost A, Pettersson S. Topical NFκB p65 antisense oligonucleotides in patients with active distal colonic IBD. A randomised, controlled pilot trial. Gastroenterology. 2002;122:A60.

29. Rutgeerts P, Reinisch W, Colombel JF et al. Preliminary results of a phase I/II study of Huzaf, an anti-IFN-γ monoclonal antibody, in patients with moderate to severe active Crohn's disease. Gastroenterology. 2002;122:A61.

30. Musch E, Andus T, Malek M. Induction and maintenance of clinical remission by interferon-beta in patients with steroid-refractory active ulcerative colitis – an open long-term pilot trial. Aliment Pharmacol Ther. 2002;16:1233–9.

31. Sandborn WJ, Sands BE, Wolf DC et al. Repifermin (keratinocyte growth factor-2) for the treatment of active ulcerative colitis: a randomized, double-blind, placebo-controlled, dose-escalation trial. Aliment Pharmacol Ther. 2003;17:1355–64.

32. Ghosh S, Goldin E, Gordon FH et al. Natalizumab Pan-European Study Group. Natalizumab for active Crohn's disease. N Engl J Med. 2003;348:24–32.

33. Hommes D, van den Blink B, Plasse T et al. Inhibition of stress-activated MAP kinases induces clinical improvement in moderate to severe Crohn's disease. Gastroenterology. 2002;122:7–14.

34. Neurath MF, Fuss I, Kelsall BL, Stuber E, Strober W. Antibodies to interleukin 12 abrogate established experimental colitis in mice. J Exp Med. 1995;182:1281–90.

35. Sandborn WJ, Targan SR. Biologic therapy of inflammatory bowel disease. Gastroenterology. 2002;122:1592–608.

36. Hugot JP, Chamaillard M, Zouali H et al. Association of NOD2 leucine-rich repeat variants with susceptibility to Crohn's disease. Nature. 2001;411:599–603.

37. Ogura Y, Bonen DK, Inohara N et al. A frameshift mutation in NOD2 associated with susceptibility to Crohn's disease. Nature. 2001;411:603–6.
38. Hampe J, Cuthbert A, Croucher PJP et al. Association between insertion mutation in NOD2 gene and Crohn's disease in German and British populations. Lancet. 2001;357:1925–8.
39. Rachmilewitz D, Karmeli F, Takabayashi K et al. Immunostimulatory DNA ameliorates experimental and spontaneous murine colitis. Gastroenterology. 2002;122:1428–41.
40. Obermeier F, Dunger N, Deml L, Herfarth H, Schölmerich J, Falk W. CpG motifs of bacterial DNA exacerbate colitis of dextran sulfate sodium-treated mice. Eur J Immunol. 2002;32: 2084–92.
41. Steidler L, Hans W, Schotte L et al. Treatment of murine colitis by *Lactococcus lactis* secreting interleukin-10. Science. 2000;289:1352–5.
42. Kruis W, Fric P, Stolte M, the Mutaflor Study Group. Maintenance of remission in ulcerative colitis is equally effective with *Escherichia coli* Nissle 1917 and with standard mesalamine. Gastroenterology. 2001;120:A127.
43. Gionchetti P, Rizzello F, Venturi A et al. Oral bacteriotherapy as maintenance treatment in patients with chronic pouchitis. A double-blind, placebo-controlled trial. Gastroenterology. 2000;119:305–9.

25
Biologics in clinical practice: safety aspects

J. C. HOFFMANN

INTRODUCTION

Although the two most common types of inflammatory bowel disease, i.e. Crohn's disease (CD) and ulcerative colitis (UC), are rarely life-threatening, it is well known that medical therapy does not give acceptable clinical results for all patients. Clearly, the use of corticosteroids in adequate doses, as well as the early use of 'classical' immunosuppressants, have increased the initial as well as the long-term response rate. However, it is estimated that the chance of having recurrent and/or a chronic active disease in a patient with CD is between 15% and 50% in the long run, in spite of best possible medical therapy[1]; therefore there is no doubt that we need more effective therapeutic agents, particularly for maintenance therapy.

When clinical studies were started in the late 1980s and early 1990s with monoclonal antibodies (mAb) directed at the CD4 molecule the hope was to interfere very specifically with bowel inflammation based on the understanding of CD at that time[2,3]. At the same time investigators started to test anti-TNF-α mAb for life-threatening diseases such as sepsis[4,5]. This new group of agents quickly revolutionized clinical research in IBD and other diseases. These agents were called biologics. Although the role of T helper cells for CD, as well as for defence against pathogens, was well established (clinical experience with AIDS) there was by and large no major fear with regard to safety. The recent experience with regard to safety problems of the anti-TNF-α mAb infliximab demonstrated that safety aspects were initially underestimated. However, before discussing the safety aspects of biologics a brief definition is required of what biologics are. The official definition from the FDA states that 'a biological product . . . is any virus, therapeutic serum, toxin, antitoxin, vaccine, blood, blood component or derivate, allergenic product, or analogous product, applicable to the prevention, treatment or cure of disease . . . derived from living sources'

Table 1   Reports of severe adverse events with lethal course in temporal relation to the application of infliximab in Germany, as reported until May 2003 to the Paul-Ehrlich Institute[19] (also Keller-Stanislawski, personal communication)

Adverse events	Crohn's disease	Rheumatoid arthritis	Graft-versus-host disease	Others
Sepsis	4	15	5	5
Myocardial infarction/ arrhythmias	1	2	—	—
Malignancy	1	—	—	—
Multi-organ failure	2	—	—	1
Pulmonary emboli	—	2	—	2
Underlying disorder	—	—	2	1
Others	2	4	6	—
Total	10	23	13	9

(www.fda.gov). In Europe the EMEA defines biologics quite differently as 'proteins and polypeptides, their derivates, and products of which they are components (e.g., conjugates). These are produced from recombinant or non-recombinant cell cultures' (http://www.emea.eu.int/pdfs/human/ich/036596en. pdf). Since a computer-designed small molecule can bind exactly at the same area of a molecule as an mAb, leading to exactly the same effects, we believe that biologics should be defined by the way they act rather than by the way they were produced. This new definition appears to be attaining increasing acceptance even in the FDA. For instance, Korwek states, in the *FDA Law Journal* in 2000, that biologics should be defined by their purpose (cure, treatment or prevention of disease), the target (through a specific immune response), and irrespective of its source[6].

SAFETY OF BIOLOGICS: THE ANTI-TNF-α STORY

The central role of the cytokine TNF-α for inflammation was discovered in the mid-1980s[7,8]. Studies in sepsis in animal models showed that anti-TNF-α mAb are effective in these models, and large clinical sepsis trails were started based on these *in-vivo* and many other *in-vitro* studies[9–11]. Unfortunately no clinical benefit was observed, nor an increase in mortality[5]. *In-vitro* studies using intestinal specimens also suggested that TNF-α should play an important role in CD[12]. At the same time studies with mice showed that TNF-α is of pivotal importance for the immune response towards mycobacteria[13] and other intracellular pathogens, such as *Listeria*[14]. Based on the *in-vitro* studies and the first positive reports from rheumatoid arthritis trials, a pilot study was published in 1995 suggesting a clinical benefit of infliximab in CD[15]. A prospective randomized trial by Targan et al. clearly demonstrated that infliximab is effective in chronic active disease; however, with only a moderate remission rate of 33% compared to 4% in the control group looking at 108 patients (19 control patients and 89 infliximab-treated patients)[16]. Based on this study, and a second study by Present et al. looking at fistulizing CD with even better results (overall 94 patients including controls)[17], the FDA granted approval for use of infliximab in patients with severe, refractory CD in August 1998, using an expedited approval process. Protocols from the FDA approval hearing in May 1998, including patients with severe forms of CD having had a dramatic response to infliximab, suggest that an emotional component was involved in this very quick unequivocal approval (www.ccfa.org/medcentral/research/basic/inflixcn.htm). It should be noted that, in contrast to the expedited approval process for zidovudin in AIDS, CD is not a life-threatening disease, and that efficacy data on only 162 treated patients were available for FDA approval and later EMEA approval in 1999 under 'exceptional circumstances'. With regard to safety only short-term safety data on this small number of CD patients were available. No statements were made with regard to the requirement of chest X-rays or mycobacterial skin testing in the US or in Europe. In 2001 Keane et al. reported on reactivation and fatal cases of tuberculosis in patients treated with infliximab[18]. As of August 2002 the data on file at Centocor state that, among previous CD study patients, the mortality rate for infliximab-treated patients was 0.9% compared to 0% in control groups. For unknown reasons this stands in contrast to lower mortality rates for infliximab-treated patients with rheumatoid arthritis and no increase in mortality in patients with sepsis. However, the data from the German registry on safety of biologics at the Paul Ehrlich Institute confirm that mortalities do occur in patients treated with infliximab[19] (also Keller-Stanislawski, personal communication). Until May 2003 there were 10 CD patients reported to have expired in temporal relation to infliximab infusions in Germany, four of whom from sepsis and another two from multiorgan failure (Table 1). At the DDW the Mayo Clinic reported that, among 500 CD patients treated with infliximab, there was a mortality rate of 2%[20]. It seems unlikely that experienced gastroenterologists performing clinical studies (data on file at Centocor) and/or working at the Mayo Clinic, lacked experience in either selecting patients or adequately treating CD patients once severe complications occur. Therefore, the data provided by the Paul Ehrlich Institute only confirm data from other sources and countries. In addition, it seems clear that severe adverse events, and even mortality, are due not only to mycobacterial infections but also to general severe immunosuppression of some CD patients. One can only speculate that some unknown factor related to CD seems to predispose a small subgroup of patients to severe, mostly infectious, complications.

LESSONS FROM ANIMAL MODELS

Although studies on the effectiveness of biologics in animal models do not always predict similar results in IBD, there are several examples demonstrating that results from animal models do sometimes predict clinical outcome. Importantly, studies in animals using a preventive approach must be distinguished from studies looking at established disease. For instance, IL-10 can prevent inflammation in several IBD animal models but is generally ineffective in established disease[21–23]. In contrast, anti-TNF-α mAb were found to be effective in established disease as well as in a preventive setting in several animal models[24,25]. Therefore, animal models can, in conjunction with *in-vitro* studies, help to select therapeutic strategies for further clinical trials.

Further, animal models can help to predict the safety profile as stated above for anti-TNF-α mAb. Useful models include murine mycobacteriosis, listerosis, and salmonellosis. For example, targeting the CD28 molecule in IBD could be dangerous, since the infectious defence towards *Listeria monocytogenes* and *Salmonella* is markedly impaired in CD28-deficient mice[26,27]. At the same time CD28-directed immunotherapies were found to be effective in IBD animal models[28,29]. This demonstrates once again that biologics are a double-edged sword with high therapeutic potential and at the same time severe immunosuppressive potential. Therefore, biologics are somewhat similar to classical immunosuppressants which do have the same problems, namely infectious complications and secondary neoplasia after long-term follow-up. The latter aspect should be a major focus of future studies, and ideally such animal model safety studies should precede even clinical pilot studies.

CONCLUSIONS

Clinical experience with so-far-available biologics has shown that most of them have acceptable short-term safety profiles. However, in contrast to the original hope, they can interfere with important immune responses, and this seems to vary in various patient populations. For instance, excess mortality has been found only in CD patients, but not in patients with rheumatoid arthritis. Animal models can help both to predict the effectiveness of biologics with regard to the inflammatory disorder and to evaluate the safety of biologics. In non-life-threatening illnesses one should be more careful to have an expedited drug-approval process. One should carefully consider whether a completely different drug-approval process is justified for biologics, since biologics seem to have similar safety problems as 'classical' immunosuppressants, namely impairment of important immune responses such as control of infections or tumour surveillance. Finally, traditional preclinical pharmacological studies seem to be as relevant for biologics as for other pharmaceutical agents, e.g. mutagenesis studies.

Acknowledgement

I thank N. Pawlowski for critical reading of the manuscript. The author is supported by the German Competence Network on IBD.

References

1. Hoffmann JC, Zeitz M. Treatment of Crohn's disease. Hepatogastroenterology. 2000;47:90–100.
2. Stronkhorst A, Tytgat GN, van Deventer SJ. CD4 antibody treatment in Crohn's disease. Scand J Gastroenterol Suppl. 1992;194:61–5.
3. Stronkhorst A, Radema S, Yong SL et al. CD4 antibody treatment in patients with active Crohn's disease: a phase 1 dose finding study. Gut. 1997;40:320–7.

4. Vincent JL, Bakker J, Marecaux G, Schandene L, Kahn RJ, Dupont E. Administration of anti-TNF antibody improves left ventricular function in septic shock patients. Results of a pilot study. Chest. 1992;101:810–15.
5. Reinhart K, Wiegand-Lohnert C, Grimminger F et al. Assessment of the safety and efficacy of the monoclonal anti-tumor necrosis factor antibody-fragment, MAK 195F, in patients with sepsis and septic shock: a multicenter, randomized, placebo-controlled, dose-ranging study. Crit Care Med. 1996;24:733–42.
6. Korwek EL. Human biological drug regulation: past, present, and beyond the year 2000. FDA Law J. 2000;50:123–50.
7. Moldawer LL, Gelin J, Schersten T, Lundholm KG. Circulating interleukin 1 and tumor necrosis factor during inflammation. Am J Physiol. 1987;253:R922–8.
8. Morimoto A, Sakata Y, Watanabe T, Murakami N. Characteristics of fever and acute-phase response induced in rabbits by IL-1 and TNF. Am J Physiol. 1989;256:R35–41.
9. Tracey KJ, Fong Y, Hesse DG et al. Anti-cachectin/TNF monoclonal antibodies prevent septic shock during lethal bacteraemia. Nature. 1987;330:662–4.
10. Mathison JC, Wolfson E, Ulevitch RJ. Participation of tumor necrosis factor in the mediation of gram negative bacterial lipopolysaccharide-induced injury in rabbits. J Clin Invest. 1988;81:1925–37.
11. Hinshaw LB, Tekamp-Olson P, Chang AC et al. Survival of primates in LD100 septic shock following therapy with antibody to tumor necrosis factor (TNF alpha). Circ Shock. 1990;30:279–92.
12. MacDonald TT, Hutchings P, Choy MY, Murch S, Cooke A. Tumour necrosis factor-alpha and interferon-gamma production measured at the single cell level in normal and inflamed human intestine. Clin Exp Immunol. 1990;81:301–5.
13. Denis M. Involvement of cytokines in determining resistance and acquired immunity in murine tuberculosis. J Leukoc Biol. 1991;50:495–501.
14. Desiderio JV, Kiener PA, Lin PF, Warr GA. Protection of mice against *Listeria monocytogenes* infection by recombinant human tumor necrosis factor alpha. Infect Immun. 1989;57:1615–17.
15. van Dullemen HM, van Deventer SJ, Hommes DW et al. Treatment of Crohn's disease with anti-tumor necrosis factor chimeric monoclonal antibody (cA2). Gastroenterology. 1995;109:129–35.
16. Targan SR, Hanauer SB, van Deventer SJ et al. A short-term study of chimeric monoclonal antibody cA2 to tumor necrosis factor alpha for Crohn's disease. Crohn's Disease cA2 Study Group. N Engl J Med. 1997;337:1029–35.
17. Present DH, Rutgeerts P, Targan S et al. Infliximab for the treatment of fistulas in patients with Crohn's disease. N Engl J Med. 1999;340:1398–405.
18. Keane J, Gershon S, Wise RP et al. Tuberculosis associated with infliximab, a tumor necrosis factor alpha-neutralizing agent. N Engl J Med. 2001;345:1098–104.
19. Andus T, Stange EF, Hoffler D, Keller-Stanislawski B. Verdachtsfälle schwerwiegender Nebenwirkungen nach Infliximab (Remicade®) aus Deutschland. Med Klin (Munich). 2003;98:429–36.
20. Colombel JF, Loftus Jr EV, Tremaine WJ et al. The safety profile of infliximab for Crohn's disease in clinical practice. Gastroenterology. 2003;124(Suppl. 1):A7.
21. Powrie F, Leach MW, Mauze S, Menon S, Caddle LB, Coffman RL. Inhibition of Th1 responses prevents inflammatory bowel disease in scid mice reconstituted with CD45RBhi CD4+ T cells. Immunity. 1994;1:553–62.
22. Herfarth HH, Mohanty SP, Rath HC, Tonkonogy S, Sartor RB. Interleukin 10 suppresses experimental chronic, granulomatous inflammation induced by bacterial cell wall polymers. Gut. 1996;39:836–45.
23. Herfarth HH, Bocker U, Janardhanam R, Sartor RB. Subtherapeutic corticosteroids potentiate the ability of interleukin 10 to prevent chronic inflammation in rats. Gastroenterology. 1998;115:856–65.
24. Powrie F, Correa-Oliveira R, Mauze S, Coffman RL. Regulatory interactions between CD45RBhigh and CD45RBlow CD4+ T cells are important for the balance between protective and pathogenic cell-mediated immunity. J Exp Med. 1994;179:589–600.
25. Neurath MF, Fuss I, Pasparakis M et al. Predominant pathogenic role of tumor necrosis factor in experimental colitis in mice. Eur J Immunol. 1997;27:1743–50.

26. Mittrucker HW, Kohler A, Mak TW, Kaufmann SH. Critical role of CD28 in protective immunity against *Salmonella typhimurium*. J Immunol. 1999;163:6769–76.
27. Mittrucker HW, Kursar M, Kohler A, Hurwitz R, Kaufmann SH. Role of CD28 for the generation and expansion of antigen-specific CD8(+) T lymphocytes during infection with *Listeria monocytogenes*. J Immunol. 2001;167:5620–7.
28. Davenport CM, McAdams HA, Kou J et al. Inhibition of pro-inflammatory cytokine generation by CTLA4-Ig in the skin and colon of mice adoptively transplanted with CD45RBhi CD4+ T cells correlates with suppression of psoriasis and colitis. Int Immunopharmacol. 2002;2:653–72.
29. Liu Z, Geboes K, Hellings P et al. B7 interactions with CD28 and CTLA-4 control tolerance or induction of mucosal inflammation in chronic experimental colitis. J Immunol. 2001;167:1830–8.

Index

Falk Symposium Series

43. Reutter W, Popper H, Arias IM, Heinrich PC, Keppler D, Landmann L, eds.: *Modulation of Liver Cell Expression*. Falk Symposium No. 43. 1987   ISBN: 0-85200-677-2*

44. Boyer JL, Bianchi L, eds.: *Liver Cirrhosis*. Falk Symposium No. 44. 1987
      ISBN: 0-85200-993-3*

45. Paumgartner G, Stiehl A, Gerok W, eds.: *Bile Acids and the Liver*. Falk Symposium No. 45. 1987   ISBN: 0-85200-675-6*

46. Goebell H, Peskar BM, Malchow H, eds.: *Inflammatory Bowel Diseases – Basic Research & Clinical Implications*. Falk Symposium No. 46. 1988   ISBN: 0-7462-0067-6*

47. Bianchi L, Holt P, James OFW, Butler RN, eds.: *Aging in Liver and Gastrointestinal Tract*. Falk Symposium No. 47. 1988   ISBN: 0-7462-0066-8*

48. Heilmann C, ed.: *Calcium-Dependent Processes in the Liver*. Falk Symposium No. 48. 1988   ISBN: 0-7462-0075-7*

50. Singer MV, Goebell H, eds.: *Nerves and the Gastrointestinal Tract*. Falk Symposium No. 50. 1989   ISBN: 0-7462-0114-1

51. Bannasch P, Keppler D, Weber G, eds.: *Liver Cell Carcinoma*. Falk Symposium No. 51. 1989   ISBN: 0-7462-0111-7

52. Paumgartner G, Stiehl A, Gerok W, eds.: *Trends in Bile Acid Research*. Falk Symposium No. 52. 1989   ISBN: 0-7462-0112-5

53. Paumgartner G, Stiehl A, Barbara L, Roda E, eds.: *Strategies for the Treatment of Hepatobiliary Diseases*. Falk Symposium No. 53. 1990   ISBN: 0-7923-8903-4

54. Bianchi L, Gerok W, Maier K-P, Deinhardt F, eds.: *Infectious Diseases of the Liver*. Falk Symposium No. 54. 1990   ISBN: 0-7923-8902-6

55. Falk Symposium No. 55 not published

55B.Hadziselimovic F, Herzog B, Bürgin-Wolff A, eds.: *Inflammatory Bowel Disease and Coeliac Disease in Children*. International Falk Symposium. 1990 ISBN 0-7462-0125-7

56. Williams CN, eds.: *Trends in Inflammatory Bowel Disease Therapy*. Falk Symposium No. 56. 1990   ISBN: 0-7923-8952-2

57. Bock KW, Gerok W, Matern S, Schmid R, eds.: *Hepatic Metabolism and Disposition of Endo- and Xenobiotics*. Falk Symposium No. 57. 1991   ISBN: 0-7923-8953-0

58. Paumgartner G, Stiehl A, Gerok W, eds.: *Bile Acids as Therapeutic Agents: From Basic Science to Clinical Practice*. Falk Symposium No. 58. 1991   ISBN: 0-7923-8954-9

59. Halter F, Garner A, Tytgat GNJ, eds.: *Mechanisms of Peptic Ulcer Healing*. Falk Symposium No. 59. 1991   ISBN: 0-7923-8955-7

60. Goebell H, Ewe K, Malchow H, Koelbel Ch, eds.: *Inflammatory Bowel Diseases – Progress in Basic Research and Clinical Implications*. Falk Symposium No. 60. 1991
      ISBN: 0-7923-8956-5

61. Falk Symposium No. 61 not published

62. Dowling RH, Folsch UR, Löser Ch, eds.: *Polyamines in the Gastrointestinal Tract*. Falk Symposium No. 62. 1992   ISBN: 0-7923-8976-X

63. Lentze MJ, Reichen J, eds.: *Paediatric Cholestasis: Novel Approaches to Treatment*. Falk Symposium No. 63. 1992   ISBN: 0-7923-8977-8

64. Demling L, Frühmorgen P, eds.: *Non-Neoplastic Diseases of the Anorectum*. Falk Symposium No. 64. 1992   ISBN: 0-7923-8979-4

64B.Gressner AM, Ramadori G, eds.: *Molecular and Cell Biology of Liver Fibrogenesis*. International Falk Symposium. 1992   ISBN: 0-7923-8980-8

*These titles were published under the MTP Press imprint.

Falk Symposium Series

65. Hadziselimovic F, Herzog B, eds.: *Inflammatory Bowel Diseases and Morbus Hirschprung.* Falk Symposium No. 65. 1992   ISBN: 0-7923-8995-6
66. Martin F, McLeod RS, Sutherland LR, Williams CN, eds.: *Trends in Inflammatory Bowel Disease Therapy.* Falk Symposium No. 66. 1993   ISBN: 0-7923-8827-5
67. Schölmerich J, Kruis W, Goebell H, Hohenberger W, Gross V, eds.: *Inflammatory Bowel Diseases – Pathophysiology as Basis of Treatment.* Falk Symposium No. 67. 1993
ISBN: 0-7923-8996-4
68. Paumgartner G, Stiehl A, Gerok W, eds.: *Bile Acids and The Hepatobiliary System: From Basic Science to Clinical Practice.* Falk Symposium No. 68. 1993
ISBN: 0-7923-8829-1
69. Schmid R, Bianchi L, Gerok W, Maier K-P, eds.: *Extrahepatic Manifestations in Liver Diseases.* Falk Symposium No. 69. 1993   ISBN: 0-7923-8821-6
70. Meyer zum Büschenfelde K-H, Hoofnagle J, Manns M, eds.: *Immunology and Liver.* Falk Symposium No. 70. 1993   ISBN: 0-7923-8830-5
71. Surrenti C, Casini A, Milani S, Pinzani M , eds.: *Fat-Storing Cells and Liver Fibrosis.* Falk Symposium No. 71. 1994   ISBN: 0-7923-8842-9
72. Rachmilewitz D, ed.: *Inflammatory Bowel Diseases – 1994.* Falk Symposium No. 72. 1994   ISBN: 0-7923-8845-3
73. Binder HJ, Cummings J, Soergel KH, eds.: *Short Chain Fatty Acids.* Falk Symposium No. 73. 1994   ISBN: 0-7923-8849-6
73B. Möllmann HW, May B, eds.: *Glucocorticoid Therapy in Chronic Inflammatory Bowel Disease: from basic principles to rational therapy.* International Falk Workshop. 1996
ISBN 0-7923-8708-2
74. Keppler D, Jungermann K, eds.: *Transport in the Liver.* Falk Symposium No. 74. 1994
ISBN: 0-7923-8858-5
74B. Stange EF, ed.: *Chronic Inflammatory Bowel Disease.* Falk Symposium. 1995
ISBN: 0-7923-8876-3
75. van Berge Henegouwen GP, van Hoek B, De Groote J, Matern S, Stockbrügger RW, eds.: *Cholestatic Liver Diseases: New Strategies for Prevention and Treatment of Hepatobiliary and Cholestatic Liver Diseases.* Falk Symposium 75. 1994.
ISBN: 0-7923-8867-4
76. Monteiro E, Tavarela Veloso F, eds.: *Inflammatory Bowel Diseases: New Insights into Mechanisms of Inflammation and Challenges in Diagnosis and Treatment.* Falk Symposium 76. 1995.   ISBN 0-7923-8884-4
77. Singer MV, Ziegler R, Rohr G, eds.: *Gastrointestinal Tract and Endocrine System.* Falk Symposium 77. 1995.   ISBN 0-7923-8877-1
78. Decker K, Gerok W, Andus T, Gross V, eds.: *Cytokines and the Liver.* Falk Symposium 78. 1995.   ISBN 0-7923-8878-X
79. Holstege A, Schölmerich J, Hahn EG, eds.: *Portal Hypertension.* Falk Symposium 79. 1995.   ISBN 0-7923-8879-8
80. Hofmann AF, Paumgartner G, Stiehl A, eds.: *Bile Acids in Gastroenterology: Basic and Clinical Aspects.* Falk Symposium 80. 1995   ISBN 0-7923-8880-1
81. Riecken EO, Stallmach A, Zeitz M, Heise W, eds.: *Malignancy and Chronic Inflammation in the Gastrointestinal Tract – New Concepts.* Falk Symposium 81. 1995
ISBN 0-7923-8889-5
82. Fleig WE, ed.: *Inflammatory Bowel Diseases: New Developments and Standards.* Falk Symposium 82. 1995   ISBN 0-7923-8890-6

Falk Symposium Series

82B. Paumgartner G, Beuers U, eds.: *Bile Acids in Liver Diseases*. International Falk
Workshop. 1995   ISBN 0-7923-8891-7

83. Dobrilla G, Felder M, de Pretis G, eds.: *Advances in Hepatobiliary and Pancreatic
Diseases: Special Clinical Topics*. Falk Symposium 83. 1995.   ISBN 0-7923-8892-5

84. Fromm H, Leuschner U, eds.: *Bile Acids – Cholestasis – Gallstones: Advances in Basic
and Clinical Bile Acid Research*. Falk Symposium 84. 1995   ISBN 0-7923-8893-3

85. Tytgat GNJ, Bartelsman JFWM, van Deventer SJH, eds.: *Inflammatory Bowel Diseases*.
Falk Symposium 85. 1995   ISBN 0-7923-8894-1

86. Berg PA, Leuschner U, eds.: *Bile Acids and Immunology*. Falk Symposium 86. 1996
ISBN 0-7923-8700-7

87. Schmid R, Bianchi L, Blum HE, Gerok W, Maier KP, Stalder GA, eds.: *Acute and
Chronic Liver Diseases: Molecular Biology and Clinics*. Falk Symposium 87. 1996
ISBN 0-7923-8701-5

88. Blum HE, Wu GY, Wu CH, eds.: *Molecular Diagnosis and Gene Therapy*. Falk
Symposium 88. 1996   ISBN 0-7923-8702-3

88B. Poupon RE, Reichen J, eds.: *Surrogate Markers to Assess Efficacy of TReatment in
Chronic Liver Diseases*. International Falk Workshop. 1996   ISBN 0-7923-8705-8

89. Reyes HB, Leuschner U, Arias IM, eds.: *Pregnancy, Sex Hormones and the Liver*. Falk
Symposium 89. 1996   ISBN 0-7923-8704-X

89B. Broelsch CE, Burdelski M, Rogiers X, eds.: *Cholestatic Liver Diseases in Children and
Adults*. International Falk Workshop. 1996   ISBN 0-7923-8710-4

90. Lam S-K, Paumgartner P, Wang B, eds.: *Update on Hepatobiliary Diseases 1996*. Falk
Symposium 90. 1996   ISBN 0-7923-8715-5

91. Hadziselimovic F, Herzog B, eds.: *Inflammatory Bowel Diseases and Chronic Recurrent
Abdominal Pain*. Falk Symposium 91. 1996   ISBN 0-7923-8722-8

91B. Alvaro D, Benedetti A, Strazzabosco M, eds.: *Vanishing Bile Duct Syndrome –
Pathophysiology and Treatment*. International Falk Workshop. 1996
ISBN 0-7923-8721-X

92. Gerok W, Loginov AS, Pokrowskij VI, eds.: *New Trends in Hepatology 1996*. Falk
Symposium 92. 1997   ISBN 0-7923-8723-6

93. Paumgartner G, Stiehl A, Gerok W, eds.: *Bile Acids in Hepatobiliary Diseases – Basic
Research and Clinical Application*. Falk Symposium 93. 1997   ISBN 0-7923-8725-2

94. Halter F, Winton D, Wright NA, eds.: *The Gut as a Model in Cell and Molecular Biology*.
Falk Symposium 94. 1997   ISBN 0-7923-8726-0

94B. Kruse-Jarres JD, Schölmerich J, eds.: *Zinc and Diseases of the Digestive Tract*.
International Falk Workshop. 1997   ISBN 0-7923-8724-4

95. Ewe K, Eckardt VF, Enck P, eds.: *Constipation and Anorectal Insufficiency*. Falk
Symposium 95. 1997   ISBN 0-7923-8727-9

96. Andus T, Goebell H, Layer P, Schölmerich J, eds.: *Inflammatory Bowel Disease – from
Bench to Bedside*. Falk Symposium 96. 1997   ISBN 0-7923-8728-7

97. Campieri M, Bianchi-Porro G, Fiocchi C, Schölmerich J, eds. *Clinical Challenges in
Inflammatory Bowel Diseases: Diagnosis, Prognosis and Treatment*. Falk Symposium 97.
1998   ISBN 0-7923-8733-3

98. Lembcke B, Kruis W, Sartor RB, eds. *Systemic Manifestations of IBD: The Pending
Challenge for Subtle Diagnosis and Treatment*. Falk Symposium 98. 1998
ISBN 0-7923-8734-1

Falk Symposium Series

99. Goebell H, Holtmann G, Talley NJ, eds. *Functional Dyspepsia and Irritable Bowel Syndrome: Concepts and Controversies.* Falk Symposium 99. 1998
ISBN 0-7923-8735-X

100. Blum HE, Bode Ch, Bode JCh, Sartor RB, eds. *Gut and the Liver.* Falk Symposium 100. 1998
ISBN 0-7923-8736-8

101. Rachmilewitz D, ed. *V International Symposium on Inflammatory Bowel Diseases.* Falk Symposium 101. 1998
ISBN 0-7923-8743-0

102. Manns MP, Boyer JL, Jansen PLM, Reichen J, eds. *Cholestatic Liver Diseases.* Falk Symposium 102. 1998
ISBN 0-7923-8746-5

102B. Manns MP, Chapman RW, Stiehl A, Wiesner R, eds. *Primary Sclerosing Cholangitis.* International Falk Workshop. 1998.
ISBN 0-7923-8745-7

103. Häussinger D, Jungermann K, eds. *Liver and Nervous System.* Falk Symposium 102. 1998
ISBN 0-7924-8742-2

103B. Häussinger D, Heinrich PC, eds. *Signalling in the Liver.* International Falk Workshop. 1998
ISBN 0-7923-8744-9

103C. Fleig W, ed. *Normal and Malignant Liver Cell Growth.* International Falk Workshop. 1998
ISBN 0-7923-8748-1

104. Stallmach A, Zeitz M, Strober W, MacDonald TT, Lochs H, eds. *Induction and Modulation of Gastrointestinal Inflammation.* Falk Symposium 104. 1998
ISBN 0-7923-8747-3

105. Emmrich J, Liebe S, Stange EF, eds. *Innovative Concepts in Inflammatory Bowel Diseases.* Falk Symposium 105. 1999
ISBN 0-7923-8749-X

106. Rutgeerts P, Colombel J-F, Hanauer SB, Schölmerich J, Tytgat GNJ, van Gossum A, eds. *Advances in Inflammatory Bowel Diseases.* Falk Symposium 106. 1999
ISBN 0-7923-8750-3

107. Špičák J, Boyer J, Gilat T, Kotrlik K, Mareček Z, Paumgartner G, eds. *Diseases of the Liver and the Bile Ducts – New Aspects and Clinical Implications.* Falk Symposium 107. 1999
ISBN 0-7923-8751-1

108. Paumgartner G, Stiehl A, Gerok W, Keppler D, Leuschner U, eds. *Bile Acids and Cholestasis.* Falk Symposium 108. 1999
ISBN 0-7923-8752-X

109. Schmiegel W, Schölmerich J, eds. *Colorectal Cancer – Molecular Mechanisms, Premalignant State and its Prevention.* Falk Symposium 109. 1999
ISBN 0-7923-8753-8

110. Domschke W, Stoll R, Brasitus TA, Kagnoff MF, eds. *Intestinal Mucosa and its Diseases – Pathophysiology and Clinics.* Falk Symposium 110. 1999
ISBN 0-7923-8754-6

110B. Northfield TC, Ahmed HA, Jazwari RP, Zentler-Munro PL, eds. *Bile Acids in Hepatobiliary Disease.* Falk Workshop. 2000
ISBN 0-7923-8755-4

111. Rogler G, Kullmann F, Rutgeerts P, Sartor RB, Schölmerich J, eds. *IBD at the End of its First Century.* Falk Symposium 111. 2000
ISBN 0-7923-8756-2

112. Krammer HJ, Singer MV, eds. *Neurogastroenterology: From the Basics to the Clinics.* Falk Symposium 112. 2000
ISBN 0-7923-8757-0

113. Andus T, Rogler G, Schlottmann K, Frick E, Adler G, Schmiegel W, Zeitz M, Schölmerich J, eds. *Cytokines and Cell Homeostasis in the Gastrointestinal Tract.* Falk Symposium 113. 2000
ISBN 0-7923-8758-9

114. Manns MP, Paumgartner G, Leuschner U, eds. *Immunology and Liver.* Falk Symposium 114. 2000
ISBN 0-7923-8759-7

Falk Symposium Series

115. Boyer JL, Blum HE, Maier K-P, Sauerbruch T, Stalder GA, eds. *Liver Cirrhosis and its Development*. Falk Symposium 115. 2000   ISBN 0-7923-8760-0

116. Riemann JF, Neuhaus H, eds. *Interventional Endoscopy in Hepatology*. Falk Symposium 116. 2000   ISBN 0-7923-8761-9

116A. Dienes HP, Schirmacher P, Brechot C, Okuda K, eds. *Chronic Hepatitis: New Concepts of Pathogenesis, Diagnosis and Treatment*. Falk Workshop. 2000   ISBN 0-7923-8763-5

117. Gerbes AL, Beuers U, Jüngst D, Pape GR, Sackmann M, Sauerbruch T, eds. *Hepatology 2000 – Symposium in Honour of Gustav Paumgartner*. Falk Symposium 117. 2000   ISBN 0-7923-8765-1

117A. Acalovschi M, Paumgartner G, eds. *Hepatobiliary Diseases: Cholestasis and Gallstones*. Falk Workshop. 2000   ISBN 0-7923-8770-8

118. Frühmorgen P, Bruch H-P, eds. *Non-Neoplastic Diseases of the Anorectum*. Falk Symposium 118. 2001   ISBN 0-7923-8766-X

119. Fellermann K, Jewell DP, Sandborn WJ, Schölmerich J, Stange EF, eds. *Immunosuppression in Inflammatory Bowel Diseases – Standards, New Developments, Future Trends*. Falk Symposium 119. 2001   ISBN 0-7923-8767-8

120. van Berge Henegouwen GP, Keppler D, Leuschner U, Paumgartner G, Stiehl A, eds. *Biology of Bile Acids in Health and Disease*. Falk Symposium 120. 2001   ISBN 0-7923-8768-6

121. Leuschner U, James OFW, Dancygier H, eds. *Steatohepatitis (NASH and ASH)*. Falk Symposium 121. 2001   ISBN 0-7923-8769-4

121A. Matern S, Boyer JL, Keppler D, Meier-Abt PJ, eds. *Hepatobiliary Transport: From Bench to Bedside*. Falk Workshop. 2001   ISBN 0-7923-8771-6

122. Campieri M, Fiocchi C, Hanauer SB, Jewell DP, Rachmilewitz R, Schölmerich J, eds. *Inflammatory Bowel Disease – A Clinical Case Approach to Pathophysiology, Diagnosis, and Treatment*. Falk Symposium 122. 2002   ISBN 0-7923-8772-4

123. Rachmilewitz D, Modigliani R, Podolsky DK, Sachar DB, Tozun N, eds. *VI International Symposium on Inflammatory Bowel Diseases*. Falk Symposium 123. 2002   ISBN 0-7923-8773 2

124. Hagenmüller F, Manns MP, Musmann H-G, Riemann JF, eds. *Medical Imaging in Gastroenterology and Hepatology*. Falk Symposium 124. 2002   ISBN 0-7923-8774-0

125. Gressner AM, Heinrich PC, Matern S, eds. *Cytokines in Liver Injury and Repair*. Falk Symposium 125. 2002   ISBN 0-7923-8775-9

126. Gupta S, Jansen PLM, Klempnauer J, Manns MP, eds. *Hepatocyte Transplantation*. Falk Symposium 126. 2002   ISBN 0-7923-8776-7

127. Hadziselimovic F, ed. *Autoimmune Diseases in Paediatric Gastroenterology*. Falk Symposium 127. 2002   ISBN 0-7923-8778-3

127A. Berr F, Bruix J, Hauss J, Wands J, Wittekind Ch, eds. *Malignant Liver Tumours: Basic Concepts and Clinical Management*. Falk Workshop. 2002   ISBN 0-7923-8779-1

128. Scheppach W, Scheurlen M, eds. *Exogenous Factors in Colonic Carcinogenesis*. Falk Symposium 128. 2002   ISBN 0-7923-8780-5

129. Paumgartner G, Keppler D, Leuschner U, Stiehl A, eds. *Bile Acids: From Genomics to Disease and Therapy*. Falk Symposium 129. 2002   ISBN 0-7923-8781-3

129A. Leuschner U, Berg PA, Holtmeier J, eds. *Bile Acids and Pregnancy*. Falk Workshop. 2002   ISBN 0-7923-8782-1

Falk Symposium Series

130. Holtmann G, Talley NJ, eds. *Gastrointestinal Inflammation and Disturbed Gut Function: The Challenge of New Concepts.* Falk Symposium 130. 2003
ISBN 0-7923-8783-X

131. Herfarth H, Feagan BJ, Folsch UR, Schölmerich J, Vatn MH, Zeitz M, eds. *Targets of Treatment in Chronic Inflammatory Bowel Diseases.* Falk Symposium 131. 2003
ISBN 0-7923-8784-8

132. Galle PR, Gerken G, Schmidt WE, Wiedenmann B, eds. *Disease Progression and Carcinogenesis in the Gastrointestinal Tract.* Falk Symposium 132. 2003
ISBN 0-7923-8785-6

132A. Staritz M, Adler G, Knuth A, Schmiegel W, Schmoll H-J, eds. *Side-effects of Chemotherapy on the Gastrointestinal Tract.* Falk Workshop. 2003
ISBN 0-7923-8791-0

132B. Reutter W, Schuppan D, Tauber R, Zeitz M, eds. *Cell Adhesion Molecules in Health and Disease.* Falk Workshop. 2003 ISBN 0-7923-8786-4

133. Duchmann R, Blumberg R, Neurath M, Schölmerich J, Strober W, Zeitz M. *Mechanisms of Intestinal Inflammation: Implications for Therapeutic Intervention in IBD.* Falk Symposium 133. 2004 ISBN 0-7923-8787-2

134. Dignass A, Lochs H, Stange E. *Trends and Controversies in IBD – Evidence-Based Approach or Individual Management?* Falk Symposium 134. 2004
ISBN 0-7923-8788-0

134A. Dignass A, Gross HJ, Buhr V, James OFW. *Topical Steroids in Gastroenterology and Hepatology.* Falk Workshop. 2004 ISBN 0-7923-8789-9